How to Survive in the 21st Century

Andrew A D Burgoyne

Previous Publications:

Unhealthy Betrayal—How the Manipulation of Science and Politics by Corporate Interests Destroys Health and Threatens the Future of Humanity. Fundamental Press, 2015.

Hijacked—How the Banking Industry, Finance, and Corporate Interests Have Hijacked our Economy and Corrupted Democracy. Fundamental Press, 2018.

How to Survive in the 21ˢᵗ Century

Copyright © 2020

Andrew A D Burgoyne

PUBLISHED BY FUNDAMENTAL PRESS

ISBN 978-0-9932539-2-8

COVER DESIGN BY SAM WALL

Health Warning

This book deals with a number of topics that are related to health issues.

Some of the topics are of a controversial nature and are purely addressed here to provoke useful debate.

This book is not intended as medical advice.

Any people with medical issues or any health conditions should consult with their doctor or their relevant medical practitioners for advice regarding treatments.

Acknowledgements

I am indebted to numerous people who have contributed information useful to this volume, in some cases people who dared speak out when others have kept silent, without all of whom this volume would have been a lot poorer, for all these people I say thank you. This is particularly the case in the field of medicine, where the pressure to conform to certain opinions is intense and challenging.

I would also like to thank my editor Shelagh Aitken PhD, for all her constructive advice and help.

Contents

Introduction

This book is not another book about health, it is about *survival.*

As I write this, we are still in social isolation due to the pandemic of Covid-19. The ramifications of this and the consequential economic shutdown and the subsequent massive bailout packages may likely impact us for generations to come. Much depends on how we chose to respond to this crisis.

This book was conceived and mostly completed before the viral outbreak and has necessitated some additional material, but the basis for how to survive in the 21st century has not changed, it has simply gained a new sense of urgency.

This book may shatter some illusions, but will hopefully reveal how we can survive what many perceive as unsurmountable problems—all manmade—but all orchestrated by irresponsible and short-sighted corporate interests.

This book explores how you can, not just become a survivor, and avoid many of the pitfalls that other less-informed people will make—but be better armed with the knowledge to help change this world in a way that can really make a difference.

Whilst we show how health is collapsing in Western countries, and, in fact, globally, few people are aware of the degree of this disaster, that has been growing independently of the current Covid-19 pandemic. Whilst we perceive sickness and ill-health, as a negative event, that mostly happens to other people, for certain corporate interests it is simply seen as an ideal money-making opportunity, and the chances are high they may have people like you in their sights.

How to Survive in the 21ˢᵗ Century

Corporations have grown more powerful than could have been imagined just a few generations ago, and their power seems to grow with each passing year, as does the wealth of those who for the most part own and operate them.

This book describes the pathological nature of corporate activity, and its direct effect on our health and our politics. We navigate through the world of propaganda and pseudoscience and reveal how serving corporate interests does not serve us but can actively destroy our health and that of our families, and not just that—but also affect the health of future generations.

Many of the problems we face are not insurmountable, the solutions are sometimes quite simple, but more significantly involve a change in thinking. Some of the solutions are beautiful and are not just staring right at us but are also right beneath our feet.

I have been researching and writing about health issues for a number of years now. I have a background in nutrition, and my research has led me to realise that our health is intimately connected to the health of the Earth, and its very fabric. Reconnecting with the Earth and the soil that feeds us is essential for our survival.

For many, the topic of health, and/or nutrition, can be confusing. Its study can involve some complex topics. We are encouraged, however, not to explore the subject of health and the many factors that contribute to it, past a superficial level—we are cautioned to leave it to the 'experts'. We show in this volume, that many of these so-called 'experts' are very people who are in the pay of corporate interests who do not care about our health and are actually undermining it.

Many of these companies have significant financial interests at stake and little interest in our health or that of our children. These same interests, however, need to conceal from the consumers of their products, the true extent of their financial interests and spend considerable sums on advertising and public relations exercises to maintain an image of corporate responsibility, portraying themselves as beneficent businesses that support health, and community welfare.

We hope to separate the wheat from the chaff and demystify some of the confusion that exists and enable you to arrive at a more informed understanding of the important issues involved, so you may avoid some of the more obvious pitfalls that exist, and help you to stay healthier and protect your family from some of the ravages of the twenty-first century.

You will find that I often use the word 'we' when writing on some topics, a habit that is related to the fact that what I write about comes from a body of knowledge: the research and writings of a wide group of researchers and various authorities to whom I refer. Also, some of the information that I offer here may challenge some of the mainstream media views that you may have been exposed to—this is because I have followed a line of research that has looked at writers who may have diverged from what most would consider the 'mainstream': people from different disciplines who have grasped some of the simple truths that others either missed or chose to ignore, and who were not afraid to air their views.

From these different writers I have assembled an understanding that reveals a troubling story that reflects the health crisis that we are currently facing, and that has a bearing on the future for us all. Whilst many may feel we are living in a world that seems to have insurmountable problems, we suggest that everything is fixable: we simply need to change our thinking and our priorities and make better-informed decisions.

How to Survive in the 21ˢᵗ Century

My previous volumes *Unhealthy Betrayal—How the Manipulation of Science and Politics by Corporate Interests Destroys Health and Threatens the Future of Humanity*, and *Hijacked—How the Banking Industry, Finance, and Corporate Interests Have Hijacked Our Economy and Corrupted Democracy*, deal with many different aspects of the way corporate interests have dominated our lives and can be considered as useful supplementary sources to this volume.

Chapter One

Problem Chemistry

Arguably one of the greatest challenges we face is maintaining health and staying alive. Most of the health issues we currently face are rooted in relatively recent history, dating from the development of industrial-scale agriculture and the industrialisation of the food supply. Much of the initial rush into the widespread use of artificial fertilizers and reliance on chemicals such as pesticides, herbicides, insecticides and fungicides in agriculture, was supported by the belief that their use was essential for the production of enough food for a growing population.

A shortage of food, however, is not the problem, as we are actually faced with an over-supply of food, but the belief still exists among many supporters of industrialised agriculture that, without massive chemical inputs, we would not be able to feed the world. This view is, of course, heavily promoted to farmers by the chemical suppliers—generally huge corporations with immense financial resources and a vast network of lobbyists, public relations people, pliant scientists and government officials.

One of the great myths of the industry is, the view that modern industrial agriculture, with its intensive chemical inputs, will help to alleviate world hunger, the same myth actively perpetuated by the promoters of genetically modified food (often the same companies). The reality, however, is somewhat different, as we revealed in a previously mentioned volume, *Unhealthy Betrayal.*[1] In this work, we revealed that the real cause of world hunger is not due to the lack of the availability of food, but predominantly, the lack of sufficient purchasing power to be able to buy the food needed to adequately sustain health or lack of access to land. This has much more to do with political economics than the ability to grow food.

Another of the great myths about industrial agriculture is that it provides cheap, affordable food. As regards to whether it is 'cheap' or not, we have to address the consequential costs of following these policies, which is a subject that is never really explored by the supporters of this system. We can examine the question in this volume, and you can be the judge of whether it is really 'cheap' or not. This is not to confuse 'cheap' with 'affordable'—the fact that quality food is beyond the reach of many people's budgets is more a testament to the dysfunctional economic system that we are lumbering under, than people's inability to choose their food sources wisely.

It is often argued that industry is simply responding to the demand for cheap food. They use the terms 'cheap' and 'affordable' sometimes together, often interchangeably when the reality is not so clear-cut. This point is discussed in another previously mentioned volume, *Hijacked.*[2] This volume discussed how our current economy evolved from its feudal roots based on the exploitation of the majority of the population, by the theft of the commons and eviction from their land. This left them unable to adequately provide for their needs and that of their families, leaving them with little purchasing power, which forced production to be exported. Whilst historically we have experienced, to some degree, rising standards of wealth that have enabled many people to improve their living standards, our current economic circumstances are increasingly favouring the already wealthy at the expense of the majority. It is, however, beyond the scope of this present volume to enlarge greatly on this important topic, for those who would like to explore this area of study, *Hijacked,* might be a useful place to start.[3]

Chemical Explosion

As regards to the ever-increasing use of chemicals in food production, such as convenience foods, ready-made meals, snacks, fast foods etc., much of it was fostered by the search for new gimmicks, and new products that would produce new profits—with little real regard for health consequences. Much of the food production was based on the rapid discovery of new chemicals; there was, and still is, intense competition among corporations vying for market dominance with new products. As income levels for many people have stagnated over time, reliance on food supplies rested on a few major corporate supermarkets, and increasingly on fast food outlets and food supplied by ever-larger corporate interests.

Initially, there was little regulation of any kind on the use of new chemicals in agricultural and food production. More than 80,000 man-made chemicals are currently used in various products created by industry, of these, very few have been tested for safety as individual chemicals and even fewer in combination with other chemicals that we are often exposed to.

In the USA, pressure eventually forced President Nixon to act to alleviate the rising concerns of many academics, doctors and individuals who were linking unrestricted chemical use with numerous emerging health issues such as the increase in cancer. Nixon founded the Environmental Protection Agency (EPA) and charged it with protecting our natural environment and public health. At the time of its inception, a large number of companies had already been established as chemical suppliers, and many of them had been spewing vast numbers of chemicals into the environment for decades. Many of these businesses were also using numerous new chemicals in food production.

Regulatory Nightmare

It has to be said that there was a huge backlash by corporate interests to prevent the creation of the EPA and, though this action failed to prevent its inception, industry pressure against any moves to regulate the chemical industry was relentless. The industry used its massive spending power to influence legislation and to fund the election of members of Congress who supported their interests. This, of course, happens just as much today as then and is not confined to the USA. We could just as easily be discussing the situation in Europe or any major Western country.

It needs to be realised that this same scenario also affected the regulation of drugs used by the medical industry and the operation of organisations such as the U.S. Food and Drug Administration (FDA), which we will discuss further later.

What becomes apparent if you research the regulatory history of these organisations, is the way, irrespective of whether we are dealing with pesticides, food chemicals, cosmetics, medicinal drugs, or any chemicals manufactured by industry, that regulation was intensely resisted and fought against every step of the way. This resulted in the situation whereby, unless you could *prove* harm, industrial corporations held the position that to prevent the use of any chemical would be an infringement of their right to do business. Of course, to *prove* harm was very difficult; in many cases it could involve studying a particular chemical and its effects, usually on animals, as it was considered unethical, to undertake research on human beings using hazardous substances. Studies, of course, took time to undertake, and often involved monitoring effects over significant periods, months and even years in some cases, before conclusions could be drawn on the safety of a particular product. This created the situation where businesses such as the tobacco industry were able to evade regulation for decades and cause numerous deaths and disabilities until eventually, the evidence of harm became so overwhelming that intervention was initiated. To this day it still cannot be *proven* (in the sense that we can supply clinical trials showing evidence) that smoking has killed a person; it was only *by association*, the sheer weight of evidence, and public pressure that eventually convinced regulators to act. The same could be said for many other products, such as lead, asbestos, DDT and PCBs.

The unifying element of this regulatory challenge mostly comes down to a battle between the competing interests of corporate profits versus public and environmental health. That is why, to this day, environmentalists are portrayed as the biggest threat to business interests and are relentlessly attacked by industry. This stems from the state of complete denial that most of the more dangerous polluters and hazardous chemical suppliers live in, with regard to the damage they create, and the burden they put on society with their actions—creating the so-called 'externalized costs' that enable them to make huge profits at our expense.

Externalizing Costs—Subsidising Corporate Recklessness

This point about externalizing costs is worthy of your attention, as it is fundamental to our wellbeing and the health of the planet. Market theory specifies that for a market to allocate efficiently, the full costs of each product must be borne by the producer and be included in the selling price: economists call this cost internalization. Externalizing some part of a product's cost to others not party to the transaction is a form of subsidy that encourages excessive production and use of the product at the expense of others. An unregulated market invariably encourages the externalization of costs because the resulting public costs become private gains to whatever company is able to get away with this practice. This is the reason large corporations dump toxins into water supplies and the environment, as it's often a much cheaper option than taking a more responsible approach, with safe disposal—the health and clean-up costs are then externalised to the public. Failure to regulate this action allows businesses to pollute our water supplies, our environment, and our bodies, with virtually no restrictions. When the onus falls on us to *prove* harm, this can be very difficult, expensive, and take inordinate amounts of time. Much of this story is further explored in *Unhealthy Betrayal.*[4]

The power of corporate influence continues to grow as corporations seek to merge and enlarge through take-overs and acquisitions, giving them immense muscle over governments and scientific institutions. The result for organisations such as the EPA is to hamstring them and inhibit their ability to effectively regulate their industry. It is well known that, when Ronald Reagan came to power, he dismantled the EPA and reduced its ability to adequately function. Dr Evaggelos Vallianatos, who worked for the EPA for more than twenty-five years described the effect on the EPA in his book, *Poison Spring— The Secret History of Pollution and the EPA* :

> He opened the door wide to corporate influence throughout the government, and especially the EPA, which began a precipitous functional decline. Reagan gave corporations the reins of power at the agency, and they immediately began tearing the EPA apart. Outside the agency, the hired political guns in Reagan's Office of Management and Budget also set about demolishing environmental protection, justifying such vandalism by the self-serving mythology of the "cost/benefit analysis," which masked a naked ideological shift toward pesticide merchants and agribusiness.[5]

Problem Chemistry

The EPA dismantled ten of its research labs, destroyed much of its library, cut its budgets for research and enforcement, slashed the number of cases filed against polluters, and sped up the pace of approvals for pesticides. Reagan appointed lawyer Anne Gorsuch (later Burford) to run the EPA and Rita Lavelle, an industry lobbyist, to run the EPA's toxic waste programs. Both understood their mission was not to empower the EPA, but to dismantle it, which they set about with zeal.

Following administrations, failed to stop the hamstringing of the EPA. In 2011, Newt Gingrich, the former speaker of the House, even called for the abolition of the EPA. Following a large movement of support for the EPA, the threat of abolition receded but was met with the threat of a cut of thirty percent of its budget, the largest cut in thirty years. This prompted the League of Conservation Voters to complain that the cut 'would jeopardize the water we drink and air we breathe, endangering the health and well-being of all Americans.' [6]

The reason this is important is it is not just something that can have serious implication for the health of all Americans: it has global implications. The U.S. EPA is considered by most other countries to be the voice of authority of what is perceived as the richest country in the world. Where countries cannot afford to test chemicals even if they wanted to, they rely on statements by the EPA as the voice of the best and most reliable science money can buy. Even in other Western countries, the EPA is held with high regard, as are their decisions when they approve chemicals. Many countries simply rubberstamp the EPA decisions. The same can be said of the U.S.FDA regarding drug releases. What this basically means is the corporate agenda drives the regulatory control of their chemicals, which is akin to the foxes guarding the chicken houses. The result means that little real protection exists against the corporate deluge of chemicals into our bodies and the environment.

We will discuss this further in the next chapters and give you an inside view of the result of the abandonment of any real oversight, and what this can mean for your health and that of your children. Before this, however, I feel it would be useful to look at the part the role of politics has to play in our health, and not just nationally, but globally.

Chapter Two

The Politicisation of Health

The story of how the theory that eating saturated fat was harmful and the cause of heart disease, because it raised our cholesterol levels and blocked our arteries, is worth discussing, as it has a direct bearing on our health today. In *Unhealthy Betrayal*, I reported on how Ancel Keys, a biologist and physiologist, introduced the theory that heart disease was caused by dietary factors that raised our cholesterol levels, and that these raised levels were caused by high levels of dietary fat—specifically the saturated fats that were found in animal products, such as in butter, cheese, and the flesh of red meats. I don't intend to explore the whole story here; I have discussed the topic in articles on my website and my aforementioned volume. To those who would like a more in-depth appraisal of this subject can I suggest you explore these sources and the referenced material for more information? [7] We will, of course, delve into this topic to some degree, as it led to the politicisation of health, initially, in the USA, via the Senator McGovern Committee.

The Cholesterol Theory Takes Root

In 1957, the American Heart Association (AHA) opposed Ancel Keys on the diet-heart issue, and produced a fifteen-page report castigating researchers which included Keys for taking 'uncompromising stands based on evidence that does not stand up under critical examination.' They further suggested; 'There is not enough evidence available to permit a rigid stand on what the relationship is between nutrition, particularly the fat content of the diet, and atherosclerosis and coronary heart disease.'

There was, however, a big campaign by the margarine and vegetable oil industries, which was subsequently supported by the American Medical Association (AMA) to win support for Keys theory. The case for condemning saturated fats reached new heights with the production of a publication announced by Senator George McGovern, the first *Dietary Goals for the United States,* which was the first Federal attempt to promote dietary guidelines for US citizens.

- The first dietary goal was to raise carbohydrate consumption to 50-60 percent of calories consumed.

- The second goal was to decrease fat consumption to 30 percent of all calories with less than 33 percent being supplied by saturated fats.

The initial response to the report at its press conference produced uproar. This prompted McGovern to hold further hearings and the production of a revised set of guidelines later that year. What McGovern really succeeded in doing, however, was to turn the whole discussion of cholesterol and saturated fats into a political issue instead of a question of science.[8]

The Politicisation of Health

The story is well worth reviewing, as it was to have far-reaching implications for our health and that of our children. A whole myth was created about the dangers of cholesterol to our health that has been shown to be based on little scientific evidence, and instead of the medical industry coming out and admitting that they got it wrong, they just keep moving the goalposts. Originally, just high cholesterol levels were supposed to be the problem, but when studies appeared to contradict this, they came up with their 'good' and 'bad' cholesterol theory. This was in competition with an alternative theory for heart disease, that the true cause was sugar and over-processed carbohydrate, as was proposed by Professor John Yudkin, a contemporary of Ancel Keys. Yudkin was head of the Department of Nutrition, Queen Elizabeth College, London, which was instituted in 1953, and regarded as the first in Europe to be devoted to undergraduate and post-graduate teaching of nutrition. Yudkin was not just a doctor, but also a highly trained biochemist, earning a PhD from Cambridge. He felt that the main culprit to health particularly heart disease, was sugar. In his research, he found that sugar consumption, raised both cholesterol levels and triglycerides in the blood, made blood platelets sticky and also raised the blood pressure—all negative signs for heart disease. He wrote about his findings in his book, *Pure White and Deadly—How Sugar Is Killing Us and What We Can Do About It,* published in 1972, in response to what he perceived was the mistaken and un-proven theory that the culprit was saturated fat.[9]

There are many people who perceive it as a battle between the powerful sugar and food industry, in combination with the oil refining and margarine industry, against the unprepared meat industry—science was simply abandoned, especially once the government of the United States declared its support for the cholesterol theory. No-one was prepared to stand up and challenge the might of this body of now-official opinion. Research grants for studying any other theories simply vanished.

Shift to Vegetable Oil Consumption

It is, however, the ramifications of this action by the politicisation of the theory that I feel is important for us to deal with here. It led to a radical shift in dietary patterns, the reduction of saturated fats was achieved by reducing red meat consumption, dairy products (particularly butter and cheese), the reduction of egg consumption, avocados, and anything that we associate with high amounts of saturated fat. It led to the development and use of highly refined vegetable oils and the abandonment of cooking with, lard, beef dripping or butter, all of which contained saturated fats. It led to the development and use of margarines which were created by hydrogenating vegetable oils, creating new man-made refined products which produced trans-fats, later found to raise bad (LDL) cholesterol levels and lower good (HDL) cholesterol levels. Eating trans-fats was found to increase your risk of developing heart disease and stroke. It was also associated with a higher risk of developing type 2 diabetes.[10]

It would be remiss of me not to discuss the introduction of vegetable oils that followed on the heels of the advice to cut down on saturated fats. Traditionally much cooking was undertaken using fats such as lard, beef dripping, butter, and ghee (clarified butter). The acceptance of the advice to cut down on saturated fats led to the food industry developing the market for vegetable oils, and for years the health benefits for the use of these new polyunsaturated oils were touted by the industry and the medical profession. More recently as the flaws in the cholesterol theory became more widely known, evidence for the so-called benefits of the change to refined vegetable oils has failed to materialise and evidence is suggesting that this move has had unforeseen consequences on our health.

Hazards of Vegetable Oils

One of the characteristics of vegetable oils, in their natural state, (without being damaged with harmful pesticides or herbicides), suggests ingesting foods containing these oils would be of benefit. They are very volatile oils and react to heat, light, and oxygen—which inside the body is exploited to benefit. Unfortunately when vegetable oils are refined these characteristics cause the oils to spoil and become rancid, as the oils are exposed to quite high temperatures in processing and are also exposed to air, and light. To help mask the rancidity, the oils are bleached and de-odorised. This tends to cause the oils to foam when used, so anti-foaming agents are often added, and xylene is often added as a stabilizer. Some oils are solvent extracted, and hexane is commonly used for this process. The problem we have here is that the damage to the oil is not easily visible, what is not seen is that many of the essential nutrients in the oil have been removed, such as the vitamin E that would protect the oil (acting as an antioxidant), and the oil now contains trans-fats and free-radical damage. This damage has an impact on our health. Free radicals are molecules with unbalanced electrons. When they enter the body they are unstable and their propensity is to become stable, which they can only achieve by stealing an electron from another molecule. When this happens inside the body, it can create a chain reaction, with each molecule in return reacting in the same way, when its own electron is stolen. These chain reactions can occur to varying degrees in the body depending on the diet, reactions of 100,000 a day are not unrealistic. The only thing that stops these free-radical chain reactions is an antioxidant, such as vitamin E or vitamin C supplied by the body—that is, it must be emphasized in a body that has adequate supplies of these vital vitamins.[11]

It is not just the effects of the trans-fats and free-radical damage that are of concern here though, the use of the oils for cooking creates further problems with the creation of hazardous products such as aldehydes, which scientists refer to as lipid oxidation products (LOPs). Warnings from the mainstream media about the hazards of consuming vegetable oils are becoming more common. Here are the comments of Robert Mendick, writing in *The Telegraph,* a UK national newspaper:

> Cooking with vegetable oils releases toxic chemicals linked to cancer and other diseases, according to leading scientists, who are now recommending food be fried in olive oil, coconut oil, butter or even lard.
>
> The results of a series of experiments threaten to turn on its head official advice that oils rich in polyunsaturated fats – such as corn oil and sunflower oil – are better for the health than the saturated fats in animal products.
>
> Scientists found that heating up vegetable oils led to the release of high concentrations of chemicals called aldehydes, which have been linked to illnesses including cancer, heart disease and dementia. [12]

Mendick refers to the work of a number of people who have raised concerns about the problems with some of the oils used. He mentions the work of Martin Grootveld, a professor of bioanalytical chemistry and chemical pathology, who reveals that 'his research showed "a typical meal of fish and chips", fried in vegetable oil, contained as much as 100 to 200 times more toxic aldehydes than the safe daily limit set by the World Health Organisation.'

Leaving aside for a moment the question of the 'safe daily limit' (the temptation is to ask 'safe for who?'), you have to realise that these people are being conservative here. If you have a known toxin, which these aldehydes are, they create damage in the body, the degree of the damage depends on many factors both known and unknown, such as; your nutritional status; your immune status; what other chemicals of significance are floating around in your system, and what the likelihood there is of a synergistic reaction with these other chemicals. Those of you that know my work will understand that this is an important issue that I am bringing to your attention, and will be further discussed in this volume. We are all individuals, we will all react differently to toxins of all kinds—this is what makes it so difficult to *prove harm,* as I have mentioned. Let us hear what Martin Grootveld, Professor of Bioanalytical Chemistry and Chemical Pathology, University of Leicester, has to say:

> LOPs [lipid oxygenation products] detectable in fried foods are both cytotoxic [toxic to living cells] and genotoxic [toxic to DNA], and currently a substantial proportion of the human population regularly consumes such toxins in Western diets. This phenomenon presents some considerable and serious public health concerns, i.e., the continuous and sometimes frequent dietary ingestion of foods deep-fried at high temperature in oxidation-prone unsaturated fatty acid (UFA)-rich CFOs [culinary frying oils] potentially increases the risks of humans to a wide variety of chronic, non-communicable human diseases (NCDs), including cardiovascular diseases (1) and cancer (2). Since polyunsaturated fatty acids (PUFAs) are much more susceptible to thermally-induced oxidation (better described as peroxidation) than monounsaturated ones (MUFAs), CFOs rich in them produce the highest levels of hazardous LOPs during frying episodes, which repetitively escalate with the unfortunately common reuse of such frying media (3,4); passage of such thermally-peroxidised, LOP-containing oils into food matrices during shallow- or deep-frying practices renders them available for human consumption. Contrastingly, saturated fatty acids (SFAs) are extremely resistant to peroxidation, and hence SFA-laden frying media such as coconut oil and animal fat (lard) generate little or no LOPs when exposed to authentic or laboratory-simulated high-temperature frying practices [usually at ca. 180 °C (3)].[13]

How To Survive in the 21ˢᵗ Century

You would be forgiven for raising the question as to whether we have simply swapped the use of a relatively cheap fat that withstands high-temperature cooking reasonably well with something far more problematic, by swapping animal fat for vegetable oils. The answer would be yes, it certainly looks like it. It looks like we have swapped a fat with, in my view, a very weak association with heart disease, to a product that is now linked to cardiovascular disease and cancer. This is not all, read on.

Mendick refers to another researcher, Professor John Stein, Oxford Emeritus Professor of Neuroscience, who claims that the fatty acids in vegetable oils are contributing to other health problems, in ways that are affecting our brains. Here is what he reveals, partly as a result of corn and sunflower oils: 'The human brain is changing in a way that is as serious as climate change threatens to be'.

'The human brain is changing in a way that is as serious as climate change threatens to be'.

Because vegetable oils are rich in omega 6 fatty acids, they contribute to a reduction in critical omega 3 fatty acids in the brain by replacing them with omega 6.

'If you eat too much corn oil or sunflower oil, the brain is absorbing too much omega 6, and that effectively forces out omega 3,' said Prof Stein. 'I believe the lack of omega 3 is a powerful contributory factor to such problems as increasing mental health issues and other problems such as dyslexia.'

He further adds: 'Health concerns linked to the toxic by-products include heart disease; cancer; "malformations" during pregnancy; inflammation; risk of ulcers and a rise in blood pressure'.[14]

The issue about brain changes regarding the use of oils high in omega six, is not, however, limited to just *our* change in oil use. The move to raise cattle on feedlots in the USA, feeding the animals diets high in grains which are used to increase the weight of the animal quickly, ready for slaughter, has led to the meat in these animals becoming both much fattier than grass-fed beef, and with a different type of fat, which is much higher in the omega-six fatty acids.

Why is this important to you? Understanding the difference between good fats, and understanding a little about essential fatty acids (EFAs), could save your life, prevent you from contracting numerous diseases, suffering from dementia, and a whole lot more. One of the major differences between the omega 3 and the omega 6 essential fatty acids is to do with inflammation. Omega 3's reduce inflammation, whereas omega 6's are known to promote inflammation. As inflammation is considered a significant aspect in many chronic diseases, we would be wise to be careful about ingesting too-high a proportion of the omega 6 fatty acids. Here is a revealing study:

> Dietary changes over the past few decades in the intake of n-6 and n-3 PUFA [polyunsaturated fatty acid] show striking increases in the (n-6) to (n-3) ratio (~15 : 1), which are associated with greater metabolism of the n-6 PUFA compared with n-3 PUFA. Coinciding with this increase in the ratio of (n-6):(n-3) PUFA are increases in chronic inflammatory diseases such as nonalcoholic fatty liver disease (NAFLD), cardiovascular disease, obesity, inflammatory bowel disease (IBD), rheumatoid arthritis, and Alzheimer's disease (AD). By increasing the

ratio of (n-3):(n-6) PUFA in the Western diet, reductions may be achieved in the incidence of these chronic inflammatory diseases.[15]

Researchers have discovered that the omega 6 essential fatty acids increase the number of markers that are known to play a role in the diseases that are mentioned, and they are all reduced by the omega 3 fatty acids. Another researcher, Dr Artemis Simopoulos, has written extensively on the benefits of omega 3 fats, here are some of her observations:

> Increased dietary intake of linoleic acid (LA) [omega 6] leads to oxidation of low-density lipoprotein (LDL), platelet aggregation, and interferes with the incorporation of EFA in cell membrane phospholipids. Both omega-6 and omega-3 fatty acids influence gene expression. Omega-3 fatty acids have anti-inflammatory effects, suppress interleukin 1beta (IL-1beta), tumor necrosis factor-alpha (TNFalpha) and interleukin-6 (IL-6), whereas omega-6 fatty acids do not. Because inflammation is at the base of many chronic diseases, dietary intake of omega-3 fatty acids plays an important role in the manifestation of disease, particularly in persons with genetic variation, as for example in individuals with genetic variants at the 5-lipoxygenase (5-LO). [16]

I have included this, not hoping to introduce too much technicality, but because she added the fact that both omega 3 and omega 6 affect gene expression, something that few people realise. She further mentions that increased intake of linoleic acid, which is an omega 6 fatty acid (as is commonly found in sunflower and safflower oils), leads to oxidation of low-density lipoprotein (LDL), platelet aggregation, and interferes with the incorporation of EFAs as in cell membrane phospholipids. This information about the oxidation of LDL, which is the supposed 'bad' form of cholesterol, is interesting because this is one of the accepted important links with heart disease. It's not simply the fact that your levels of LDL are linked with heart disease, it is now more widely accepted that it is the *oxidised* form of LDL that is the real issue. This is significant, and I bring it to your intention here that one of the biggest culprits involved in the oxidation of LDL, is sugar. Both sugar and over-processed carbohydrates are associated with this effect on LDL. So could Professor Yudkin have been right all this time some of you may ask? Personally, I think he was right. What I believe for certain is that over-processed carbohydrates, and especially sugar, are responsible for a much greater role in the deterioration of our health than anybody gives credit for. The added point Dr Simopoulos makes is that excess LA also interferes with the incorporation of EFAs in cell membrane phospholipids. This has been mentioned before by a number of researchers.

What might be helpful to understand, is that our cell walls are made up of essential fatty acids. They form a bilayer of phospholipids that maintain the integrity of the cell. These essential fatty acids are called 'essential', as they have to be obtained from the diet, the body cannot create them. The quality of integrity is also affected by the ingestion of damaged fats. When the body is faced with either; an excess level of the wrong fats, damaged fats, oxidised fats, or simply a serious lack of good fats, the body has to make do. It doesn't have the ability to convert an omega 6 to an omega 3 or repair seriously damaged fats, it simply tries to use what is there. The result is that some cells simply no longer function the way they are supposed to.

It is worth stressing this point that the cell membranes which are composed of essential fatty acids (EFAs) are less able to maintain the cell integrity in a number of ways. One of the important ways is by maintaining oxygen levels. One of the first questions a nutritionist is likely to need to know of a patient, is what are their energy levels like? The energy levels can give some indication as to the cellular state, people with good energy levels are considered to be functioning well, when the levels drop this indicates a drop in cellular metabolism for one reason or another. Aside from the drop in energy levels that we can expect when the cells are not able to maintain adequate oxygenation if the levels drop too low, we are at risk of much more serious health issues. Dr Otto Warburg, a brilliant physician, who some rank, as the greatest biochemist of the 20ᵗʰ century, discovered what he believed was the prime cause of cancer, and that was his observation that when a cell's oxygen level drops too far (below one third of the normal level for oxygen) that the cell will become cancerous. This story in itself deserves a much wider audience, as it is too little known. Warburg and his discovery were ignored, more, due to the political issues than the science. Brian Scott Peskin introduces this story with his book, *The Hidden Story of Cancer.* [17]

Increase in Over-processed Carbohydrates

The move away from reliance on fats and the reduction of the consumption of red meat led to the increase in the consumption of grains, in particular highly processed carbohydrates such as wheat and all the white flour products such as white bread, pasta, pizza, cakes, biscuits and a whole host of products, many of which had in addition, high levels of sugar. The food industry, it must be said, was keen to embrace the move to the consumption of refined flour products as they were inexpensive, easy to manipulate, and provided a whole array of highly profitable items.

The food industry adapted to the new food guidelines by utilising the increasing knowledge gained from food scientists, who were discovering just how addictive sugar was, and just what levels would work best to get consumers to buy more of their products. They had discovered that the combination of sugar and salt was a real winner, and with the inclusion of fat in many circumstances made the perfect trio. They had discovered what people in the industry referred to as the 'bliss point', where the optimum levels of the combinations of sweet and salty existed. They found that younger people, for example, preferred things sweeter and saltier than their peers, which enabled more accurate targeting to their consumers. Companies like Nestlé were experimenting with the distribution of fat globules, and the various shapes and sizes that would give the best 'mouth feel' to maximise the success of their sales. They discovered that children could develop their taste for salt at four or five months of age, but the liking for sweet-tasting foods appeared from their very first introduction to food or drink. They also discovered that the more sugar was eaten, the more it seemed to be craved. The addiction was not simply a psychological addiction, animal research came to the same conclusions. A researcher, Anthony Sclafani, fed a group of rats with sugar-laden Froot Loops, a 'breakfast cereal' made by Kellogg, he found that they developed such a craving for sugar that they would take risks just to get hold of it. When it was withdrawn they would experience withdrawal symptoms. Other scientists at Princeton found the same situation, withdrawal signs included chattering jaws. Other researchers found that rats addicted to heroin or cocaine would choose sugar water in preference to either of these two drugs and within two days would convert their addiction from heroin or cocaine to sugar.[18]

With the heat off sugar, however, the food industry felt free to experiment in the creation of food products that would deliver good returns. Using cheaply produced processed carbohydrates as one of the starting points would deliver a fantastic array of marketable products. This led to some creative thinking and the re-invention of what one might call 'breakfast'. When John Harvey Kellogg first produced flaked cereal at Battle Creek, it was his brother, Will, who added the sugar to it. John Kellogg did not approve, so his brother went solo and so was born Kellogg's Toasted Cornflakes. Other's followed suit, so much so that Battle Creek turned into a cereal boom town. By 1911 there were more than 108 different brands of cereal being manufactured there, the majority with different amounts of sugar added, from 25 percent in some cereals to more than 75 percent. Following massive marketing campaigns, these products were to become a staple breakfast for many children, especially in the USA.[19]

As the food industry developed new products, the tendency was to use the new vegetable oils and fats, the new margarines, and hydrogenated oils—use of the animal fats was curtailed.

These changes to our dietary habits had significant effects on our health, particularly on our weight which introduced a whole host of other problems, some of which we will explore in the next chapter

Chapter Three

Hiding Sweet Poison

According to a report in *The Lancet* in 2010, being overweight and obesity were estimated to cause 3·4 million deaths, and the rise in obesity has led to widespread calls for regular monitoring of changes in overweight and obesity prevalence in all populations. They tell us that worldwide, the proportion of adults with a body-mass index (BMI) of 25 kg/m² or greater increased between 1980 and 2013 from 28·8% to 36·9% in men, and from 29·8% to 38·0% in women. They further tell us that the prevalence has increased substantially in children and adolescents in developed countries; 23·8% of boys and 22·6% of girls were overweight or obese in 2013. [20]

The rise in diabetes is inexorably linked to the rise and prevalence of obesity. According to the World Health Organisation (WHO), the number of people with diabetes had risen from 108 million in 1980 to 422 million by 2014, and the global prevalence of diabetes among adults over 18 years of age had risen from 4.7% in 1980 to 8.5% in 2014. WHO also informs us that diabetes prevalence has been rising more rapidly in middle and low-income countries, which is, in my view, predictable if you consider that junk food based on over-processed carbohydrates are cheap compared to quality protein and quality fruit and vegetables.

They also point out that diabetes is a major cause of blindness, kidney failure, heart attacks, stroke, and lower-limb amputation, and that in 2016 an estimated 1.6 million deaths were directly caused by diabetes. They also inform us that another 2.2 million additional deaths were attributable to high blood glucose in 2012 and, of those, almost half of all the deaths attributable to high blood glucose occur before the age of 70 years. WHO suggests that diabetes was the seventh leading cause of death in 2016. [21] As regards to deaths attributed to high glucose, they are not suggesting that by having high glucose you will die, merely that statistically the 2.2 million that died all had high blood glucose; they may have died from a heart attack, but high blood glucose was reported. This is interesting in that it is linked to the condition known as metabolic syndrome that will be discussed in this chapter.

The evidence of the move to a diet based on highly processed carbohydrates can be seen in the obesity figures and the epidemic of diabetes. One curious notion about weight gain and the medical profession is its adherence to the almost complete denial of the role of carbohydrates, particularly over-processed carbohydrates, in weight gain of the human population. If you were to ask a vet, or any knowledgeable person in the agricultural industry, about how to increase weight in animals, the advice would invariably be to increase the amount of cereals in the animal's diet. It has been known for decades that the way to increase weight is by feeding animals (which includes humans) on cereals.

Blame the Victim

You may wonder why it is that we are bombarded with the idea that weight gain in people is all to do with the amount you exercise and the number of calories that you consume. It's the calories and exercise dummy! Except that it is not! There is very little scientific evidence to support this view. What we have here is the classic 'blame the victim' routine that is the basic ploy of corporatocracy: to put the cause of a problem, particularly health problems, onto the victim—instead of having to be confronted with their role in the cause of whatever disaster they are creating. In this case, we have an obesity crisis and a diabetes epidemic, and a whole host of problems created by the consumption of sugar, in all its forms, and from the consumption of over-processed carbohydrates.

To blame these crises on the victims is, in my view, as obscene, as it would be to blame the victims of cancer for the cancer epidemic or victims of heart disease for the heart disease epidemic. We do know that there are factors that can influence our health: exercise, for example, has been shown to improve the health status of most people studied; being a non-smoker, we also know improves our likely health status. With regards to exercise, there is very little supporting evidence to suggest that it is the best way to lose weight. Where it is of great benefit and helps us maintain health is due to its ability to maintain a healthy heart, improve oxygenation and cleansing of the cells, improve energy levels, and improve lymphatic drainage—which helps the body cleanse itself and get rid of toxins—all of which are good reasons to include some form of exercise in your life.

From the moment that the US government, made saturated fats the enemy and produced guidelines suggesting its populace increase the level of carbohydrate and reduce saturated fats, it enabled the food industry to embark on developing a whole new range of foods from inexpensive refined carbohydrates. Denying the result of this development, and its impact on the health of society by blaming obesity and all the terrible health consequences of this disease on the victims is not just being ignorant of the science that exists, it is an insult to all the people who are harmed.

The Insidious Effects of Sugar and Processed Carbs

One of the problems with the whole cholesterol myth—and myth is what it is—is that research has focused for the last 60 years on virtually ignoring the harmful effects of sugar and processed carbs to study the cholesterol issue. Even so, some research has been undertaken that has revealed the many ways that sugar in its various guises can impact our health. In this chapter we can review some of the evidence that shows the impact it is having on our health. Firstly, it is important to understand some of the sources of sugar that impact our health. Below is a table listing some of the guises sugar come in, it is not exhaustive however, it is simply a selection. Alcohol, for example, is not listed here, but it is still, in all its guises, sugar albeit fermented sugar. It still has a negative effect on our health, not just due to the fact that the alcohol, as we all know, is a poison to the body, although one that we may find appealing on occasion. When consumed in excess of 50 grams a day (approximately three glasses of wine), it is considered over our toxic threshold. Whereas someone consuming excess sugar via sweetened drinks will often visibly look overweight, excess alcohol intake may not increase body fat *visibly*. It can however still create a fatty liver. According to Dr Robert Lustig, professor of Pediatric Endocrinology at the University of California, 'The difference between alcoholic fatty liver disease and non-alcoholic fatty liver disease lies only in the terminology—the effect on the body is the same'.[22]

Agave nectar	Barbados sugar	Barley malt	Beet sugar
Blackstrap molasses	Brown sugar	Buttered syrup	Cane juice crystals
Cane sugar	Caramel	Carob Syrup	Castor sugar

Confectioner's syrup	Corn syrup	Corn syrup-solids	Crystalline fructose
Date sugar	Demerara sugar	Dextran	Dextrose
Diastatic malt	Diastase	Ethyl maltol	Evaporated cane juice
Florida crystals	Fructose	Fruit juice	Fruit juice concentrate
Galactose	Glucose	Glucose solids	Golden sugar
Golden syrup	Grape sugar	High-fructose corn syrup	Honey
Icing sugar	Invert sugar	lactose	Malt syrup
Maltodextrin	Maltose	Maple syrup	Molasses
Muscovado sugar	Organic raw sugar	Panocha	Raw sugar
Refiner's syrup	Rice syrup	Sorghum syrup	Sucrose
Sugar	Treacle	Turbinado sugar	Yellow sugar

Table I: Various Names for Sugar Added to processed Food. Lustig 2013.

It might be useful to review some of the effects of ingesting sucrose, the form of sugar that historically we were most exposed to. Sucrose is made up of two types of sugar, glucose and fructose. The components affect the body in different ways. When we consume refined sucrose, the glucose is released very quickly into the body which spikes the blood glucose levels which is a problem for the body. In response to this challenge, the body releases the hormone, insulin, which helps to convert the glucose into glycogen in the liver, which is a form of liver starch. Excess glucose is converted to fat (as triglycerides) for storage in the liver and the muscles. This reduces the blood sugar level and helps bring it back to normal, and return the body to homeostasis (which effectively is its most harmonious state). The fructose component, which does not directly affect the blood sugar levels in the same way, is sent directly to the liver where it is processed into fat, a triglyceride. Some is stored in the liver, and any excess is shipped out so as to not overload the liver and impair its function.

The problem we face with consuming such levels of processed sugar as is happening in our population is that our bodies were not designed to deal with the amounts currently consumed. Prior to the relatively recent introduction of refined sugar into the diet, our ancestors were only exposed to fructose from eating fruit in season, or honey on rare occasions. You would have to eat very large amounts of fruit to compare with the intake of an average sugar-loaded beverage, something that was unlikely to occur. I have previously reported on the obesity epidemic, a growing problem in our society, particularly among the young.[23] Concerns exist about the levels of sugar consumed by children, and the rising levels of obesity in children, particularly associated with the consumption of sugar-laden drinks and the consequences for their future health. There are increasing numbers of studies showing the harmful effects on children of sugar consumption. A study by Welsh et al. raises concerns for their future health with the following comments:

> Consumption of added sugars among US adolescents is positively associated with multiple measures known to increase cardiovascular disease risk.
>
> Cardiovascular disease (CVD) is a leading cause of morbidity and mortality among US adults. Whereas atherosclerosis and CVD occur

later in life, their risk factors, including lipid disorders, diabetes mellitus, and obesity are increasingly identified among adolescents and even children. Currently, 32% of US children and adolescents aged 2 to 18 years are overweight or obese. Though CVD among children is rare, an increase in risk factors at younger ages and their apparent tendency to track into adulthood highlights the need for early and effective prevention efforts.

Our results demonstrate that intake of added sugars is positively associated with known cardiovascular risk factors when controlling for other characteristics. We found increased dyslipidemia (lower HDLs and higher LDLs and triglyceride levels) among adolescents.[24]

Another study by Stanhope et al. found similar issues and more:

In epidemiological studies, consumption of sugar and/or sugar-sweetened beverages has been linked to the presence of unfavorable lipid levels, insulin resistance, fatty liver, type 2 diabetes, cardiovascular disease, and metabolic syndrome.[25]

A Harvard School of Public Health review of articles and sugary drinks reveals that a study that followed 40,000 men for two decades found that those who averaged one can of a sugary beverage per day had a 20% higher risk of having a heart attack or dying from a heart attack than men who rarely consumed sugary drinks. Another study, this time on women, the Nurses' Health Study, which tracked the health of nearly 90,000 women over two decades, found that women who drank more than two servings of sugary beverage each day had a 40 percent higher risk of heart attacks or death from heart disease than women who rarely drank sugary beverages. They also found that people who consume sugary drinks regularly—1 to 2 cans a day or more—have a 26% greater risk of developing type 2 diabetes than people who rarely have such drinks. They also found the risks are even greater in young adults and Asians.[26]

How To Survive in the 21ˢᵗ Century

Increasing numbers of doctors are critical of the levels of sugar in people's diets. Dr Aseem Malhotra, an internationally renowned cardiologist, believes that poor diet is actually responsible for more disease than smoking, alcohol and physical inactivity combined. He suggests the component of the western diet that most needs to be targeted is sugar. He writes: 'Unlike fat and protein, refined sugars offer no nutritional value and, contrary to what the food industry wants you to believe, the body does not require any carbohydrate from added sugar for energy. Thus it is a source of completely unnecessary calories.' He is critical of the food industry's denial of sugar's role in obesity and its failure to acknowledge the multitude of scientific studies to the contrary. He is greatly concerned about the serious increase of diabetes that he obviously links to sugar consumption: 'Of all the chronic diseases, type 2 diabetes, which is entirely preventable, is perhaps the most damaging. Diabetes increases the risk of heart attack, stroke, kidney failure, eye disease and leg amputations. Up to half of all diabetic patients go on to suffer acute or chronic pain, and two-thirds will ultimately develop dementia. The direct and indirect costs to the UK of diabetes is over £24bn and projected to approach £40bn by 2030. If we do nothing, this will cripple the NHS [UK's National Health Service].'[27]

Professor Simon Capewell, an expert in clinical epidemiology at the University of Liverpool is leading a health campaign in the UK to cut sugar from people's diets, which he feels is fuelling Britain's obesity epidemic. He suggests 'Sugar is the new tobacco. Everywhere, sugary drinks and junk foods are now pressed on unsuspecting parents and children by a cynical industry focussed on profit not health.'[28] An apologist for the sugar industry tried to argue that sugar is essential to food. Professor Capewell counters 'It is not. He would have been more accurate in saying sugar is essential to food industry profits and lining the pockets of its co-opted partners.' Professor Capewell teamed up with Dr Aseem

Hiding Sweet Poison

Malhotra in a non-profit campaign called Action on Sugar which compared sugar and tobacco:

> How does sugar compare to tobacco? A teaspoon of sugar or one cigarette will not harm you. But over time, the habit can be fatal. Unlike Big Tobacco, Big Sugar deliberately targets children. And added sugar has become so pervasive within the food environment that we can't avoid it even if we wanted to. It is thus not simply a matter of personal choice. But perhaps most disturbing of all the similarities is the financial and political muscle that both industries have exerted to try and protect their profits, at the expense of our health. It's time to wind back the harms of too much sugar, reverse the "diabesity" epidemic and the unspeakable suffering it causes. It's time for Action On Sugar.[29]

You may be wondering why it is if sugar is so damaging to our health that more has not been made of this issue. That is a valid question and deserves some explanation before we dig a little further into some of the science behind this.

Corporate Cover-up

We previously mentioned that Ancel Keys, the physiologist, who proposed the cholesterol theory of heart disease in 1957, was funded by the sugar industry and did not receive universal acceptance for his theory. What later came to light was the extent to which the sugar industry influenced public understanding. Researchers have recently revealed just to what extent this occurred in documents from the Sugar Research Foundation:

> Early warning signals of the coronary heart disease (CHD) risk of sugar (sucrose) emerged in the 1950s. We examined Sugar Research Foundation (SRF) internal documents, historical reports, and statements relevant to early debates about the dietary causes of CHD and assembled

findings chronologically into a narrative case study. The SRF sponsored its first CHD research project in 1965, a literature review published in the *New England Journal of Medicine,* which singled out fat and cholesterol as the dietary causes of CHD and downplayed evidence that sucrose consumption was also a risk factor. The SRF set the review's objective, contributed articles for inclusion, and received drafts. The SRF's funding and role was not disclosed. Together with other recent analyses of sugar industry documents, our findings suggest the industry sponsored a research program in the 1960s and 1970s that successfully cast doubt about the hazards of sucrose while promoting fat as the dietary culprit in CHD. Policymaking committees should consider giving less weight to food industry–funded studies and include mechanistic and animal studies as well as studies appraising the effect of added sugars on multiple CHD biomarkers and disease development.[30]

It has only been since 1984 that the *New England Journal of Medicine* has required authors to disclose all conflicts of interest. Prior to this time most corporate interests, including the sugar industry, were able to freely sway opinion and manipulate science unbeknown to the general public, and officialdom. There is, of course, much more to this story we have simply revealed one item in their shenanigans. For now, we can make sure you are better informed about metabolic syndrome, something that affects many people, most of them unaware of it.

Metabolic Syndrome

Dr Lustig, the renowned paediatric endocrinologist we have already referred to, in his volume, *Fat Chance—The bitter truth about sugar,* sends us warning that the levels of sugar consumption in western diets are causing serious harm, and much of the harm goes unrecognised. He mentions that twenty percent of the obese population has a normal metabolic profile, whereas up to forty percent of normal-weight people have an abnormal metabolic profile, and he suggests 'Knowing where you stand is crucial to taking steps to prolong your life.' Whilst obesity is associated with a whole host of problems, the fact that normal-weight people can have an abnormal metabolic status is significant. He explains the significance:

'You don't die of obesity; you die of the diseases that "travel" with it. It's these metabolic decompensations that make obesity the scourge that it is. Diabetes, hypertension, heart disease, cancer, and dementia—the things that kill you are collectively packaged under the concept of "metabolic syndrome."' He suggests that metabolic syndrome may soon overtake smoking as the leading cause of heart disease worldwide, with the problem 'increasing at alarming rates and translates into fifteen to twenty years of life lost.'[31]

I first wrote about metabolic syndrome, in *Unhealthy Betrayal,* and reported the work of Gerald Reaven M.D., who wrote about it in his own volume as Syndrome X. He listed a number of factors associated with what we now refer to as 'metabolic syndrome';

1. Impaired glucose tolerance.
2. High insulin levels (hyperinsulinemia).
3. Elevated triglycerides (blood fats).
4. Low HDL this is referred to as the "good" cholesterol.
5. Slow clearance of fat from the blood.
6. Smaller, more-dense LDL, often referred to as the "bad" cholesterol particles.
7. Increased propensity of the blood to form clots.
8. Decreased ability to dissolve blood clots.
9. Elevated blood pressure (hypertension).[32]

All these factors are associated with a much greater risk of heart disease. One of the main features is impaired glucose tolerance, with accompanied high insulin levels. Many believe that this situation is arrived at by excessive dietary uptake of over-processed carbohydrate, particularly sugar. The sugar ingestion provokes an insulin response to deal with the impending blood sugar onslaught, and with repeated dietary uptake of quickly absorbed carbohydrates (absorbed as glucose in the body), the body becomes resistant to the elevated insulin levels. This results in ever-higher levels of insulin being produced and released to deal with the continuous onslaught of glucose. Insulin signals certain cells to "open their doors" to blood sugar by attaching to specially designated receptors on the cell's surface. As the cells become resistant, they no longer respond to insulin's instructions. Unable to flow into designated cells, blood sugar accumulates in the bloodstream.

Elevated triglycerides were something that Professor Yudkin had already observed when he fed rats sugar: 'We found that the amount of triglyceride in the blood was enormously and rapidly increased when rats ate sugar.' He also found that the livers of the rats became enlarged by some 25 %. He also noted that it produced an increase in blood pressure and a change in the properties of blood platelets. The platelets were found to clump together more and become sticky ('aggregated'). He also noted in his studies using chickens, that their aortas were affected by fatty deposits, in 46 percent of the chickens fed sugar. Yudkin also studied the effects of sugar on people, and noted in one study of nineteen young men, the same increase in blood triglycerides, the same stickiness of the blood platelets, and, further, he found the rise in blood pressure proportional to the quantity of sugar in the diet. Yudkin's view of sugar has proved to be a warning that society has ignored at its peril:

As for sugar, the most relevant fact is that every one of the abnormalities seen in coronary heart disease and in diabetes can be produced by the inclusion of sugar in the diet.[33]

Dr Lustig draws our attention to one of the factors of metabolic syndrome, and that is one of the dangers of having excess insulin floating around in the body, as in hyperinsulinemia: it is associated with the development and growth of various forms of cancer. If you add the understanding that cancer itself utilises sugar to grow, you can see why it may be prudent to avoid such a product (and also over-processed carbohydrates), particularly if you have cancer, and if you don't have cancer, perhaps minimise your use, unless you feel lucky.

There are other aspects of excess glucose in the body that are worth bringing to your attention. Dr Lustig is concerned with the effects on the liver, where excess glucose is turned into glycogen. His concern is with the metabolism of excess energy: excess fats, excess protein, alcohol, or fructose, all of which are processed by the liver into fat—and which need to be transported out of the liver or these fats will 'muck up the works'. He suggests anything that drives liver fat accumulation, is a potential driver of metabolic disease. One of the problems with diets high in over-processed carbohydrates is not just the visible excess weight that people can carry, it's the less visible internal fat that accumulates around the organs, such as the liver and kidneys, leading to compromised function.

Lustig suggests that the liver problem is a serious dilemma for the body, but he believes that the accompanying problem with the creation of reactive oxygen species (ROS) adds to the body's problem with maintaining health. This situation is created when glucose is metabolised in the mitochondria (the energy creators in the cells) where glucose is transformed into adenosine triphosphate (ATP), the body's energy molecule. The cells are generally protected from normal metabolic creation of ROS products by the peroxisome, which is full of antioxidants and is situated next to the mitochondria for this very reason. However, when excess glucose and fructose are ingested, excess ROS products are created, and much more so when fructose is ingested in excess. ROS products can create havoc in the body: they damage cell functioning, and even destroy the cell, or as Dr Lustig suggests 'the cells crap out, and when enough cells give up, you've got the basis for metabolic syndrome.' [34]

Another way sugar and over-processed carbs cause havoc in the body is by the creation of advanced glycated end-products (AGEs). They are formed by the process of glycation, where a glucose molecule attaches itself to, for example, a protein molecule, without the critical benefit of an enzyme to orchestrate the reaction. Enzymes play an essential role in living organisms to regulate chemical reactions to ensure they conform to the metabolic program that they were designed for. Without this guidance, haphazard unions can be formed that can persist and create unforeseen consequences, which can multiply if abnormal levels of glucose persist. These AGEs can bind to other AGEs continuously through what is referred to as 'cross-linking' creating unforeseen chemical reactions. This can happen to haemoglobin, creating glycated haemoglobin, as happens with diabetics. It can happen in the eyes where AGEs are known to accumulate, causing cataracts and other eye problems. They can affect kidney function, the linings of the arteries, and nerve endings. Whilst AGEs are known to accumulate with our advancing years, the AGE acronym, is appropriate, in that their creation can seriously advance the ageing process. As regards to heart disease, regarded as the number one killer globally, AGEs and the glycation process also play a critical role in this disease. LDL, the low-density lipoprotein that has been labelled the 'bad' cholesterol, has been found to be particularly susceptible to oxidation by ROS and glycation, and it is this oxidised form of LDL that is associated with coronary heart disease.[35] Confusion exists regarding the whole LDL theory linking LDL with coronary heart disease due to the fact that in the majority of cases there is a complete failure to specifically identify whether the LDL in question is the damaged and oxidized version or simply normal LDL. Studies of people with normal LDL, that has not been oxidised, do not support the heart disease theory. A study by Ravnskov et al., in January 2018, which was a comprehensive review of the literature challenged the view that cholesterol was the culprit and particularly LDL. [36]

Dangers of Statins

Whilst on the subject of advanced ageing products, one of the tragedies of the 21st century, could be considered to be the way the medical industry steered away research from looking at the dietary implications of the greater consumption of sugar and over-processed carbohydrates, into the use of pharmaceutical products to supposedly deal with the consequential problems of such a disastrous diet. The use of statins is one example that I believe will be shown not to have been a benefit to humanity, but a negative impact on health—albeit a great money maker for the pharmaceutical industry.

I first wrote on the danger of statins in *Unhealthy Betrayal,* [37] where I reported the works of a number of researchers and doctors alarmed at the side effects of such drugs. In the above comprehensive review that we have referred to the authors made the following observations:

> For half a century, a high level of total cholesterol (TC) or low-density lipoprotein cholesterol (LDL-C) has been considered to be the major cause of atherosclerosis and cardiovascular disease (CVD), and statin treatment has been widely promoted for cardiovascular prevention.

However, there is an increasing understanding that the mechanisms are more complicated and that statin treatment, in particular when used as primary prevention, is of doubtful benefit.

The authors challenged three recently published large reviews and found falsifications and misleading information:

> The authors of three large reviews recently published by statin advocates have attempted to validate the current dogma. This article delineates the serious errors in these three reviews as well as other obvious falsifications of the cholesterol hypothesis.
>
> Our search for falsifications of the cholesterol hypothesis confirms that it is unable to satisfy any of the Bradford Hill criteria for causality and that the conclusions of the authors of the three reviews are based on misleading statistics, exclusion of unsuccessful trials and by ignoring numerous contradictory observations.[38]

A few years ago, Uffe Ravnskov and his colleagues published a review of 19 studies where the authors had measured cholesterol in more than 68,000 people and followed them for several years. Ravnskov reveals that at follow-up, they found that those with the highest level of 'bad' LDL-cholesterol lived the longest. He points out that in one of the studies the authors even found that those with high LDL-cholesterol lived longer than those on cholesterol-lowering treatment. This goes against what many have been preaching, and he further made a number of points:

1. Almost all studies have found that people with low cholesterol become just as atherosclerotic as people with high cholesterol.

2. Numerous studies have found that high cholesterol is not a risk factor for women or elderly people.

3. The small benefit from the statin trials is independent of the amount by which cholesterol is lowered.

4. Whereas the drug industry claims that serious side effects from statin treatment are extremely rare, numerous independent researchers have documented that more than 25% may suffer from side effects including muscular damage, type 2 diabetes, liver damage, hearing loss, Alzheimer's, dementia, Parkinson's disease, depression, nerve damage, kidney failure or cancer.

5. Very few with inherited high cholesterol (familial hypercholesterolemia) die from heart disease and the cause is not their high cholesterol. Furthermore, people with this abnormality are protected against cancer and infectious diseases.

6. After the introduction of new regulations by health authorities in Europe and the US according to which all trial data have to be made public, no statin trial has been successful.

7. Statin use is not associated with the incidence or the mortality of heart disease; neither in the US nor in Europe. [39]

No doubt for some of you these statements come as a surprise, they are nevertheless, views that are shared by a significant body of opinion.

Duane Graveline, M.D., suffered what is referred to as transient global amnesia that he believed was caused by taking a statin called Lipitor, in 1999. He suffered a second attack when he re-started the drug a year later. At first, he was reluctant to believe that the statin could be responsible, which is why he started taking it again. He says that he reverted to being a thirteen-year-old high school student, with no memory of the rest of his life, that of being a married man with children and a wife. Whilst these attacks only lasted twelve hours or so, by 2003 he had noted the gradual onset of unusual tiredness, and weakness, and that minimal exercise was followed by uncomfortable aching in his lower back and legs as if they had been strained excessively. In three years he went from a physically fit man to what he referred to as a 'doddering old man.' This experience provoked him to look further into statins, and his research led him to extensive writing about what he perceived as the dangers of statin use. In his book, *The Dark Side of Statins,* he discusses many of the problems associated with statin use that is based on their inhibition of the mevalonate pathway, which as reductase inhibitors, inhibits cholesterol production, but also affects other critical components such as the production of dolichols and Co-enzyme Q10 (CoQ10), selenoprotein, Rho proteins, and disruption of normal phosphorylation. Further explanation of some of these vital processes are discussed below.

Disrupting the mevalonate pathway to address a perceived cholesterol imbalance has been compared to cutting down an entire tree just to remove a bad apple—it is simply a very risky manoeuvre, with many unforeseen consequences. CoQ10 is a really important antioxidant essential to the normal functioning of energy production in the mitochondria. With CoQ10 impairment, irreversible DNA damage can occur from excessive build-up of superoxide and hydroxyl radicals, which CoQ10 is uniquely placed to prevent. The situation is further compounded by the inhibition of dolichols which are vital to the repair of mitochondrial DNA mutations in our daily lives. Damage to DNA by deletions and substitutions have to be identified, excised and finally replaced with the correct form so we can continue to function. Our dolichols are vital in this process, in that each step of our mitochondrial DNA correction requires specific glycoprotein-derived enzymes which are mediated by the dolichols. Dolichols orchestrate this entire process of glycoprotein synthesis, which statins have long been known to inhibit.[40]

We know that the American Heart Association (AHA) and the American Medical Association (AMA) has bought into the whole cholesterol myth propagated by Ancel Keys, who we understand was funded by the sugar industry. They also bought the statin drug treatment program promoted by people like Daniel Steinberg, who published *The Cholesterol Wars*, in 2007, which enthusiastically supported and promoted the whole cholesterol theory, in the face of mounting evidence that it was based on unsound science. He also promoted the use of cholesterol-lowering drugs, like statins, that were based on fungal toxins so toxic that early attempts to use them led to disastrous outcomes.

It is estimated that approximately 70 million Americans and over 200 million people worldwide are taking statins. A significant and growing number of doctors are becoming aware that the science is not just shaky, it is increasingly seen as distinctly lacking. Unfortunately with such vast amounts of money involved the industry can use its clout and key opinion leaders to publish meta-studies spinning the statistics to their advantage, and then assailing the medical profession with the 'evidence' of how great statins are for us all. What they are unable to do, however, is to make water flow uphill, or explain how we are expected to swallow the idea that the destruction of mevalonate, which is integral to the production of such important molecules as Co-Q10, will not lead to cellular destruction and loss of energy. It is beyond the scope of this book to get into an in-depth discussion of this important topic, I can only allude to some of the major health implications and suggest that those of you interested consult further from the sources I quote. Here, for example, is a quote from James B. Joseph, and Hannah Yoseph, MD, from their book *How Statin Drugs Really Lower Cholesterol—And Kill You One Cell at a Time*, which gives the story of statin development starting in the late 1950s, and revealing some of the science behind this development: 'One biochemical pathway that a pharmaceutical drug should never touch is the mevalonate pathway. Leave our cells' reproductive, rejuvenating and life-restoring cycles alone, thank you very much! There is a simple word for healthy cell cycles: life'.

One biochemical pathway that a pharmaceutical drug should never touch is the mevalonate pathway. Leave our cells' reproductive, rejuvenating and life-restoring cycles alone, thank you very much! There is a simple word for healthy cell cycles: life.

Statins which are reductase inhibitors disable reductase which converts food into mevalonate which, as the genius Marvin D Siperstein discovered is required for DNA synthesis, cell growth and replication. The Yosephs who discuss Siperstein's work make the comment 'Despite the magnitude of the find that neither DNA nor cells can replicate without an intact mevalonate pathway, his work remains largely ignored.' The significance of this is better expressed by their explanation of how important cell replication is:

> Dead cells slough off our skin, hair and eyes and out our bowel tract, urethra and sweat. Every single cell in our body dies. In normal cycles, cells reproduce by splitting and cloning themselves. As they die and slough we do not miss them. Statins eventually result in the consequence of our cells being unable to replace themselves. Take a statin and cells stop reproducing. Death accelerates one cell at a time.

Cell metabolism is how cells utilise oxygen and the food we eat, it's how cells breathe, anything that obstructs this process suffocates the cells—and

Hiding Sweet Poison

CoQ10 is as essential to metabolism as oxygen. Cells that have a very high demand for CoQ10 are muscle cells, especially the heart muscle. Dr Yoseph mentions that this is why muscle cell damage (myopathy) and muscle cell death (rhabdomyolysis) are the most commonly reported statin injuries. She quotes Peter Langsjoen MD: 'We are now in a position to witness the unfolding of the greatest medical tragedy of all time. Never before in history has the medical establishment knowingly created a life threatening nutrient deficiency in millions of otherwise healthy people. [41]

We are now in a position to witness the unfolding of the greatest medical tragedy of all time. Never before in history has the medical establishment knowingly created a life threatening nutrient deficiency in millions of otherwise healthy people.

CoQ10 has a critical role to play in energy conversion in the electron transport chain (ETC) where electrons are pumped through a series of mechanisms to create energy in the mitochondria. Understanding that there are approximately ten thousand ETCs per mitochondria and that various cells have from hundreds to thousands of mitochondria *per cell,* you can understand how a reduction in the availability of the essential nutrient CoQ10 can have a huge impact on the availability of energy in the body. This does not just impact our ability to be able to function adequately on a physical level, it can also impact on other levels. The egg cell, for example, has a huge number of mitochondria, approximately 100,000, which cannot create a new embryo successfully without adequate supplies of energy. CoQ10 being an antioxidant can prevent oxidation of low-density lipoprotein that some associate with heart disease. It has other less well-known benefits, muscle relaxation, for example, takes more energy

(ATP) than muscle contraction, when ATP is lacking, muscles remain tenser and our blood pressure increases (it has been known for some time that CoQ10 taken as a supplement can reduce blood pressure). CoQ10 reduces the 'stickiness' of blood platelets and can help prevent clots from forming which makes it important in general maintenance of good health. To give you some idea of the importance of CoQ10 in energy production, it is believed that 10 per cent of the human body is mitochondria.[42] This is by no means the only important use of CoQ10, I have merely introduced some aspects of its use to enable you to realise the huge impact that introducing a drug like a statin into your body that impairs the synthesis of CoQ10, and dolichols can have, and further how it can have a many-faceted effect on your health outcome.

Mindless Intervention

It's not just the physical body that requires energy, the brain consumes 20% of the body's energy supply, 20% of the available oxygen, and is particularly vulnerable to free radical damage (due to its rich oxygen supply and high fatty acid content). One potent free radical, called peroxynitrite (formed from nitric oxide) oxidises lipids in the membranes of nerve cells. It generates the highly toxic by-product hydroxynonenal (HNE), which is found in excess quantities in multiple brain regions of Alzheimer's patients. HNE kills brain cells, not only directly but indirectly by making them more susceptible to excitotoxicity. We know that CoQ10 (and vitamin E) can protect cell membranes from lipid peroxidation and that CoQ10 has been found to reduce peroxynitrite damage and HNE formation in the bloodstream. [43] Whilst the brain only comprises 2 % of our body weight, it is composed of 25 % of the body's cholesterol, and myelin, the white matter that insulates brain circuits, is made from tightly-wound membranes containing 75% of the brain's cholesterol. Cholesterol also helps guide developing nerve endings to their destinations on "lipid rafts". If the brain is too low in cholesterol, its membranes, synapses, myelin and lipid rafts can't form or function properly, reducing the brain's ability to function affecting mood regulation, learning, and memory. The neurologist Dr David Permutter informs us of a recent study available on the NIH Public Access site, where researchers showed that in the elderly, the best memory function was observed in those with the highest levels of cholesterol. Low cholesterol is associated with an increased risk for depression and even death.[44]

You should be able to see from the foregoing that, statin intervention can have a very significant effect on many of our bodily systems, and perhaps understand why there are so many doctors who could miss many of the side effects as simply old age creeping in, albeit at a much faster than normal pace. Uffe Ravnskov, MD, PhD, in his book, *Fat and Cholesterol are Good for You*, accuses the cholesterol campaign of 'Medical Quackery of the first order,' and further quotes the eminent American physician and scientist George Mann who called it "the greatest scientific deception of this century, perhaps any century." As regards to the use of statins, he suggests 'they may destroy your muscles and your mind, make you impotent and produce cancer.' [45]

Much more could be said on the disastrous work of statins. For those of you who would like more information, there are sources on my website www.fundamental-health.com aside from material that I have referenced here. For now, I will leave the last word to some of the doctors and scientists who have dared to speak the truth about cholesterol, a product that is absolutely essential to your health and wellbeing.

The idea that high cholesterol levels in the blood are the main cause of CVD is impossible because people with low levels become just as atherosclerotic as people with high levels and their risk of suffering from CVD is the same or higher. The cholesterol hypothesis has been kept alive for decades by reviewers who have used misleading statistics, excluded the results from unsuccessful trials and ignored numerous contradictory observations.[46]

We have revealed how political intervention into the science of health has led to the promotion of a false theory that has led to huge consequences for our health both with regards to the food industry's development of highly processed carbohydrates (made with damaged vegetable fats, synthetic salt, and their sugar-laden drinks—most of which contain further added chemicals and colourings), and the medical industry's response to the creation of drug treatments for what are obviously metabolic conditions. Metabolism refers to the dietary eating habits, the inclusion of drinks, the air that we breathe, the chemicals were are exposed to—the entire spectrum of chemicals that the body has to process to maintain our health and, of course, this would include the various forms of radiation exposure. This metabolic challenge will be the subject of the next chapter.

Chapter Four

Surviving Metabolic Carnage

There is no known method for measuring or predicting a "safe" level of exposure to any carcinogen below which cancer will not result in any individual or population or group. That is, there is no, basis for the threshold hypothesis which claims that exposure to relatively low levels of carcinogens is safe and therefore justifiable.[47]

Samuel S. Epstein, Professor Emeritus of Occupational and Environmental Medicine, University of Illinois, and world cancer expert. 1926-2018.

In my previous volume, *Unhealthy Betrayal,* [48] I related how someone in the higher echelons of industry suggested that environmentalists and nutritionists represented the greatest threat to profits that industry faced. As a nutritionist, I can see how such a statement could be made, in the face of the rising levels of pollution that were being dumped on the human population and the environment. Forcing industry to take responsibility for their actions, and the health consequences of their pollution would, of course, reduce their profit margins as we mentioned in the first chapter, and in some cases might make what they do unprofitable. The question then would surely be, if their business creates such problems for health if they were to act responsibly, that their business plan would not be viable, do we really need this kind of business? One of the great cries of industry faced with challenges to their irresponsible pollution would be 'Jobs! There will be a loss of Jobs! More layoffs!' Surely the creative potential of humanity is better than is belied by this facile plea. Why can't we create better employment for our population than this? This would be a better question, and one I would be happy to answer, but not in this volume: this question would be better dealt with by dealing with the dysfunctional economic system that is collapsing in debt. This topic was explored in a previous volume, *Hijacked.* [49] In this section, however, we will look at some of the metabolic consequences of the failure of the regulatory systems to protect our health and the environment we live in.

Cancer Blindness

One thing that is fundamentally important to understand is that business interests and *your* interests are not the same, and that to maintain the enormous levels of profits that the pharmaceutical industry is making—it is essential to them that you do not make the connection between the massive health disaster were are currently facing—and both the chemical pollutants that are causing this disaster and how industry profits by treating this disaster with drugs, radiation, and surgery. We hope to help you in this volume understand how not to become just another early victim, to this social disaster.

One of the most obvious results of the chemical onslaught of the last century is the dramatic and inexorable rise of cancer incidence. According to Cancer Research UK, there were 17 million new cases of cancer worldwide in 2018, with 9.6 million deaths, and they predict that worldwide there will be 27.5 million new cases of cancer each year by 2040. They also mention that UK mortality is ranked higher than that of two-thirds of the rest of the countries in the world and predict that one in two people will develop cancer at some point in their lives in the UK. [50] That's a pretty dismal report on the state of health of our society, particularly from a supposedly leading industrial society. Surely we can do better than this.

Samuel S. Epstein, Professor Emeritus of Occupational and Environmental Medicine, University of Illinois (died 18 March 2018), and world cancer expert was a critic of the U.S. National Cancer Institute and the American Cancer Society, and a thorn in the side of the less-responsible side of industry. He criticised the cancer societies for their failure to recognise the true extent of the role of chemical exposure in the workplace in the creation of cancer, and their abject failure to devote anything but the absolute minimal resources to the study of occupational or environmental sources of carcinogens. This tragedy has unfortunately changed little: few cancer charities seem to dare to challenge corporate interests and acknowledge the fact that we have released more than 100,000 chemicals into our lives and the environment, for which there are serious consequences.

In his volume, *The Politics of Cancer Revisited,* in a section on how to prevent cancer, he wrote regarding food: 'Your dietary choices and habits are clearly important. Some diets may reduce your cancer risk, while others may increase it. This is, however, an area where caution and common sense must be exercised, especially as the facts are incomplete, and the consumer is caught between opposing viewpoints. Industry, on the one hand, dismisses as hysterical any questions on the safety or carcinogenicity of food, while on the other hand public interest groups emphasize the carcinogenic hazards of many food additives and contaminants.' He brings to our attention the 1978 report "Cancer-causing Chemicals in Food," by the American government's Subcommittee on Oversight and Investigations of the House Committee on Interstate and Foreign

How To Survive in the 21ˢᵗ Century

Commerce which was very critical of the oversight of the EPA, the FDA, and the USDA of the food system.[51] I quote some of the report below:

> The attached report by the Subcommittee on Oversight and Investigations reviews the Federal Government's efforts to protect the public from potentially dangerous amounts of pesticide residues in food. It focuses on the activities of the Environmental Protection Agency (EPA), Department of Agriculture (USDA), and the Food and Drug Administration (FDA) with regard to pesticide tolerance setting, residue monitoring, and enforcement of statutes designed to keep unhealthy levels of pesticides from being deposited on or in food products.

> The subcommittee concludes that these programs are inadequate. As a result, American consumers cannot be sure that the meat, poultry, fruits and vegetables they buy are not tainted with potentially dangerous pesticide residues.

> We all have to eat. Because of the nature of chemical contaminants, we are forced to rely on the Federal government to protect us against potentially dangerous chemicals we cannot see, smell or taste. Our examination leads us to believe that we cannot rely on the Federal government to protect us.

> We found for instance that the EPA (1) continues to approve tolerances for potentially carcinogenic, mutagenic, and teratogenic pesticides which result in residues in or on food; has set tolerances for some of these pesticides without complete safety data; (3) has exempted some potentially dangerous pesticides from its tolerance requirements which end up in or on food; (4) uses an inadequate and outadated statistical base for setting tolerance levels; (5) often does not know what level of pesticide residue usually results from the use of a product; and (6) bases its approval of pesticides merely on industry-supplied safety data which often does not fully examine the potential hazard posed by the pesticide.

In sum, the Subcommittee concludes that EPA's tolerance setting program is abysmal and needs a complete overhaul.

Additionally, the Subcommittee is alarmed with the inadequate monitoring and enforcement programs of USDA and FDA. The Subcommittee found that even when meat was found to be contaminated with dangerously high levels of toxic pesticides neither USDA nor FDA could stop these products from reaching the dinner table. This is an appalling state of affairs which cannot be allowed to continue. [52]

You would be forgiven for thinking that this report had a serious effect on the power and influence of the pesticide industry, who, as I reported earlier, had infiltrated the EPA, and turned it into a 'toothless tiger'. The sad fact is that things just deteriorated further, and the remorseless onslaught of cancer has continued and even increased—and is still increasing!

I regard the failure to acknowledge the occupational exposure to chemicals, and food-borne chemical exposure as a kind of blindness: if you don't look, you will never find anything. If you don't supply funding to undertake any serious studies to evaluate these risks, you can then say 'Well there is no evidence to support the view that industrial chemicals are responsible for society's massive demise of health.' Fortunately studies have been undertaken in spite of the intransigence of organisations like the EPA, the FDA, and their European counterparts that can help us see behind the charade of regulatory oversight.

Marie-Monique Robin, an award-winning journalist and film-maker, informs us that in the European Union (EU) every year 220,000 tons of pesticides are released into the environment: 108,000 tons of fungicides, 84,000 tons of herbicides, and 21,000 tons of insecticides. She suggests that if you add the 7,000 tons of "growth regulators"—hormones that are designed to shorten grain stalks—that it means approximately one pound of active substances for every European citizen. She points out that France has the lion's share, with its 80,000 tons annually, being the EU's largest user and ranking fourth-largest globally after the USA, Brazil and Japan. Robin also informs us that France, in 2008, led cancer incidence with 360.6 cases per 100,000 people, ahead of Australia (360.5), Canada (335) and Argentina (232). But to illustrate the way the figures demonstrate just how cancer incidence is linked to the industrialised countries, she also gives the figures for India (92.9), Bolivia (101), and Niger (68.6), all countries with much lower use of pesticides.

Robin investigated the causes for our current health disaster and published her findings in her book, *Our Daily Poison—From Pesticides to Packaging, How Chemicals Have Contaminated the Food Chain and Are Making Us Sick*. She mentions how Dominique Belpomme, was the first French cancer specialist to publicly declare that cancer is, above all, an "environmental disease created by man", in 2004. She cites a lot of research documenting the incidence of non-Hodgkin's lymphoma (NHL), Parkinson's disease, brain and prostate cancer in the agricultural community, for example, where the incidence for these conditions is much higher amongst farmers who apply the pesticides, and agricultural workers that spray them. She also cites a lot of research documenting the raised incidence of leukaemia and NHL among their children, and the higher levels of breast cancer among the wives of the pesticide users. She also points out how people who regularly treat their house plants with pesticides have twice the likelihood of developing cerebral tumour. She cites studies that looked at pesticide levels in children and revealed that by simply changing to an organic diet, their levels of organophosphorus pesticide dropped to practically undetectable levels after ten days. In another study, conducted over four consecutive seasons, twenty-three children between the ages 3-11 changed their diets several times. Each time, regardless of the season, the level of pesticides measured in their urine disappeared in less than ten days after switching to organic food.[53]

Chemical Body Burden

In my first book, *Unhealthy Betrayal,* I discussed some of the research that examined the chemical levels in the human population, something we refer to as the 'chemical body-burden'. The EPA has conducted surveys into this since 1976, analysing human adipose tissue. I reported on their 1982 study where they looked for 54 different chemicals, all environmental toxins. They were shocked to find that five of the toxins were found in every subject tested and they included the dioxin (OCCD), and the solvents xylene, ethylphenol, styrene, and 1,4-dichlorobenzene at worrying levels. They further found; another three dioxins, benzene, toluene, chlorobenzene, ethylbenzene and DDE (a breakdown product of DDT), in 91-98 per cent of samples. They also found PCBs (polychlorinated biphenyls) in 83 per cent of samples and beta-BHC in 87%. 76% of the people analysed had levels in excess of 25,000ng of total toxic compounds per gram of fat and contained at least 20 toxic compounds.[54]

Personally, I find the studies that examine the chemical content of human beings useful, they are an accurate reflection of our toxic exposure and indicate the degree that we are either succeeding or failing to protect people from harm—the consequences for our health being difficult to predict. The Environmental Working Group is a non-profit, non-partisan organization dedicated to protecting human health and the environment, and one of the things they do is monitor health. One of the most vulnerable groups is children, particularly younger children, new-borns and, even more critically, the foetus as yet unborn. In July 2005 they released a report that monitored cord blood from new-borns. This would obviously give some idea of the health status of the new-born and the challenges that it faces. Here is what they had to say:

> Not long ago scientists thought that the placenta shielded cord blood — and the developing baby — from most chemicals and pollutants in the environment. But now we know that at this critical time when organs, vessels, membranes and systems are knit together from single cells to finished form in a span of weeks, the umbilical cord carries not only the building blocks of life, but also a steady stream of industrial chemicals, pollutants and pesticides that cross the placenta as readily as residues from cigarettes and alcohol. This is the human "body burden" — the pollution in people that permeates everyone in the world, including babies in the womb.[55]

The study, done in collaboration with Commonweal, involved researchers from two major laboratories analysing samples of umbilical cord blood from ten babies born in US hospitals in 2004. The study revealed a total of 287 chemicals in the group, with an average of 200 industrial chemicals and pollutants. Here is what they had to say about this study:

> *Of the 287 chemicals we detected in umbilical cord blood, we know that 180 cause cancer in humans or animals, 217 are toxic to the brain and nervous system, and 208 cause birth defects or abnormal development in animal tests. The dangers of pre- or post-natal exposure to this complex mixture of carcinogens, developmental toxins and neurotoxins have never been studied.*

We cannot over-emphasize the significance of this statement. All the studies that have been undertaken have been directed at studying one chemical or another as an isolated ingredient on our lives, and decisions have been made that, at a certain level of exposure—it has been deemed "acceptable", and has been given universal usage as the "acceptable daily intake" (ADI) level. Among the chemicals found were numerous pesticides, consumer product ingredients and the waste products from burning coal, gasoline and garbage. This range of chemicals included eight perfluorochemicals used as stain and oil repellents from fast food packaging, clothes and textiles—also including the Teflon chemical perfluorooctanoic acid (PFOA), which was characterized as a likely human carcinogen by the EPA's Science Advisory Board. Dozens of widely used brominated flame retardants and their toxic by-products added to the toxic brew in these infant's blood samples. The researchers emphasized some of the reasons that early exposure was considered so much more dangerous to mothers with a growing foetus and growing children:

> Chemical exposures in the womb or during infancy can be dramatically more harmful than exposures later in life. Substantial scientific evidence demonstrates that children face amplified risks from their body burden of pollution; the findings are particularly strong for many of the chemicals found in this study, including mercury, PCBs and dioxins. Children's vulnerability derives from both rapid development and incomplete defence systems:
> - A developing child's chemical exposures are greater pound-for-pound than those of adults.
> - An immature, porous blood-brain barrier allows greater chemical exposures to the developing brain.
> - Children have lower levels of some chemical-binding proteins, allowing more of a chemical to reach "target organs."
> - A baby's organs and systems are rapidly developing and thus are often more vulnerable to damage from chemical exposure.

- Systems that detoxify and excrete industrial chemicals are not fully developed.

- The longer future life span of a child compared to an adult allows more time for adverse effects to arise. [56]

The Centers for Disease Control and Prevention (CDC) initiated a study that examined blood and urine samples of 2,400 volunteers in 2001 measuring the residues of 27 chemical products in the volunteers. In 2005 this was followed by a further study which included 116 products, followed by another study in 2005 looking at 148 products, and a further study in 2009 looking at 212 products.

Findings in the Fourth Report indicated widespread exposure to commonly used industrial chemicals; such as polybrominated diphenyl ethers (fire retardants) found in the serum of nearly all National Health and Nutrition Examination Survey (NHANES) participants; bisphenol A (BPA), found in plastics (polycarbonates) and epoxy resins, a known endocrine disruptor, was found in more than 90 per cent of people tested. Another widespread contaminant was perfluorinated chemicals such as perfluorooctanoic acid (PFOA), used in heat-resistant non-stick cookware. Acrylamide was found to be another widespread pollutant, created when cooking carbohydrates at high temperatures, such as in French fries, cereals such as cornflakes, and it is found in tobacco smoke.

A good number of pesticides and their breakdown products were discovered, including the persistent organochlorine DDT and its breakdown product DDE, which were still present although they have been banned from use in the USA since 1972. What is notable is that *all* the chemicals looked for were found in the 2,400 volunteers. It begs the question as to 'how many man-made chemicals do we actually carry in our bodies?' I am assuming that nobody actually knows.[57]

It begs the question as to 'how many man-made chemicals do we actually carry in our bodies?'

Just to add a note of interest as we have mentioned non-stick cookware chemicals permeating most of the population, pressure by the Environmental Working Group (EWG) forced the EPA to act on their revelations in a petition regarding the Teflon maker DuPont, who for years had been hiding information that its products caused cancer, birth defects and other serious health problems:

Today the Environmental Protection Agency (EPA) announced it will fine Teflon maker DuPont $16.5 million for two decades' worth of covering up company studies that showed it was polluting drinking water and newborn babies with an indestructible chemical that causes cancer, birth defects and other serious health problems in animals. The chemical is in the blood of over 95 percent of Americans.

The EWG, however, were not celebrating, they pointed out the derisive nature of the fine, $16.5 million, which is less than a half of a percent of DuPont's after-tax profits from the Teflon product when averaged out over the 20-year cover-up. It moved the EWG President, Ken Cook, to ask the question:

"What's the appropriate fine for a $25 billion company that for decades hid vital health information about a toxic chemical that now contaminates every man, woman and child in the United States? What's the proper dollar penalty for a pollutant that will never break down, and now finds its way into polar bears in the Arctic and human babies in their mothers' wombs? We're pretty sure it's not $16 million, even if that is a record amount under a federal law that everyone acknowledges is extremely weak.

In an administration that habitually favors polluting industries, this fine, at the very least, should have prompted DuPont to apologize to the public for its actions. What we've heard instead is a company lawyer dismissing the settlement as nothing more than business as usual, with no expression of having failed its obligation as a corporate citizen."[58]

This is an important point. It offers the illusion of action by the EPA, whilst in an economic sense, it simply reinforces the message that it's ok to pollute the planet, harm citizens with awful illnesses like cancer, and merely pay a small fine, like a small tax on your profits. No problem, its business as usual!

In December 2003 the World Wide Fund for Nature (WWF), as part of their DetoX campaign took blood samples from 47 volunteers from 17 European countries, comprising of 39 members of the European Parliament (MEPs), 4 observers, a former MEP and 3 WWF staff members. They were analysed for 101 predominantly persistent, bioaccumulative and toxic man-made chemicals. Every volunteer was shown to be contaminated by a cocktail of hazardous chemicals. The chemicals tested for included 12 organochlorine pesticides (including DDT and Lindane), 45 polychlorinated biphenyls (PCBs), 21 polybrominated diphenyl ether (PBDE) flame retardants, 8 phthalates and 13 perfluorinated chemicals.

The average number of chemicals detected was 41, with one person registering 54 of the chemicals they were studying. The chemical found in the highest concentration was the phthalate DEHP (Di Ethyl Hexyl Phthalate), a known endocrine disruptor and reproductive toxicant. The chemical found with the highest median concentration was p,p-DDE, the breakdown product of DDT, the pesticide that has been banned in the EU since 1983 and known as a persistent organic pollutant. Deca-BDE a suspected neuro-toxic chemical used as a flame retardant was found at the highest concentration so far detected in human serum, at a level that was considered "most alarming of all", as it was found to be ten times higher than the highest levels measured in workers normally exposed to the product. Thirty-four per cent of the volunteers were contaminated with Deca BDE. Here are some of their main conclusions:

> The survey highlights the ubiquitous contamination of every single person tested, even non-occupationally exposed people.
>
> The detection of the phthalate DEHP and 7 different perfluorinated chemicals in every single person tested is very significant, as it illustrates that chemicals that have not been phased out, are contaminating us to the same extent as older, banned chemicals such as DDT, HCB and PCBs. We have shown that the chemicals that industry insists are safe are in fact accumulating in our bodies in the same way as hazardous chemicals have in the past.
>
> The findings demonstrate the nonsense of industry's insistence that their chemicals are under 'adequate control' (despite the fact that the vast majority of which have no safety data). WWF believes that historic data, reinforced by the findings in this survey, show that industry have failed to protect everyday consumers from exposure to their hazardous chemicals and also highlights that it is impossible to adequately control chemicals that are persistent and bioaccumulative.
>
> WWF believes that the best way to stop this ongoing chemical contamination and the threat to future generations is to prevent the manufacture and use of chemicals that are found in elevated concentrations in biological fluids such as blood and breast milk.[59]

How To Survive in the 21ˢᵗ Century

Personally, I do not feel that it is possible to overemphasise the gravity of the previous conclusion by WWF. In my view, it is sheer madness to pollute the body of a woman to such an extent that her blood and breast milk is laden with chemicals that are known carcinogens, endocrine disruptors, and immune destroyers, and expecting to build a healthy population. Even if you look at it from a purely economic standpoint: to simply judge the wealth of a nation by its GDP (gross domestic product), without taking into account the health costs of the chemical onslaught, the ecological damage, health damage, the lost days of work, the working lives lost to death—is a kind of economic blindness—like the cancer blindness.

WWF believes that the best way to stop this ongoing chemical contamination and the threat to future generations is to prevent the manufacture and use of chemicals that are found in elevated concentrations in biological fluids such as blood and breast milk

---

Before we leave this topic of the body burden, Marie-Monique Robin, in her book *Our Daily Poison,* reports on a French study by Future Generations (Générations Future) that analysed the daily food intake of a ten-year-old child. They analysed three typical meals which included five fresh fruits and vegetables, included some dairy products, fish, water and some snacks. According to *Le Monde,* "The results were damning." The researchers found 128 residues, 81 chemical substances--which included 42 classified as possible or probable carcinogens, and 5 substances classified as certain carcinogens, as well as 37 probable endocrine disruptors. The biggest source of chemicals came from the salmon steak for dinner, a fish recommended by many as it is an oily fish, rich in omega-3 essential fatty acids. It contained 34 detected chemical residues.[60]

Rachel Carson, a marine biologist, warned of the dangers of the persistent organic pesticides such as DDT in the early 1960s, with her book *Silent Spring,* where she reported on the massive environmental disaster unfolding at that time, with birds dying in massive numbers, where the bald eagle, was almost driven to extinction. She warned that many of these toxic substances were able to persist in the environment, and those that were fat-soluble were taken up and stored in animal bodies, such as the salmon mentioned above. Her work has been attributed to starting the environmental movement, for which she was severely attacked and ridiculed by the chemical industry. [61]

Following in her footsteps was Theo Colborn, a senior scientist with the WWF, who was discovering the problems with hormone-disrupting chemicals and new persistent chemicals. She was witnessing falling sperm counts in the human population and widespread infertility problems and other serious damage to wildlife. She reported on a large number of hormone disruptors, and in particular the large chemical families such as the 209 compounds classified as PCBs, the 75 dioxins and the 135 furans 'which have a myriad of documented disruptive effects', some of which I reported in *Unhealthy Betrayal.*[62] One of the most dangerous chemicals, the dioxin 2,3,7,8-tetrachlorodibenzo-p-dioxin (TCDD), is associated with Agent Orange, one of the herbicides and defoliants used in Vietnam. Now it is accepted as the most probable agent responsible for the birth defects in the children of Vietnam veterans and the continuing birth defect problems affecting the southern Vietnamese population to this day. Dioxins are produced in the manufacture of phenoxy herbicides, such as 2,4,5-T (now banned) and 2,4-D, and also in wood pulp mills as a bleach for paper production, in the manufacture of polyvinyl chloride (PVC) products, the burning of crop residues (one of the major emitters are sugar mills), manufacture of wood preservatives etc.

Theo Colborn, in *Our Stolen Future,* wrote about some of the ways the chemical deluge was disrupting the health of animals and people, and she echoed Carson's warning about the persistence of some of the nastier pollutants, dioxins, and PCBs among them. She noted that the PCB concentrations increased in the colder regions of the north, and concentrations of PCBs had multiplied by 3 billion times as they moved up the Arctic food chain into animals at the top such as polar bears. She observed:

> Like polar bears, humans share the hazards of feeding at the top of the food web. The persistent synthetic chemicals that have invaded the great bear's world pervade ours as well.
> Humans also carry PCBs and other persistent chemicals in their body fat, and they pass this chemical legacy on to their babies. Virtually anyone willing to put up the $2,000 for the tests will find at least 250 contaminants in his or her body fat, regardless of whether he or she lives in Gary, Indiana, or a remote island in the South Pacific. You cannot escape them.

She wrote extensively about the hazards facing humanity with its obsession with releasing chemicals that were little understood, into the environment that we all have to live in, and realised that the most vulnerable were the as yet unborn, and infants with little-developed immune systems:

> While prenatal exposure seems to pose the greatest hazard, health specialists also worry about the chemicals passed on in breast milk because some sensitive developmental processes continue in the weeks immediately after birth. During breast feeding, human infants are exposed

to higher concentrations of these chemicals than at any subsequent time in their lives. In just six months of breast feeding a baby in the United States and Europe gets the maximum recommended dose of dioxin, which rides through the food web like PCBs and DDT. The same breast feeding baby gets five times the allowable daily level of PCBs set by international health standards for a 150 pound adult.[63]

Theo Colborn discovered that dioxin was dangerous at infinitesimally small doses, diluted in the parts per trillion it was able to damage the male reproductive development by giving 'a single hit' to the mother, one drop! She also found that the Eskimo children were taking in five times the level of dioxin of Canadian and American children.

As is predictable with persistent pollutants such as PCBs and dioxins, the Inuit continue to be affected by them, as large marine animals are still part of their diet, and still have high contaminant loads. Katherine Brieger, informs us that the toxic cocktail of their food being laced with PCBs, DDT, mercury, and other toxic chemical pollutants is taking its toll on the population, impairing the immune system, altering neurological development, and producing children with lower birth weight—further, the children frequently present with motor control problems, low IQs, and poor memory. She also reports that numerous studies of PCBs in humans have found increased rates of melanomas, liver cancer, gall bladder cancer, biliary tract cancer, gastrointestinal tract cancer, brain cancer, and a potential link to breast cancer.[64]

Eventually, the EPA concluded the TCDD's acute toxicity kills animals at "lower levels than any other man-made chemical." E G Vallianatos, who worked for the EPA for more than twenty-five years, adds: 'in addition, TCDD initiates and promotes cancer at a potency 17 million times greater than that of benzene, 5 million times greater than carbon tetrachloride, and a hundred thousand times greater than PCBs. It also bioaccumulates in animals at dramatic rates: twenty thousand times greater than benzene, six thousand times greater than carbon tetrachloride, and four times greater than PCBs.' The agency clean-up crews were warned to be exceptionally cautious whenever they detected dioxin contamination above one part per billion. Vallianatos notes that whilst this sounds like a small amount: 'One part TCDD per trillion—which is a thousand times smaller than 1 part per billion—it is still toxic enough to mutate living entities such as chicken embryos.'

Vallianatos says that despite the mounting evidence the chemical giants still continued to deny problems associated with their products and continued to demonize anyone at the EPA who suggested that these compounds be regulated. He reports how Monsanto had dumped 30-40 pounds of dioxin a day into the Mississippi River from 1970—1977 and sold products contaminated with dioxin for more than thirty years. Cate Jenkins, another EPA scientist, found Monsanto studies had significant deficiencies in both their design and conclusions. She concluded the studies had been tampered with and sent a memo to Raymond C. Loehr, chairman of the executive committee of the Science Advisory Board of the EPA, suggesting that the Monsanto studies were fraudulent. 'It was eventually discovered that Monsanto subverted its own dioxin studies by covering up the neurological diseases suffered by workers exposed to the compound; excluding workers with cancer from its studies, and even adding dioxin-exposed workers to the "control" group of its studies.'[65]

It was eventually discovered that Monsanto subverted its own dioxin studies by covering up the neurological diseases suffered by workers exposed to the compound; excluding workers with cancer from

its studies, and even adding dioxin-exposed workers to the "control"
group of its studies.

Acceptable Daily Intake and Maximum Residue Limits

There are many critics of our chemical regulatory systems. One of the common criticisms made is due to the way that they have established the system of using the acceptable daily intake (ADI) of a poisonous food additive and the 'maximum residue limit' (MRL) for a poisonous pesticide. How this is established affects decisions as to what level of exposure we are likely to face. The ADI is based on what is referred to as the no-observed-adverse-effect (NOAEL) level. This is where experiments are carried out on animals that are exposed to reducing levels of exposure to a *single* toxin until there is no *apparent* effect. Then it has been decided that simply reducing this level by a factor of 100 would suffice to be regarded as a safe dose. The way MRLs are arrived at is more arbitrary, more a political decision which can vary from product to product, country by country.

Robin informs us that when the European Commission led a vast program to harmonise the standards between the twenty-seven member states in 2008, it led to an increase in the authorized pesticide residue levels of up to 1,000 times higher for 65 percent of the pesticides used. She suggested that the program provoked Greenpeace to criticise the levels, specifically for children, for apples, pears, and grapes which suggested that "10% of the set acceptable levels are potentially dangerous for children." She interviewed Erik Millstone, professor, of the University of Sussex, regarding the use of such tools as the ADI. He suggested that he did not consider it a scientific tool. It introduced the concept of 'acceptability'. He raised the question "'Acceptable', but for whom?" He points out that those benefiting from the use of the chemical products are always businesses, not consumers and makes the observation: "So it is consumers taking the risk, and businesses reaping the benefit."[66]

Cocktail Effect Blindness

What is important to understand here is that all these so-called 'acceptable' levels are all based on individual chemicals of one sort or another. Yet what we have already shown you is that we are all exposed to innumerable toxins in our food and the environment that we live in, and we *all,* without exception have a *range of toxins* floating around in our bodies. And the simple fact is there is *no-one* who knows what kind of synergy is occurring with the mixtures we all carry for the simple reason that few if any studies are done to find out. What studies have been undertaken point to some dramatic interplays between some of the chemicals in our 'cocktail.'

André Leu, in his volume, *Poisoning Our Children—The Parent's Guide to the Myths of Safe Pesticides* points out one of the great myths about pesticides is based on the assumption that once a chemical degrades it disappears and becomes harmless. He points out that a substantial number of agricultural pesticides— such as organophosphates like diazinon, malathion, chlorpyrifos, and dimethoate—become even more toxic when they break down. Some of the oxon metabolites of organophosphates, for example, can be up to 100 times more toxic than the original pesticide. When dimethoate, widely used as a fruit fly treatment, breaks down in food, it can become 300 per cent more toxic. Aside from the problem with the breakdown products, another problem with the orthodox review process is that they only review laboratory-grade products. So, for example, when they reviewed Monsanto's most popular pesticide, Roundup, they ignored the other ingredients in the product formulation, often referred to as 'inerts'. The problem here according to Leu, is there are numerous studies that show that Roundup is more toxic than its active ingredient, glyphosate, and these studies link the pesticide to a whole range of health problems. The health problems include cancer, placental cell damage, miscarriages, stillbirths, endocrine disruption, and damage to organs such as the liver and kidneys. He mentions that French scientists have shown that one of the "inert" adjuvants in Roundup, the polyethoxylated tallowamine POE-15, adds considerably more to the levels of toxicity. [67]

In a study in 2013, Robin Messange, Séralini and others studied the toxicity of nine pesticides, comparing active principles and their formulations. Here is what they had to report:

> Pesticides are used throughout the world as mixtures called formulations. They contain adjuvants, which are often kept confidential and are called inerts by the manufacturing companies, plus a declared active principle, which is usually tested alone. We tested the toxicity of 9 pesticides, comparing active principles and their formulations, on three human cell lines.
>
> Fungicides were the most toxic from concentrations 300–600 times lower than agricultural dilutions, followed by herbicides and then insecticides, with very similar profiles in all cell types. Despite its relatively benign reputation, Roundup was among the most toxic herbicides and insecticides tested. Most importantly, 8 formulations out of 9 were up to *one thousand times more toxic* [my emphasis] than their active principles. Our results challenge the relevance of the acceptable daily intake for pesticides because this norm is calculated from the toxicity of the active principle alone. Chronic tests on pesticides may not reflect relevant environmental exposures if only one ingredient of these mixtures is tested alone. [68]

Only testing the active ingredient is not only bad science, it is also totally irresponsible. The reason the inert adjuvants accompany the active ingredient is to enhance the action and therefore the effectiveness of the product in question. In another study, Theo Colborn writes regarding her concern about harm done that is not immediately perceived. Here are some of her observations:

> The U.S. Environmental Protection Agency's (EPA) Office of Pesticide Programs (OPP) estimated that 891 pesticide active ingredients were registered in 1997 (Aspelin and Grube 1999) and that 888 million pounds of pesticide active ingredients were used in the United States in 2001 (Kiely et al. 2004). Few of these chemicals are applied alone but rather are applied in formulations using different combinations of several pesticide active ingredients (MeisterPRO 2004). It is not uncommon for many classes of pesticides, such as insecticides, herbicides, and fungicides, to be used on the same crop. In the case of insecticides, an adjuvant is often added to the formulations to enhance the intensity of the lethal effect. In the case of herbicides, due to the increasing incidence of plant tolerance to a specific pesticide, some formulations now have as many as three active ingredients.

> Each active ingredient has a specific mode of action for controlling a pest, and each active ingredient has its own possible side effects on the wildlife and humans exposed to it. It is impossible to determine the cumulative risk posed to wildlife and humans as the result of releasing vast amounts of pesticide mixtures into the environment.

> In this article I challenge the protective value of current pesticide risk assessment strategies in light of the vast numbers of pesticides on the market and the vast number of possible target tissues and end points that often differ depending upon timing of exposure. Because of the uncertainty that will continue to exist about the safety of pesticides, it is apparent that a new regulatory approach to protect human health is needed.

> In conclusion, an entirely new approach to determine the safety of pesticides is needed. It is evident that contemporary acute and chronic

toxicity studies are not protective of future generations. The range of doses used in future studies must be more realistic, based on levels found in the environment and human tissue. In this new approach, functional neurologic and behavioral end points should have high priority, as well as the results published in the open literature. In every instance, the impacts of transgenerational exposure on all organ systems must be meticulously inventoried through two generations on all contemporary-use pesticides and new pesticide coming on the market. To protect human health, however, a new regulatory approach is also needed that takes into consideration this vast new knowledge about the neurodevelopmental effects of pesticides, not allowing the uncertainty that accompanies scientific research to serve as an impediment to protective actions. [69]

If her advice was to be followed, it would doubtless transform the health of society in so many ways, not just the reduction of cancer, but so many other conditions, many not necessarily obviously associated with pesticide exposure. It would also transform the world of pseudo-science that we currently labour under into something more akin to science we could actually respect.

The Precautionary Principle

In *Unhealthy Betrayal*, I reported on the Wingspread Statement on the Precautionary Principle, signed by a group of international scientists, doctors, lawyers, government officials, and others, following the meetings that took place over 23rd to 25th January in Racine, Wisconsin in the USA in 1998. They were meeting in response to growing concerns regarding the unrestrained use of chemicals that were creating environmental and health concerns. It is worth repeating here:

> The release and use of toxic substances, the exploitation of resources, and physical alterations of the environment have had

substantial unintended consequences affecting human health and the environment. Some of these concerns are high rates of learning deficiencies, asthma, cancer, birth defects and species extinctions; along with global climate change, stratospheric ozone depletion and worldwide contamination with toxic substances and nuclear materials.

We believe existing environmental regulations and other decisions, particularly those based on risk assessment, have failed to protect adequately human health and the environment - the larger system of which humans are but a part.

We believe there is compelling evidence that damage to humans and the worldwide environment is of such magnitude and seriousness that new principles for conducting human activities are necessary.

While we realize that human activities may involve hazards, people must proceed more carefully than has been the case in recent history. Corporations, government entities, organizations, communities, scientists and other individuals must adopt a precautionary approach to all human endeavors.

Therefore, it is necessary to implement the Precautionary Principle: When an activity raises threats of harm to human health or the environment, precautionary measures should be taken even if some cause and effect relationships are not fully established scientifically.

In this context the proponent of an activity, rather than the public, should bear the burden of proof.

The process of applying the Precautionary Principle must be open, informed and democratic and must include potentially affected parties. It must also involve an examination of the full range of alternatives, including no action. [70]

The precautionary principle is not something that has taken priority in regulatory approach. In 2010, the president's Cancer Panel raised concerns in their Annual Report about the failure of current regulatory authorities:

The Panel was particularly concerned to find that the true burden of environmentally induced cancer has been grossly underestimated. With nearly 80,000 chemicals on the market in the United States, many of which are used by millions of Americans in their daily lives and are un- or understudied and largely unregulated, exposure to potential environmental carcinogens is widespread. One such ubiquitous chemical, bisphenol A (BPA), is still found in many consumer products and remains unregulated in the United States, despite the growing link between BPA and several diseases, including various cancers.

Environmental health, including cancer risk, has been largely excluded from overall national policy on protecting and improving the health of Americans. It is more effective to prevent disease than to treat it.

Industry has exploited regulatory weaknesses, such as government's reactionary (rather than precautionary) approach to regulation. Likewise, industry has exploited government's use of the flawed and grossly outdated Doll and Peto methodology for assessing "attributable fractions" of the cancer burden due to specific environmental exposures. This methodology has been used effectively by industry to justify introducing untested chemicals into the environment. [71]

Aside from the above reports that should urge us to use more caution than we currently do with regard to our unbridled embrace of the use of man-made chemicals of virtually any composition—there is one anecdote that I also reported in my previous volume that I feel is worth repeating briefly. It concerns Dr Frances Kelsey of the FDA and the drug thalidomide that was given to expectant mothers to supposedly combat morning sickness. As we now know this drug caused appalling birth defects: children born without arms or legs, hands sprouting from the shoulders and even worse deformations, affecting more than eight thousand children in forty-six countries. America, however, was one of the countries that did not suffer as badly as it could have, mostly due to the exercising of the precautionary principle by Dr Kelsey. Apparently, she was very sceptical about the use of this drug, particularly its possible side effects. She also found the clinical trials supplied by Richardson-Merrell for their new drug application (NDA) woefully inadequate. On top of this, she was hearing reports of the side effect peripheral neuritis (in the British Medical Journal December 1960). She rejected their application and asked for more information. Merrell sent through another application, which she again did not approve; she informed Merrell that she was aware of the neuritis coming out of Europe and accused Merrell of hiding this effect. By November 1961, reports of birth defects were surfacing in Germany and Australia. Merrell, in the end, withdrew their application in April 1962. Dr Kelsey was honoured by President John F. Kennedy for her role in saving America from what could have been an immense tragedy. [72]

Science for Sale

Dr Kelsey is one of America's unsung heroines; most people have never heard of her. She represents scientific integrity and was doing her job in actually protecting the American public from disaster by a member of the Big Pharma family trying to impose another drug, with no proven value on the community, with absolutely shoddy trials. One of the criticisms often made of the application process, whether it is for a drug or a pesticide or a chemical ingredient for the food industry, is that the regulators rely almost entirely on industry-supplied studies. The studies and data supplied cannot be independently checked, and generally, the studies are accepted as accurate and truthful. It's only in retrospect that we find out how badly flawed the whole process is. I reported in *Unhealthy Betrayal* on the discovery of blatant fraud in the mid-1970s, which involved the scandal of Industrial Bio-Test Laboratories (IBT), the nation's largest toxicological laboratory. IBT conducted 35-40 per cent of all toxicological testing in the United States at that time.

Dan Fagin and Marianne Lavelle of the Center for Public Integrity, reveal some of the story in their book *Toxic Deception-How the Chemical Industry Manipulates Science, Bends the Law and Endangers Your Health:*

> The lab was exposed as a fraud in April 1976 when Adrian Gross, an alert FDA Pathologist, started asking questions after he saw a rat study of the arthritis drug Naprosyn that looked too good to be true. In the ensuing months, federal regulators found evidence that dozens of its studies had been faked. Among other transgressions, sick animals were listed as healthy or were not included in order to achieve favourable test results. Some reports were total fabrications based on no study at all. Ultimately, hundreds of studies were declared invalid.

Dowell Davis, an FDA pharmacologist who was part of the investigative team, thought it was the worst case of fraud he had come across; "They were hell-bent on providing their clients with favourable reports. They did not care about good science. It was about money. They really had what was an assembly line for acceptable studies." In three cases, the investigators wrote in an internal memo, there was evidence that Monsanto executives knew that the studies were faked but sent them to the FDA and the EPA anyway. One of the staff at the laboratory, Paul Wright, had been a research chemist at Monsanto before he went to work at IBT in 1971 as its chief rat toxicologist. Wright's protocols for the three studies for Monsanto were riddled with mistakes. If you think that this was simply an isolated example, albeit on a large scale, you would be wrong. In another celebrated case, this time involving Craven Laboratories, Inc., of Austin, Texas, it was caught faking pesticide studies. Craven was a top residue testing lab for guess who? Yep, you got it—Monsanto (as well as DuPont and other pesticide manufacturers). It was discovered that Craven had faked studies on more than 20 pesticides used on more than 50 food crops. The chemical companies were not charged for their part in either affair nor did they have to re-submit their products for fresh reviews due to the discovery of the faked work. [73]

Whilst industry always complains about the cost and kicks up a hullabaloo about the process of getting a chemical or drug approved, the reality is that they have basically set the agenda, they call the shots. They have infiltrated the very organisations that are supposed to regulate them, and they so terrorize the scientists in their respective industries, that few feel able to stand up to them. But by far, the most problematic industry that has been able to evade any form of real regulation has been the genetic engineering industry, the subject of our next chapter

Chapter Five

Genetically Modified Crops and Food

It is not my intention to unnecessarily burden you with negative information: my hope is to sufficiently inform you of what is perceived as some of the more important challenges threatening your health and that of those whom you care about—yet at the same time suggest that there are surprisingly elegant and beautiful solutions to many of the problems we face. I am overly optimistic about humanity's future—but I also feel that a better-informed public is an essential ingredient to generate real change. The next topic that of genetically modified food is, in some ways, the classic scenario, where propaganda and half-truths dominate the advance of corporate interests masquerading as real science. Some have compared the dangers of releasing modified organisms with unknown potential into the food chain and the environment as playing Russian roulette with humanity and even life on Earth as we know it. Jeffrey Smith, for example, even named one of his books *Genetic Roulette*, which is a useful book for more information on this topic.[74] The fact that this industry has been allowed to develop with virtually no oversight or regulation is considered irresponsibility of the greatest magnitude by many and should be a concern to all of us.

It is very difficult to ascertain to what degree genetically modified products are impacting health, as there are few studies undertaken on this topic. The way that the genetic modification of our food has been able to escape any proper scrutiny or oversight is all to do with politics and very little to do with science. In 1992   the FDA released their 'Statement of Policy: Foods Derived from New Plant Varieties', which expressed their position on the new science of genetic engineering with their relationship with agricultural crops and foods. Below is the view of their stance taken:

> FDA believes that the new techniques are extensions at the molecular level of traditional methods and will be used to achieve the same goals as pursued with traditional plant breeding. The agency is not aware of any information showing that foods derived by these new methods differ from other foods in any meaningful or uniform way, or that, as a class, foods developed by the new techniques present any different or greater safety concern than foods developed by traditional plant breeding.[75]

For many, this was an extraordinary position to take in the face of such vast uncertainty in a science that was at that time very little understood. It was, however, perceived by various US administrations that the industry might serve to become a significant contributor to the US economy, and for this reason, was given such a favourable status. An article in the *New York Times,* January 25th, 2001 revealed how the White House was working behind the scenes to help Monsanto, which was perceived as being in the vanguard of the biotechnology movement at that time. The article discussed the outcome of a meeting between four Monsanto executives and the White House:

Genetically Modified Crops and Food

It was an outcome that would be repeated, again and again, through three administrations. What Monsanto wished for from Washington, Monsanto — and, by extension, the biotechnology industry — got. If the company's strategy demanded regulations, rules favored by the industry were adopted. And when the company abruptly decided that it needed to throw off the regulations and speed its foods to market, the White House quickly ushered through an unusually generous policy of self-policing.

Even longtime Washington hands said that the control this nascent industry exerted over its own regulatory destiny — through the Environmental Protection Agency, the Agriculture Department and ultimately the Food and Drug Administration — was astonishing. [76]

Generally Recognised as Safe for Whom?

In *Unhealthy Betrayal*, I included reports from a number of sources who offered warnings on the blind adoption of genetically engineered products with little or no oversight. One of the sources was from Henryk Behr, who ordered some tryptophan from a British company, Biovea, in September 2010. Writing in 2011, he describes how one hour after taking a second prescribed dose of 500mg tryptophan, in his words "the gates of hell opened and they have not closed to this day." He is now suffering with what has been referred to as Eosinophilia Myalgia Syndrome (EMS) which is considered a very rare and untreatable autoimmune condition and is considered incurable. He relates how his life went from a happy and contented busy family life to a life of sitting on a couch in severe pain every day, where he can no longer play with his children, or even watch television. He complains of being unable to sleep more than two hours a night for the last seven months, is unable to perform sexually, and sometimes even unable to walk. He now suffers from severe depression. He attributes his decline to the fact that his tryptophan was created with genetically engineered bacteria. He mentions that several other companies had been producing L-Tryptophan without using genetically engineered bacteria—and had experienced no problems with it, in total contrast to the genetically engineered GE version.[77]

The gates of hell opened and they have not closed to this day

---

Problems like Henryk Behr experienced with genetically modified organisms were not new to the Japanese; research undertaken in Japan in 1995 had already identified serious issues with genetically engineered yeast when they discovered an accumulation of a highly toxic compound that did not exist in non-engineered cells. Their comments make sober reading:

> The results presented here indicate that, in genetically engineered yeast cells, the metabolism is significantly disturbed by the introduced genes or their gene products and the disturbance brings about the accumulation of the unwanted toxic compound MG in cells. Such accumulation of highly reactive MG may cause damage in DNA, thus suggesting that the scientific concept of `substantially equivalent' for the safety assessment of genetically engineered food is not always applied to genetically engineered microbes, at least in the case of recombinant yeast cells. In order to apply recombinant yeast cells to practical fermentation processes, the safety level of MG in cells should be established.
>
> Thus, the results presented may raise some questions regarding the safety and acceptability of genetically engineered food, and give some credence to the many consumers who are not yet prepared to accept food produced using gene engineering techniques. [78]

Steven M. Drucker is a public interest attorney, who initiated a lawsuit that forced the U.S. FDA to divulge its files on genetically engineered foods. He wrote an excellent volume called *Altered Genes Twisted Truth—How the Venture to Genetically Engineer Our Food Has Subverted Science, Corrupted Government, and Systematically Deceived the Public.* It's a useful place to start if you would like more information on this important topic. He mentions that the CDC established that in the USA between 5,000 and 10,000 people were stricken with EMS and around 1,500 have been permanently disabled by it.

Steve Drucker believes that the FDA is acting contrary to U.S. law, in the way that the industry has escaped any real regulatory oversight, he believes 'GE foods were not being freed from extraneous burdens; they were being illegally exempted from the central provisions of one of the nation's most important consumer protection statutes.' It has been argued that genetically engineered food has been awarded GRAS status, meaning it has been accepted as being Generally Recognized As Safe, a status awarded by the FDA. Drucker argues that this status cannot be legally awarded to genetically engineered food as it is unable to demonstrate "reasonable certainty" that the substance is not harmful under its intended conditions of use. It also has to demonstrate that it is the "same quantity and quality". Drucker quotes a number of sources that were critical of not just the FDA's action but the principle of allowing genetically altered products into the food chain without the ability to prove they are safe. He quotes, for example, Professor Liebe Cavalieri at Washington D.C., where he addresses the idea that genetic engineering is no different from traditional plant breeding as "simplistic, if not downright simple-minded", and that it was "disgraceful" that eminent scientists should engage in trying to support the very idea. Drucker quotes volumes of evidence that support the view that genetically engineered products should be seriously controlled, I will mention one more source that he refers to, that of an editorial in the prestigious UK medical journal, *The Lancet.* In its editorial headed "Health risks of genetically modified foods," it stated that there are "good reasons to believe that specific risks may exist," and that "governments should never have allowed these products into the food chain without insisting on rigorous testing for effects on health." [79]

The American Academy of Environmental Medicine added its general concern about genetically modified organisms (GMOs) in food with the following caution:

> Because GM foods pose a serious health risk in the areas of toxicology, allergy and immune function, reproductive health, and metabolic, physiologic and genetic health and are without benefit, the AAEM believes that it is imperative to adopt the precautionary principle, which is one of the main regulatory tools of the European Union environmental and health policy and serves as a foundation for several international agreements.[80]

Their urge for caution was echoed in a 2001 report by the Expert Panel of The Royal Society of Canada, which took the view that '(a) it is "scientifically unjustifiable" to presume that GE foods are safe and (b) the "default presumption" for every GE food should be that the genetic alteration has induced unintended and potentially hazardous side effects.' They further recommend that a national research program be established to monitor the long-term effects of GM organisms on the environment, and both human, and on animal health and welfare.[81]

As regards to the idea that genetically modified crops are 'substantially equivalent', an analysis by T. Bøhn et al. in 2013 on soybean crops cultivated in Iowa, USA, looked at precisely this point. They analysed conventionally grown soybeans, organically grown soybeans and genetically modified, glyphosate-tolerant soy (GM-soy). They found that the organic soybeans had the healthiest profile, with more total protein, zinc, and sugars, and less saturated fat and total omega-6 fatty acids. Aside from the nutritional differences, the GMO soybeans contained high residue levels of glyphosate and aminomethylphosphonic acid AMPA (mean 3.3 and 5.7 mg/kg, respectively). AMPA is one of the breakdown products of glyphosate, considered more persistent and linked to liver disease and excessive cell division in the bladder. [82]

> The concept of 'substantial equivalence' (i.e., close nutritional and elemental similarity between a genetically modified (GM) crop and a non-GM traditional counterpart) has been used to claim that GM crops are substantially equivalent to, and therefore as safe and nutritious as, currently consumed plant-derived foods. However, we argue that compositional studies that have overlooked (not measured) pesticide residues contain serious shortcomings. Chemical residues, if present, are important because (i) they are clearly a part of a plant's composition, and (ii) they may add toxic properties to the final plant product either by itself or by affecting the plant metabolism. This is particularly relevant for herbicide-tolerant varieties.

> Using 35 different nutritional and elemental variables to characterise each soy sample, we were able to discriminate GM, conventional and organic soybeans without exception, demonstrating "substantial non-equivalence" in compositional characteristics for 'ready-to-market' soybeans.

> We argue that pesticide residues should have been a part of the compositional analyses of herbicide tolerant GM plants from the beginning. Lack of data on pesticide residues in major crop plants is a serious gap of knowledge with potential consequences for human and animal health.[83]

The use of glyphosate has risen exponentially following the introduction of GMO crops. Dr Vandana Shiva, the world-renowned biologist and author, reporting from the epicentre of transgenic soy, Cordoba, Argentina, informs us how the spraying of the herbicide glyphosate sold under Monsanto's brand name Roundup has increased:

> Three hundred million liters of glyphosate are being sprayed annually. That translates into five litres per person—the highest in the world. Cordoba is also the epicenter of a health crisis and children are paying the highest price. Cancer rates and birth defects have exploded. Six to seven percent of the children being born suffer from malformations.

She also makes a point regarding the 'substantial equivalence' that is worth your attention: 'The false claim of substantial equivalence by the biotechnology industry has blocked the scientific research that would assess the difference. Science has been supplanted by propaganda'.[84]

The false claim of substantial equivalence by the biotechnology industry has blocked the scientific research that would assess the difference. Science has been supplanted by propaganda.

Some Dangers of Genetically Modified Food

Dr Arpad Pusztai, a geneticist and a specialist in biotechnology for over 35 years, was undertaking research for the Rowett Research Institute in Scotland. Pusztai was considered the world's leading expert on lectins and the genetic modification of plants—and was considered an enthusiast in his field. Pusztai had undertaken a study whereby potatoes had been modified with a lectin that was supposed to act as a natural insecticide. He had been feeding rats on a diet of GM potatoes and found that rats fed for more than 110 days on this diet showed marked developmental changes. He found that the GMO rats had remarkably smaller liver, heart, and even brain sizes and further that they demonstrated weaker immune systems. However, he made the mistake of airing his research and his views on the popular UK ITV program *World In Action* in August 1998. In this, he referred to his research on the genetically modified potatoes and mentioned he had discovered "slight growth retardation, and an effect on the immune system." He further added: 'If I had the choice I would certainly not eat it". He demanded tighter rules over GM foods and warned: "I find it's very unfair to use our fellow citizens as guinea pigs. We have to find guinea pigs in the laboratory." Initially, he was congratulated for his work by his immediate boss. But, within 48 hours, this 68-year-old researcher was effectively fired, along with his wife who had been a researcher with Rowett for more than 13 years. He was told that he was never to speak to the press again about his research, nor was his research team, under threat of legal action. His papers were seized and his research team was disbanded. In the following weeks, his reputation was attacked and his work ridiculed.[85]

That began a controversy that put him in conflict with the biotech industry, the scientific establishment, and both the US and UK governments, as was revealed some years later by Andrew Rowell:

> Now, five years on, there are disturbing claims that this distinguished scientist was the victim of behind-the-scenes manoeuvring at the highest political level. Some of the allegations are truly explosive. They raise profound questions about the extraordinary network of relationships between senior Labour figures and the biotech companies. They also throw new light on why the multi-billion-pound GM industry continues to press ahead in the face of huge public opposition.[86]

This eminent researcher, who had worked for the Rowett Institute for more than thirteen years, had been given permission to undertake the TV interview. It was said that the huge backlash against him was orchestrated at the highest level politically. His work was attacked and his reputation impugned, but some 30 leading scientists leapt to his defence. [87] In spite of the fact that Pusztai was revealing preliminary evidence of his trial, albeit quite damning evidence, it remains the most in-depth GMO feeding study ever published. In my view, it says a lot about an industry that has refused point-blank to publish any long-term feeding studies of its products and has to hide behind political protection instead of any real scientific scrutiny, and which lives in a state of complete denial as to the harm that its products create.

Dr Amy Dean and Jennifer Armstrong, M.D., writing an article on genetically modified foods in American Academy of Environmental Medicine, reviewed much of the information on the development of genetically modified food. They explain one of the methods of gene insertion:

> According to the World Health Organization, Genetically Modified Organisms(GMOs) are "organisms in which the genetic material (DNA) has been altered in such a way that does not occur naturally." This technology is also referred to as "genetic engineering", "biotechnology" or "recombinant DNA technology" and consists of randomly inserting genetic fragments of DNA from one organism to another, usually from a different species. For example, an artificial combination of genes that includes a gene to produce the pesticide Cry1Ab protein (commonly known as Bt toxin), originally found in Bacillus thuringiensis, is inserted into the DNA of corn randomly. Both the location of the transferred gene sequence in the corn DNA and the consequences of the insertion differ with each insertion. The plant cells that have taken up the inserted gene are then grown in a lab using tissue culture and/or nutrient medium that allows them to develop into plants that are used to grow GM food crops.

Genetically Modified Crops and Food

They further reveal a number of alarming problems that have been introduced with exposure to the genetic modifications:

> Natural breeding processes have been safely utilized for the past several thousand years. In contrast, "GE crop technology abrogates natural reproductive processes, selection occurs at the single cell level, the procedure is highly mutagenic and routinely breeches genera barriers, and the technique has only been used commercially for 10 years."

> Despite these differences, safety assessment of GM foods has been based on the idea of "substantial equivalence" such that "if a new food is found to be substantially equivalent in composition and nutritional characteristics to an existing food, it can be regarded as safe as the conventional food." However, several animal studies indicate serious health risks associated with GM food consumption including infertility, immune dysregulation, accelerated aging, dysregulation of genes associated with cholesterol synthesis, insulin regulation, cell signaling, and protein formation, and changes in the liver, kidney, spleen and gastrointestinal system...The strength of association and consistency between GM foods and disease is confirmed in several animal studies.

They also point out that GM foods are specifically associated with certain conditions:

> Multiple animal studies show significant immune dysregulation, including upregulation of cytokines associated with asthma, allergy, and inflammation. Animal studies also show altered structure and function of the liver, including altered lipid and carbohydrate metabolism as well as cellular changes that could lead to accelerated aging and possibly lead to the accumulation of reactive oxygen species (ROS). Changes in the kidney, pancreas and spleen have also been documented. A recent 2008 study links GM corn with infertility, showing

a significant decrease in offspring over time and significantly lower litter weight in mice fed GM corn. This study also found that over 400 genes were found to be expressed differently in the mice fed GM corn. These are genes known to control protein synthesis and modification, cell signaling, cholesterol synthesis, and insulin regulation. Studies also show intestinal damage in animals fed GM foods, including proliferative cell growth and disruption of the intestinal immune system.[88]

The U.S. Department of Agriculture has reported that 94 percent of soybean and 91 percent of cotton crops were genetically modified by 2014. Currently, up to 90 percent of domestic corn acres are planted with herbicide-tolerant seeds. Currently, of U.S. cotton acres, 85 percent are genetically engineered, with what is referred to as 'insect-resistant crops', which contain genes from the soil bacterium Bt (Bacillus thuringiensis) and produce insecticidal proteins and insect-resistant seeds.[89]

Some consider that the way that GE companies have hijacked one of the organic farmer's tools by using the bacterium, Bacillus thuringiensis, to combat attack by certain caterpillars on their brassica crops, for example, as possibly compromising one of their most useful tools. Jonathan R. Latham, PhD, the biologist and geneticist, has concerns as to the development of GMOs, and the use of this organism concerns him:

> Aside from grave doubts about the quality and integrity of risk assessments, I also have specific science-based concerns over GMOs. These concerns are mostly particular to specific transgenes and traits.
>
> Many GMO plants are engineered to contain their own insecticides. These GMOs, which include maize, cotton and soybeans, are called Bt plants. Bt plants get their name because they incorporate a transgene that makes a protein-based toxin (sometimes called the Cry toxin) from the bacterium Bacillus thuringiensis. Many Bt crops are

Genetically Modified Crops and Food

"stacked," meaning they contain a multiplicity of these Cry toxins. Their makers believe each of these Bt toxins is insect-specific and safe. However, there are multiple reasons to doubt both safety and specificity. One concern is that Bacillus thuringiensis is all but indistinguishable from the well known anthrax bacterium (Bacillus anthracis). Another reason is that Bt insecticides share structural similarities with ricin. Ricin is a famously dangerous plant toxin, a tiny amount of which was used to assassinate the Bulgarian writer and defector Georgi Markov in 1978. A third reason for concern is that the mode of action of Bt proteins is not understood (Vachon et al 2012); yet, it is axiomatic in science, that effective risk assessment requires a clear understanding of the mechanism of action of any GMO transgene so that appropriate experiments can be devised to affirm or refute safety. All this is doubly troubling because some Cry proteins are toxic towards isolated human cells (Mizuki et al., 1999).

A second concern follows from GMOs being often resistant to herbicides. This resistance is an invitation to farmers to spray large quantities of herbicides, and many do. As research recently showed, commercial soybeans sold today routinely contain quantities of the herbicide Roundup (glyphosate) that its maker, Monsanto, once described as "extreme" (Bøhn et al 2014).

This concern about the levels of pesticides is shared among many researchers and the public alike. The proponents of genetically modified food, do not give the higher use of insecticides as one of their main reasons for their development, even though it is quite obviously so when you look at the USDA figures. Another concern expressed by a number of scientists about genetic modification is the possibility of introducing unwanted by-products, novel substances that have led to unforeseen yet serious consequences. Dr Latham:

> A yet further reason to be concerned about GMOs is that most
> of them contain a viral sequence called the cauliflower mosaic virus

97

(CaMV) promoter (or they contain the similar figwort mosaic virus (FMV) promoter). Two years ago, the GMO safety agency of the European Union (EFSA) discovered that both the CaMV promoter and the FMV promoter had wrongly been assumed by them (for almost 20 years) not to encode any proteins. In fact, the two promoters encode a large part of a small multifunctional viral protein that misdirects all normal gene expression and that also turns off a key plant defence against pathogens. EFSA tried to bury their discovery. Unfortunately for them, we spotted their findings in an obscure scientific journal. This revelation forced EFSA and other regulators to explain why they had overlooked the probability that consumers were eating an untested viral protein. [90]

This would not be the first occasion that changes to the plant structure had aspects that went unnoticed for decades by the very geneticists who were supposedly in charge of their development. The current rage for using the CRISPR-Cas9 enzyme for altering DNA has already been found to introduce hundreds of unintended mutations, which prompted researchers to warn: 'More work may be needed to increase the fidelity of CRISPR--Cas9 with regard to off-target mutation generation before the CRISPR platform can be used without risk.' [91] Dr Shiva suggests that currently, it is technically not possible to make single (and only a single) genetic change to a genome using CRISPR and to ensure that it has done so.[92]

Reasons for the Development of Genetically Modified Food

Reasons that are given for the development of genetically modified food, usually suggest the more altruistic myths behind their use, such as to solve world hunger, create better-tasting or more-nutritious food, better resistance to disease, higher yields etc. Here's is Dr Latham's view, one that is pretty universal among researchers:

Genetically Modified Crops and Food

> Science is not the only grounds on which GMOs should be judged. The commercial purpose of GMOs is not to feed the world or improve farming. Rather, they exist to gain intellectual property (i.e. patent rights) over seeds and plant breeding and to drive agriculture in directions that benefit agribusiness. This drive is occurring at the expense of farmers, consumers and the natural world. US farmers, for example, have seen seed costs nearly quadruple and seed choices greatly narrow since the introduction of GMOs. The fight over them is thus not of narrow importance. Their use affects us all.[93]

In January 2002, Catholic Cardinal Peter Turkson accused the merchants of the genetic engineering of crops of 'breeding economic dependence and a new form of slavery'. As regards to the claim that GMOs were necessary to feed the world: 'It is a scandal that nearly 1 billion people suffer from hunger', Cardinal Turkson said, 'especially since there is more than enough food to feed the whole world'. He further elaborated:

> There would be no need for such crops if African growers had access to fertile land that was not destroyed, devastated or poisoned by the stockpiling of toxic waste and if growers were able to benefit from the fruits of their labors by being allowed to set aside enough seeds for planting the next year and not be forced to continually buy genetically modified seeds from abroad.[94]

In *Unhealthy Betrayal,* I pointed out how world hunger was nothing to do with lack of food, as we live in a world with an overabundance of food—but more to do with the lack of purchasing power to pay for the food—which is more directly determined by political economics than food production. We previously discussed how in South America, for example, due to massive indebtedness that was purposely inflicted on these countries, food was being exported simply to pay the interest charges on immense debts while many of the populace went hungry. Currently, most of the GMO crops in South America are for export.[95]

Frances Moore Lappé and Joseph Collins, in their book *World Hunger—10 Myths,* expressed the situation with regard to access to adequate food: 'Hunger has thus become for us the ultimate symbol of powerlessness…Certainly, the cause is not scarcity. The world is awash with food…Put most simply, the root cause of hunger isn't a scarcity of food, it's a *scarcity of Democracy.*' [96] This conclusion is well-supported by the rest of their volume, and further in both of my previous volumes, *Unhealthy Betrayal,* and *Hijacked,* for those who would like further amplification of this important observation. For now, I intend to try and keep to factors that more directly have implications for your health while at the same time addressing some of the mythology that supports the genetic modification of food and the industrialisation of agriculture and food supplies.

One of the products that the biotech industry and its supporters have promoted for decades has been their GMO product Golden Rice, which they have suggested was the urgently required solution for treating vitamin A deficiency that causes so many problems, such as xerophthalmia, a progressive eye disorder causing night blindness and leading to damage of the cornea, due to deficiency of vitamin A. Proponents of GE Golden Rice have suggested that this product was the solution, as it was supposed to have higher levels of beta carotene, a precursor to vitamin A, engineered into the rice grain. However, Allison Wilson, PhD, and Jonathon Latham, PhD, revealed that this has not appeared to be accepted by the FDA:

> But, in a surprising twist, the US Food and Drug Administration (FDA) has concluded its consultation process on Golden Rice by informing its current developers, the International Rice Research

Genetically Modified Crops and Food

Institute (IRRI), that Golden Rice does not meet the nutritional requirements to make a health claim.

The FDA letter, posted 25th May 2018 (FDA 2018b), further states 'the concentration of β-carotene in GR2E rice is too low to warrant a nutrient content claim.'

Wilson and Latham also mention an FDA memo that gives the beta-carotene content of unmilled Golden Rice GR2E as ranging from 0.50-2.35ug/g, which they point out is both low and variable. They suggest that with comparison to beta-carotene levels in non-GMO foods such as fresh carrot (13.8-49.3ug/g); Asian greens (19.74-66.04 ug/g), and spinach (111ug/g), that it just doesn't measure up. They further mention:

'FDA notes the mean value of beta-carotene for GR2E is 1.26ug/g. This is, paradoxically, less beta-carotene than the 1.6ug/g measured for the original iteration of Golden Rice.'

On top of this mediocre level of beta carotene, they further mention that it is a very unstable version that dissipates with storage even in the short-term. They note that studies showed that after only three weeks that the beta-carotene content of Golden Rice GR2E was reduced by 40% after ten weeks only retained 13% of its original level.[97]

In Africa, vitamin A deficiency has been addressed by planting foods that are higher in beta-carotene, such as the orange coloured sweet potato, as opposed to the white more traditionally-planted variety. The orange colour is from beta-carotene. The Peru-based International Potato Center and its partners have developed and disseminated more than 130 orange-fleshed sweet potato varieties across Africa and Asia, reaching 5 million households.

Another of the reasons given for the development of genetically engineering plants was to make them more resilient to insects, which would supposedly increase yields, and perhaps reduce the need for harmful pesticides.

It is worth bringing to your attention another attempt by the industry to create what works out to be a systemic poison produced from the Bacillus thuringienisis, mentioned earlier, that has been genetically engineered into the plant itself, such as Bt cotton. Bt cotton has been planted in India, which was where the first reports emanated regarding allergic reactions to handling the plants. Reports of 100 cases of allergies from two villages in India surfaced in 2004, and 150 cases in 2005 from the same villages, producing itching in all parts of the body, followed by red patches, redness of the eyes, [and] swelling of [the] face and hands. More severe reactions were reported in other areas, leading to one woman being hospitalised. For some people, the symptoms persisted for five to six months, with a serious discharge from the face, where the skin became dark, almost black in colour.[98]

Jeffrey Smith reported on 1,820 deaths among sheep that grazed on Bt cotton plants after harvest. In one village, the death rate from 42 herds was 25% (651 out of 2,601 animals). Traditionally after harvesting the cotton, the plants have been fed to the sheep. In this instance, following ingesting the Bt cotton crop, within two or three days the animals appeared dull and inactive, developing coughs with nasal discharge, with death following in five to seven days. The following year some farmers refused to feed the crop remains to their animals and the animals were fine, but those who continued to feed the Bt crop remains to their animals had the same reoccurrence and their animals died. The Animal Health Centre (AHC) undertook post mortems on some of the animals and found "black patches in the small intestines, enlarged bile duct and liver with discolouration, and accumulation of pericardial fluid." [99]

Genetically Modified Crops and Food

You may not feel that the issue with Bt cotton concerns you, as you are not likely to encounter this particular problem. What you may not be aware of is how this technology is being used in plants that humans consume such as aubergines, and corn (maize). Some scientists have warned that the human gut biome could be turned into a pesticide factory, because the Bt toxin is now a systemic plant toxin, with no off switch. According to the biotech industry, the Bt pesticides introduced into GMO crops are natural proteins whose toxic activity extends to only a narrow group of species, and can, therefore, be safely eaten by humans. Is this really the case? Let's explore this further. According to Jonathon Latham, PhD., the commercial Bt toxins differ greatly from their natural predecessors which were insoluble crystals that had to be eaten then dissolved in the gut of the target organism, usually a caterpillar, then processed by the gut enzymes in a precise sequence. Once processed this way, the much smaller molecule attaches to the receptors in the gut and makes holes in its membranes. This causes the victim to be digested from the inside by the contents of its own gut, which now includes the Bacillus thuringiensis.

Latham believes that the differences of commercial GMO Bt toxins are important, as they are more toxic, and are active against many more species than the natural forms of Bt toxins. He found many of the GMO toxins to be truncated proteins that were able to make hybrid molecules that do not exist in nature. Some of them mutate to replace specific amino acids it seemed that the GMO plant invariably altered the BT toxins. He found that of the 23 Bt commercial lines analysed all had at least two major alterations, most had many alterations. He, therefore, felt it was wrong of biotech companies to call their GMO Bt proteins natural as they do, it was misleading and scientifically wrong. He believes that the GMO Bt toxins are potentially hazardous to an unknown range of organisms. The pollen grains, for example, have been shown to kill swallowtail butterflies.[100]

Monsanto and the EPA swore that the genetically engineered corn would only harm insects and that the Bt toxin would be completely destroyed in the human digestive system and would not have any impact on consumers. However, in May 2011, doctors at Sherbrooke University Hospital in Quebec found Bt toxin in the blood of pregnant women. They discovered Bt toxin in 93 percent of the pregnant women they tested and found it in 80 percent of the umbilical blood in their babies. They also tested non-pregnant women and discovered 67 percent of them tested positive for the toxin. According to Dr Joseph Mercola: 'These shocking results raise the frightening possibility that eating Bt corn might actually turn your intestinal flora into a sort of living pesticide factory, essentially manufacturing Bt toxin from within your digestive system on a continuing basis'.

These shocking results raise the frightening possibility that eating Bt corn might actually turn your intestinal flora into a sort of living pesticide factory, essentially manufacturing Bt toxin from within your digestive system on a continuing basis.

Dr Mercola suggests that this scenario is very plausible:

If this hypothesis is correct, is it then also possible that the Bt toxin might damage the integrity of your digestive tract in the same way it damages insects? Remember, the toxin actually ruptures the stomach of insects, causing them to die. The biotech industry has insisted that the Bt toxin doesn't bind or interact with the intestinal walls of mammals (which would include humans). But again, there is peer-reviewed published research showing that Bt toxin does bind with mouse small intestines and with intestinal tissue from rhesus monkeys.

He suggests that this could result in a rise in gastrointestinal problems, food allergies, autoimmune diseases, and childhood learning disorders. Aside from this impact on human health, it seems that, in fact, the Bt toxin is creating a new generation of insects that are becoming resistant to it, and a new generation of insect larvae is eating the roots of genetically-engineered corn intended to be resistant to such pests.

Dr Mercola believes that the failure of Monsanto's genetically modified Bt corn could be "the most serious threat ever to a genetically-modified crop in the U.S." Bt corn accounts for 65 percent of all corn grown in the US, which could mean billions of dollars at stake. [101]

A further report studied the effect of Bt toxin on human lymphocytes, and found it toxic to these tissues, using toxin isolated from Bt cotton.[102]

Genetic Engineering—Unnecessary Technology?

The question has to be asked, whether genetic engineering is a useful development that has a real benefit to offer humanity, or whether it is another misplaced adventure with a technology that history might show was a dangerous development leaving a harmful legacy to humanity. It could be compared with atomic energy. We know that atomic energy development was directly due to the decision to create a nuclear weapons potential, and the creation of the atom bomb. Much of the secrecy around this industry was thought necessary to enable weapons development. Unfortunately, the secrecy continues to exist to such a degree that today the atomic energy development still wishes to project itself as "green energy", as opposed to probably the most dangerous pollution yet devised by mankind, leaving an unparalleled legacy of wastes that will exist as a threat for more than 24,000 years—that to this day has not been addressed. Genetic engineering, whilst it definitely has the potential to leave a legacy that in some ways could be comparable, in that it could unleash a genetic timebomb that could endure forever—it, however, does not have the excuse for secrecy that atomic energy had due to the weapons program, but nevertheless has the same degree of concealment, distortion of the truth, and blind arrogance.

You could argue, however, that the GM industry is simply using the tools of corporate culture, much like the pharmaceutical industry and pesticide industry, which thrives on the existence of a massive public relations exercise, and government funding program to ensure that it gets what it wants, irrespective of the harm it does to humanity. Perhaps I am being really dumb here, and I am living under an illusion that business can actually co-exist with humanity and actually serve the greater interests of humanity—the truth may be that we are all simply numbers of dumb consumers, who need to be led to the trough to feed on whatever garbage, either material or intellectual that corporate business interests deign to throw at us. After all, don't the same companies that poison us with their pesticides, also poison us with their food additive chemicals, and then when we are made sick by this overdose get us to buy their drugs to supposedly treat the symptoms of this onslaught?

I have yet to come up with one reason to support genetic engineering. No doubt they will try to label me as another Luddite, someone who can't move with the future, someone prejudiced and ignorant who wishes to prevent 'progress'. My problem, if you can call it that, is that I think for myself, I question what I am being fed, whether it is information or actual food. My advice to you is to do the same. I hope to give you enough information so that you will be able to decide for yourself, what foods will really produce health, what information to accept as reliable, and how to recognise what is simply more industry propaganda. I hope to supply you with the resources to understand that the world we live in is a world of abundance there is enough food for everyone. In fact, organic agriculture, and regenerative agriculture are increasing the ability to produce food without harmful chemicals at an incredible rate—more on this in chapter nine.

One of the great myths that genetic engineering proponents would like us to swallow is the idea that their industry could provide tastier, more nutritious food. Let me dispel that myth by explaining one of the great truths about food production. Call it the "garbage in—garbage out" principle that goes something like this. If you choose to grow crops on depleted soils exhausted of many of the nutrients that supply health and vigour, growth simply supported by synthetic fertilizers and you feed your animals on this poor quality food, which lacking in nutrients, such as essential minerals and vitamins, and that can be further loaded with toxic man-made chemicals, do you expect these creatures to thrive? Hopefully, you realise this will not produce health. The question that follows is whether you think that eating these animals would be expected to provide healthy nourishment, and thereby endow health to its human consumer? The answer is the same: it is garbage in garbage out! There are a great number of people who do not seem to appreciate this simple principle, and treat their own bodies like a garbage receptacle, pouring all kinds of rubbish into themselves, simply because they can. The body is a remarkable thing it can endure mistreatment for a considerable period of time before the dire lack of essential nutrients and the onslaught of garbage causes the energy levels to drop, and the immune system to barely function, so that inflammation builds and eventually, they succumb to an illness of one form or another. This does not have to be humanity's future. There are exciting developments afoot: read on.

To create quality nutritious food, you need to feed the correct nutrients to the recipient, whether it is an animal or a plant. Industrialised agriculture has discovered that plants will *seem* to survive quite well on water and sunlight once established, and with a minimal input of fertiliser will grow sturdily enough with the application of pesticides, herbicides and fungicides the plant will survive to reach a market, and return a profit of sorts to the grower. The product however will be lacking in numerous essential minerals, vitamins, and other beneficial nutrients and will doubtless contain residues of pesticide treatment. Its organic counterpart is generally supported by a superior soil, with more nutrients for the maintenance of plant life, and minimal chemical inputs. However, to generate vibrant health we need to grow crops on soils that are alive with a rich biological component a truly fertile soil—more on this in chapter nine. The taste of such plants would be reflected in the variety of the plant chosen and the richness of the soil structure. I have yet to see any genetically engineered planting to be offered a really supportive soil structure, without pesticide inputs or artificial fertilizers. I believe that the chances of this happening are minimal to non-existent. Numerous reports also detail how animals, given the choice will simply not eat GMO crops: their senses tell them this is not good food. There is, however, a real lack of studies looking at the effect of consuming the various genetically modified foods that play a part in our diets. The only decent studies undertaken have revealed significant worries. With such a complete lack of reliable information, we are left in the position of being guinea pigs for the GMO industry. Therefore my advice would be to avoid any form of genetically modified food like the plague.

Chapter Six

Harvesting Sickness

We have reviewed a number of factors that are having a direct impact on the health of our respective societies. That has included the man-made chemical explosion into our lives via food products from the food industry, pesticides, herbicides and fungicides from the agricultural industry; environmental sources of exposure from various industries; and in more recent years, the assault from the genetical engineering industry. What is lacking from our analysis is a review of the way the pharmaceutical industry has been galvanized to appear to deal with the consequences—that is the demise of our health and the explosion of chronic disease we are confronted with. In this chapter, we will look at this response and the effect of the medical industry itself on our health. Before we do, I feel it will be useful to help you understand the size of the problem we are facing with the chemical onslaught and its ramifications on your health and for future generations.

When the European Union introduced its comprehensive review of chemicals in 2007, called the Registration Evaluation and Authorization of Chemicals (REACH), which was initially based on chemicals that were imported into the EU (estimated at more than 1000 metric tonnes per year), more than 143,000 chemicals were *pre-registered*. This is a phenomenal amount by any standards and of course, is reflected in the experience of America. The USA, in 2010, in their introductory letter in the US President's Cancer Panel's Annual Report, had this to say regarding chemical exposure of US citizens:

> The Panel was particularly concerned to find that the true burden of environmentally induced cancer has been grossly underestimated. With nearly 80,000 chemicals on the market in the United States, many of which are used by millions of Americans in their daily lives and are un- or understudied and largely unregulated, exposure to potential environmental carcinogens is widespread.

The EU information suggests the number of chemicals may be much higher in the US than the panel estimated; nevertheless, their comments on agricultural chemicals, should give pause for concern:

> Pesticides (Insecticides, Herbicides, and Fungicides) Nearly 1,400 pesticides have been registered (i.e., approved) by the Environmental Protection Agency (EPA) for agricultural and non-agricultural use. Exposure to these chemicals has been linked to brain/central nervous system (CNS), breast, colon, lung, ovarian (female spouses), pancreatic, kidney, testicular, and stomach cancers, as well as Hodgkin and non-Hodgkin lymphoma, multiple myeloma, and soft tissue sarcoma. Pesticide-exposed farmers, pesticide applicators, crop duster pilots, and manufacturers also have been found to have elevated rates of prostate cancer, melanoma, other skin cancers, and cancer of the lip.
>
> Approximately 40 chemicals classified by the International Agency for Research on Cancer (IARC) as known, probable, or possible human carcinogens, are used in EPA-registered pesticides now on the market.[103]

The President's Cancer Panel also revealed that the Department of Agriculture's Pesticide Data Program, in its most recent report (which analyzed 11,683 food samples, conducting an average of 105 tests on each sample representing more than 1.22 million analyses in total), found that only 23.1% of samples had zero pesticide residues detected, 29.5 percent had one residue, and the remainder had two or more. This suggests that approximately half the foods in the USA have a mixture of chemical residues.

Dr Vandana Shiva, world-renowned biologist and author of numerous books, refers to a World Health Organization (WHO) report concerning the global epidemic of non-communicable chronic diseases that expresses serious concerns regarding this development: "Non-communicable diseases (NCDs), such as heart disease, stroke, cancer, chronic respiratory diseases and diabetes, are the leading cause of mortality in the world. This invisible epidemic is an under-appreciated cause of poverty and hinders the economic development of many countries. The burden is growing—the number of people, families and communities afflicted is increasing." Dr Shiva makes an important point regarding their source: 'You cannot catch these diseases from other people. You will not get cancer, heart disease or diabetes from sitting next to people with these diseases. The multiple causes are environmental, which means that we can prevent them by changing our habits, food water etc. to avoid the environmental exposures that cause them'.

You cannot catch these diseases from other people. You will

not get cancer, heart disease or diabetes from sitting next to people

with these diseases. The multiple causes are environmental, which

means that we can prevent them by changing our habits, food water
etc. to avoid the environmental exposures that cause them. [104]

What needs to be emphasized here is these diseases are all fundamentally *metabolic diseases,* which means the solutions to them have to address the chemical assault that causes the metabolic processes of the body to fail, and to assist the body in restoring metabolic homeostasis with such things as nutritional support and, importantly, reassessing what food we eat. Whilst intervention using drugs in the short-term may assist, drugs by their very nature cannot restore metabolic homeostasis; they can only ameliorate symptoms—the root cause of the disease process being unchanged and ignored.

If you take a simple example of a person who becomes addicted to eating a lot of junk food with lots of pasta, pizza, doughnuts, sugar-based treats, and desserts, sweetened beverages etc., a diet that would continuously spike their insulin to very high levels—this would eventually lead to prediabetes, and then diabetes. Treating someone like this with drugs would not reverse the disease process; it may delay the process somewhat, but it will not cure it. A radical shift in the diet—removing all the highly-processed carbohydrates could. It is, however, not common knowledge among doctors that you can reverse type 2 diabetes with diet. Dr Jason Fung, in his book *The Diabetes Code,* reveals how he has been successfully reversing diabetes of many type 2 sufferers for a number of years, and is as good a source as any to help understand how this is achievable. For many people, however, the disease process can be more complex, and more challenging to fix. We hope to address this point with some further examples.

Transgenerational Effects

One of the concerns for many researchers is the effects of so many chemicals and their possible harmful interreactions, particularly in younger children who have not developed adequate immune systems for dealing with them and especially the developing embryo. Mohan Manikkam reports on an example that involved small amounts of common insect repellent, plasticizers, and jet fuel residues during pregnancy that led to permanent changes in the germline—these are the first cells that lead to the formation of sperm or egg production cells in the fetus. The researchers found that changes were passed on and inherited by future generations.

> The epigenetic transgenerational actions of various environmental compounds and relevant mixtures were investigated with the use of a pesticide mixture (permethrin and insect repellant DEET), a plastic mixture (bisphenol A and phthalates), dioxin (TCDD) and a hydrocarbon mixture (jet fuel, JP8).
>
> The plastics, dioxin and jet fuel were found to promote early-onset female puberty transgenerationally (F3 generation). Spermatogenic cell apoptosis [cell death] was affected transgenerationally. Ovarian primordial follicle pool size was significantly decreased with all treatments transgenerationally.[105]

Whilst research into the environmental effects of man-made chemicals has been sorely neglected, there are, some researchers who have been able to look into this phenomena, and not just into the effects on the current population but, by looking at the transgenerational effects, see how we are actually affecting *future* generations. Whilst this area of study may be in its relative infancy, the implications are profound and should concern us all. If environmental influences can effect such fundamental changes, it brings into question the whole concept as to what 'genetic inheritance' really means and makes it even more imperative that we clean up our act, both by massively reducing our exposure to hazardous man-made chemicals and developing more creative solutions to these challenges. One of the big changes in our understanding of the ability of chemicals in our environment to affect development came with the eventual realization of the human genome project. The fruit fly genome was decoded and found to have 13,000 genes; the flea genome was decoded and found to have 30,000. What caused total consternation was discovering that the human genome came in at approximately 20,000 genes, placing our genetic makeup somewhere between the flea and a fruit fly. This shocked everybody, such a dismally low number representing human complexity. It is only now being appreciated that we are not simply controlled by our DNA, and that our RNA has a much more important role than previously understood. It seems we have a more adaptable biological system, but we are also uniquely vulnerable to exposure to manmade chemicals than we were previously assumed to be. We must accept that pregnant women have to be better protected and also acknowledge that the very future of mankind is at stake.

Here are the views of Michael K Skinner and his associates on this very subject:

> Environmental factors such as toxicants, nutrition, and stress all have been shown to promote the epigenetic transgenerational inheritance of disease and phenotypic variation. One of the first observations in mammals involved the actions of the agricultural fungicide vinclozolin on a gestating F0 generation female promoting transgenerational disease in the F3 and F4 generation progeny [note F1 is first-generation, F2 is second-generation, F3 is third-generation, etc.]. This was found to be mediated in part through differential DNA methylation regions (termed epimutations) in the sperm that are transmitted between generations and correlate with transgenerational disease phenotypes. Transgenerational

disease was found in the testis, ovary, kidney, prostate, and mammary gland. Subsequently, a large number of toxicants (plastics, pesticides, hydrocarbons), nutritional abnormalities (high fat and caloric restriction), and stress (social and aversion) have been shown to promote the transgenerational phenomenon. Epigenetic transgenerational inheritance has now been observed in plants, flies, worms, fish, mice, rats, pigs, and humans.

No doubt the idea that these effects can be linked back four generations to a single moment of exposure will come as a surprise to many. Hopefully, it will give people a little more food for thought. Here is Michael Skinner's understanding of the situation: 'The predominant current view for the origin and evolution of disease considers genetic mutations as the primary molecular mechanism involved. Environmental impacts on the epigenome that have the ability to promote genetic mutations extend these previous views and help clarify how the environment may have direct impact on disease etiology and on the origins of phenotypic and genotypic variation in evolutionary processes.'

The predominant current view for the origin and evolution of disease considers genetic mutations as the primary molecular mechanism involved. Environmental impacts on the epigenome that have the ability to promote genetic mutations extend these previous views and help clarify how the environment may have direct impact on disease etiology and on the origins of phenotypic and genotypic variation in evolutionary processes.[106]

One of the problems we are faced with regarding the disease symptoms that many of us may be confronted with is that they are not easily perceived as linked to our previous actions. If we eat junk food, for example, we may feel fine at the time of consumption and feel that there has been no detrimental effect; it's only via research by others or the passage of time, that the consequences can be understood. Of course, it is much more difficult for people to understand this particular lesson when there are huge advertising campaigns and public relations exercises by food companies who seek to profit from our ignorance, suggesting that their food is great to consume. It is much much more difficult when the effects occurred when you were in the womb and as a result you may be faced with autism, serious learning difficulties, or even just diminished abilities. The cost of these problems, however, in their emotional, and social nature on families, as well as financial cost, can be substantial for society.

Poisoning Us is a Costly Business

According to Philippe Grandjean, adjunct professor of Environmental Health at Harvard School of Public Health, and Philip Landrigan, professor of the Children's Environmental Health Center, Mount Sinai School of Medicine, disorders of neurobehavioural development affect 10 -15% of all births. And this is only part of what they refer to as 'The global, silent pandemic of neurodevelopmental toxicity'. They note that 201 chemicals have been reported to cause injury to the nervous system in adults, and more than 1000 chemicals have been reported to be neurotoxic in animals. They are concerned about the levels of chemicals that are found in both umbilical cord samples and mother's milk.

> Neurodevelopmental disabilities, including autism, attention-deficit hyperactivity disorder, dyslexia, and other cognitive impairments, affect millions of children worldwide, and some diagnoses seem to be increasing in frequency. Industrial chemicals that injure the developing brain are among the known causes for this rise in prevalence. In 2006, we

did a systematic review and identified five industrial chemicals as developmental neurotoxicants: lead, methylmercury, polychlorinated biphenyls, arsenic, and toluene. Since 2006, epidemiological studies have documented six additional developmental neurotoxicants—manganese, fluoride, chlorpyrifos, dichlorodipheny-trichloroethane, tetrachloroethylene, and the polybrominated diphenyl ethers. Pesticides mentioned, each with supporting references, were: Acetamiprid, amitraz, avermectin, emamectin, fipronil (Termidor), glyphosate, hexaconazole, imidacloprid, tetramethylenedisulfotetramine.

In *Unhealthy Betrayal,* I reported on some of the lessons learned from the way industry's efforts to downplay the dangers of lead, and in particular its effects on children, caused significant damage to their brains. Grandjean and Landrigan gave some of their experience with lead:

> Joint analyses that gathered data for lead-associated IQ deficits from seven international studies support the conclusion that no safe level of exposure to lead exists. Cognitive deficits in adults who had previously shown lead-associated developmental delays at school age suggest that the effects of lead neurotoxicity are probably permanent. Brain imaging of young adults who had raised lead concentrations in their blood during childhood showed exposure-related decreases in brain volume. Lead exposure in early childhood is associated with reduced school performance and with delinquent behaviour later in life.

There has been a reported dramatic increase in attention-deficit hyperactivity disorder (ADHD) in children. Grandjean and Landrigan both linked this to a number of factors: 'For example, an increased risk of attention-deficit hyperactivity disorder has been linked to prenatal exposures to manganese, organophosphates, and phthalates. Phthalates have also been linked to behaviours that resemble components of autism spectrum disorder. Prenatal exposure to automotive air pollution in California, USA has been linked to an increased risk for autism spectrum disorder.'

They also suggested that consequential brain damage could be compared with traumatic brain injury:

> Developmental neurotoxicity causes brain damage that is too often untreatable and frequently permanent. The consequence of such brain damage is impaired CNS [central nervous sytem] function that lasts a lifetime and might result in reduced intelligence, as expressed in terms of lost IQ points, or disruption in behaviour. A recent study compared the estimated total IQ losses from major paediatric causes and showed that the magnitude of losses attributable to lead, pesticides, and other neurotoxicants was in the same range as, or even greater than, the losses associated with medical events such as preterm birth, traumatic brain injury, brain tumours, and congenital heart disease.

What I found particularly interesting from their study was the estimated costs to society. I have argued for some time now that, industry's claim that properly regulating industrial chemicals would be expensive to society, that it would raise the cost of food, for example—a huge distortion of reality—more directly due to how the cost is apportioned. Grandjean's analysis is a useful assessment:

> Loss of cognitive skills reduces children's academic and economic attainments and has substantial long-term economic effects on societies. Thus, each loss of one IQ point has been estimated to decrease average lifetime earnings capacity by about €12 000 or US$18 000 in 2008 currencies. The most recent estimates from the USA indicate that the annual costs of childhood lead poisoning are about US$50 billion and that the annual costs of methylmercury toxicity are roughly US$5 billion. In the European Union, methylmercury exposure is estimated to cause a loss

of about 600,000 IQ points every year, corresponding to an annual economic loss of close to €10 billion.

They additionally added that in the USA, the murder rate fell sharply 20 years after the removal of lead from petrol, which they referred to as 'a finding consistent with the idea that exposure to lead in early life is a powerful determinant of behaviour decades later. Although poorly quantified, such behavioural and social consequences of neuro-developmental toxicity are potentially very costly'.

They further emphasized the way prevention of damage is cost-effective:

> Prevention of developmental neurotoxicity caused by industrial chemicals is highly cost-effective. A study that quantified the gains resulting from the phase-out of lead additives from petrol reported that in the USA alone, the introduction of lead-free petrol has generated an economic benefit of $200 billion in each annual birth cohort since 1980, an aggregate benefit in the past 30 years of over $3 trillion. [107]

We have reviewed a lot of evidence suggesting that man-made chemicals released into the environment and our food supplies are impacting our health in numerous ways. On top of that, we have looked at the way the politicization of health has impacted the food supply and our eating habits. We have shown how the very organizations set up to protect us have been subordinated to the interests of industry, generally large corporations whose sole *raison d'être* is to make money out of us. The 'health' industry is worth billions. In 2014, total pharmaceutical revenues worldwide had exceeded one trillion U.S. dollars for the first time.[108] By 2018, the global market for pharmaceuticals reached $1.2 trillion and is predicted to reach $1.5 trillion in 2023.[109]

How To Survive in the 21ˢᵗ Century

What must be understood from these vast figures, is that sickness is generating vast wealth for some people. If you extrapolate the kind of analysis provided by Professors, Grandjean and Landrigan across the whole health spectrum, not just the health effects of cognitive decline, it must also be apparent that the costs to society, aside from the immense personal and social costs, have to be generating equally vast figures, in fact, substantially more. It must be self-evident that the incentive to prevent or even cure disease would not be in the interests of such a profitable industry. In purely economic terms you are looking at a massive transfer of wealth from a large proportion of society to a very small minority (most shares are held by the top 1% of the population), leaving a huge burden on society—that is the burden of a sick population—a population that will have a reduced ability to add to the productive potential and will require resources for their ongoing care. In a purely economic sense, this system can only lead to the complete bankruptcy and collapse of society if allowed to continue its present course.

The Failure of Medicine

One of the problems we have created by allowing corporate interests to dictate policy, by using their excessive profits to buy influence in various political systems, to control scientific research, manipulate university studies, to indoctrinate populations with their public relations campaigns and advertising, to create pseudo-scientific justification for the use of their products—all of which I explore in-depth in *Unhealthy Betrayal*—is it creates a world divorced from real science, divorced from the very people who could help restore health and the creation of a reality that has led to the greatest impoverishment of society, comparable in some respects to slavery.

This pervasive influence has been so corrosive and has existed for such a long time that it has corrupted all the institutions that we rely on for delivering us health, so much so that the pharmaceutical industry is one of the leading industries that now cause us harm.

Dr Ray Strand, in his book *Death By Prescription*, warned us (in 2003) that adverse drug reactions to *properly* prescribed medication led to more than 100,000 deaths per year, which made it the fourth leading cause of death in America. He further reported that if you added the further 80,000 deaths caused by improperly prescribed or administered medication, adverse drug events become the number-three leading cause of death in America, behind heart disease and cancer. He compares this substantial loss of life to the 56,000 Americans that were killed in the Vietnam War. He wonders why this health catastrophe does not inspire the population to demand urgent reform.[110]

In his book, he explores much of the information about the way drugs are poorly regulated, poorly understood, and lead to such epidemic problems. He cites a number of studies that estimate that 5 % of all hospital admissions are the result of adverse drug events and that the odds of a problem with medication increases once a person *enters* the hospital. Most people during their hospital stay receive an average of ten different drugs, and the more critically ill can receive upwards of 38 different drugs during their hospitalization. He draws our attention to the fact that all drugs are synthetic (not derived from natural substances) and by their very nature are basically toxic. All of them have to be broken down in the body and excreted; many of them share the same excretion pathway, by the same enzyme system in the liver such as the cytochrome P450 system. Problems can arise when more than one drug is taken that shares this same metabolic system, as it can create a situation where the drugs' effects are greatly amplified leading to unsuspected and serious consequences.

The situation can be compounded by a patient seeing more than one physician, currently, nearly 50% of patients do, often times a specialist in their relevant field. Dr Strand mentions that specialists tend to prescribe more potent medications, usually in combination with several other medications. He suggests that it is not uncommon to see patients that are taking anywhere between 8 and 20 different drugs at the same time. Consequently more powerful medications pose a much more serious risk. Part of the problem, as he sees it, is that as we see more specialists, we risk receiving more fragmented care, as communication between the various specialists and the primary care physician breaks down.

To illustrate the problem with drug interactions he lists all the drugs that interact with Coumadin (warfarin), a commonly prescribed blood thinner. He lists 74 drugs that amplify the effects and 13 that decrease the effects. He also lists 78 drugs that are known to use the P450 enzyme system. He gives the example of a physician prescribing Prozac and Zoloft (two anti-depressants) together: because they both use the cytochrome P450 system, the drugs will actually enhance each other's effect in the body possibly leading to serotonin syndrome (serotonin excess). If you add an MAO inhibitor (monoamine oxidase inhibitor) the effect can be further amplified, leading to possibly disastrous consequences.

Dr Strand cites a personal story that is worth repeating here regarding a patient of his, the young daughter of a colleague who had developed pneumonia and needed hospitalization. He started her on an antibiotic for her pneumonia and acetaminophen for her fever, nausea and vomiting. On the third day, her blood tests were showing evidence that her liver was being damaged, and she was becoming jaundiced. She continued to rapidly deteriorate, so they discontinued all her medication. She was shipped by air ambulance to the University of Minnesota's Children's hospital where she could get more specialist care. A scan revealed severe liver damage. The pediatric gastroenterologist informed Dr Strand that the cause of her liver necrosis was due to "a severe reaction to acetaminophen." He was told that the combination of the Erythromycin and acetaminophen can cause significant stress on anyone's liver. Thankfully her life was spared and she recovered.[111]

I am sure for many of you to learn that adverse drug events have led many people to find that the medical profession is now regarded as the third leading cause of death in America may come as a shock. There are, however, some doctors who feel the situation is even worse than this if you add statistics for medical errors. In *Death By Medicine,* written by a number of doctors, they suggest: 'It is now evident that the American medical system is the *leading* cause of death and injury in the US.'[112] They reveal that the reason they decided to publish, what is a severe critique of medicine, is 'to call attention to the failure of the American medical system.' They review in some detail the defects of the current practice of healthcare in the USA in particular, with the hope of bringing much-needed reform:

> By exposing these gruesome statistics in painstaking detail, we provide a basis for competent and compassionate medical professionals, such as the courageous Dr. David Graham, to recognise the inadequacies of today's system and at least attempt to initiate meaningful reforms.

Dr Graham who they refer to is the FDA Associate Director for Science and Medicine in the FDA's Office of Drug Safety, who testified before Congress after spending twenty years with the FDA on some of the problems he faced. They quote some of his testimony that I feel is worth repeating:

> During my career, I believe I have made a real difference for the cause of patient safety. My research and efforts within the FDA led to the withdrawal from the US market of Omniflox, an antibiotic that caused haemolytic anemia; Rezulin, a diabetes drug that caused acute liver failure; FenPhen and Redux, weight loss drugs that caused heart valve injury; and

123

PPA (phenylpropanolamine), an over-the-counter decongestant and weight loss product that caused hemorrhagic stroke in young women.

My research also led to the withdrawal from outpatient use of Trovan, an antibiotic that caused acute liver failure and death. I also contributed to the team effort that led to the withdrawal of Lotronex, a drug for irritable bowel syndrome that causes ischemic colitis; Baycol, a cholesterol-lowering drug that caused severe muscle injury, kidney failure and death; Seldane, an antihistamine that caused heart arrhythmias and death...

Dr Graham discusses further examples of the challenges he faced at the FDA, I will offer one more example, that of the drug Vioxx, by Merck, a disaster to health that I previously reported on in *Unhealthy Betrayal*. Here he is reporting on his concerns in 2004: 'We are faced with what may be the single greatest drug safety catastrophe in the history of this country or the history of the world. We are talking about a catastrophe that I strongly believe could have, should have, been largely or completely avoided. But it wasn't, and over 100,000 Americans have paid dearly for this failure. In my opinion, the FDA has let the American people down, and sadly, betrayed a public trust.' [113]

We are faced with what may be the single greatest drug safety catastrophe in the history of this country or the history of the world. We are talking about a catastrophe that I strongly believe could have, should have, been largely or completely avoided. But it wasn't, and over 100,000 Americans have paid dearly for this failure. In my opinion, the FDA has let the American people down, and sadly, betrayed a public trust.

Harvesting Sickness

I have no wish to enter the debate as to whether the medical industry is the first or third leading cause of death, suffice it to agree that we do, however, acknowledge we have a serious problem here that deserves our attention. What I feel can be useful, is looking at what most of the critics of current medical practice have to say that we can use to benefit us all. What seems prevalent in all critics is the way the pharmaceutical industry has been able to control and manipulate the very organizations set up to regulate their industry to the detriment of our health. Whilst it is beyond the scope of this present volume to undertake an in-depth look at this problem (much of this is dealt with in a previous volume, *Unhealthy Betrayal*)[114], some discussion would be useful to understand the scale of the challenge we face.

Dr Strand suggests that in 1960 there were only 650 medications available in the USA, and by 2003 had increased exponentially to more than 8,000. Estimates vary to some degree, but the general consensus is that currently there are in excess of 10,000 drugs on the market.[115] Of these, very few have been seriously reviewed for safety. Dr Strand believes that physicians can only hope to understand the most common and basic problems of drug interactions with so many on the market, and he believes that as more drugs are taken the risk goes up exponentially. He informs us that over 16,000 patients each year die from the use of prescription and over-the-counter nonsteroidal anti-inflammatories (NSAIDs), and further that this class of drugs were responsible for more than 100,000 hospital admissions in 2002 due to intestinal bleeding. Of these admissions, many were due to patient's over-the-counter use.

Dr Marcia Angell, former editor in chief of the *New England Journal of Medicine,* wrote a critical book about the pharmaceutical industry in 2004, *The Truth About Drug Companies—How They Deceive Us and What to Do About It.* Writing from the viewpoint of someone who has been intimately connected with the industry, her views have some authority when she suggests that the industry is failing us all:

> The combined profits for the ten drug companies in the Fortune 500 ($35.9 billion) were more than the profits for all the other 490 businesses put together ($33.7 billion) [in 2002]. Over the past two decades, the pharmaceutical industry has moved very far from its original high purpose of discovering and producing useful new drugs. Now primarily a marketing machine to sell drugs of dubious benefit, this industry uses its wealth and power to co-opt every institution that might stand in its way, including the US Congress, the FDA, academic medical centers, and the medical profession itself.[116]

Dr Angell is not alone in this criticism; Dr Peter Gøtzsche, a specialist in internal medicine and co-founder of the Cochrane Collaboration, has also published a volume critical of the pharmaceutical industry called *Deadly Medicines and Organised Crime—How Big Pharma has Corrupted Healthcare*. In this volume, he compares many of the actions of the pharmaceutical industry to organized crime, and many would agree that the comparison is justified. He begins with some examples of the lies and deceit that is typical of the industry by simply Googling the pharmaceutical company's name with 'fraud' and after getting between 0.5 and 27 million hits taking one of the first examples for review.

He cites the example of how in 2012 Pfizer agreed to pay $60 million to settle a US federal investigation into bribery overseas. He points out that Pfizer wasn't only accused of bribing doctors, but also hospital administrators and drug regulators in several countries in Europe and Asia. The investigators found that Pfizer sought to hide the bribery by listing the payments as legitimate expenses, such as training, freight and entertainment. He mentions that Pfizer didn't admit or deny the allegations, which he points out is routine practice when drug companies settle allegations of fraud. He gives another example, that of Hoffman-La Roche, based in Switzerland, which he suggested was one of the largest corporate fraudsters worldwide in the 1990s. Apparently, high-level Roche executives led a cartel that, according to the US Justice Department's antitrust division, "was the most pervasive and harmful criminal antitrust conspiracy ever uncovered." Dr Gøtzsche elaborates on the investigators' findings:

> Top executives at some of the world's biggest drug companies, largely from Europe and Asia, met secretly in hotel suites and at conferences. Working together in a coalition they brazenly called 'Vitamins Inc.', they carved up world markets and carefully orchestrated price increases, in the process defrauding some of the world's biggest food companies.

Dr Gøtzsche points out that at the time this conspiracy was running Roche had revenues of $3.3 billion alone in the US and that during this time the conspirators 'gradually and artfully raised the prices of raw vitamins, so as not to attract notice; they also rigged the bidding process.'[117]

Gøtzsche also draws our attention to what he describes as the largest healthcare fraud settlement in US history, whereby GlaxoSmithKline (GSK) pleaded guilty to having marketed a number of drugs illegally for off-label use. The drugs included Wellbutrin (bupropion, an antidepressant), Paxil (paroxetine, an antidepressant), Advair (fluticasone + salmeterol, an asthma drug), Avandia (rosiglitazone, a diabetes drug), and Lamictal (lamotrigine, an epilepsy drug). Gøtzsche mentions that the Justice Department had charged a former vice president and top lawyer for Glaxo a year earlier with making false statements and obstructing a federal investigation into illegal marketing of

Wellbutrin for weight loss. The indictment accused the vice president of lying to the FDA, denying that doctors speaking at company events had promoted Wellbutrin for uses not approved by the agency, and of withholding incriminating documents. Gøtzsche further informs us:

> The company paid kickbacks to doctors, failed to include certain safety data about rosiglitazone in reports to the FDA, and its sponsored programmes suggested cardiovascular *benefits* from Avandia despite warnings on the FDA approved label regarding cardiovascular risks. Avandia was withdrawn in Europe in 2010 because it increases cardiovascular deaths.[118]

Dr Gøtzsche's book is an extensive critique of the pharmaceutical industry and its domination of both the regulatory process and the medical industry. Doctors rely on the information they are given by the industry to be accurate. He makes the point: 'The fact that drugs are dangerous and should be used with caution means that the ethical standards for those who do research on drugs and market them should be very high.'

There are a great many researchers and doctors who have been trying for a number of years to draw attention to the way the whole direction of medicine has been hijacked by the interests of large corporate interests. I hope to give you enough information to help you realize that it is not simply a matter of a few bad apples or a few over-critical medical researchers.

Dr John Abramson, in his book *OVERDO$ED AMERICA—The Broken Promise of American Medicine. How the Pharmaceutical Companies are Corrupting Science, Misleading Doctors, and Threatening Your Health*, felt compelled to write about what he saw as the failure of medicine because it really mattered to him:

Harvesting Sickness

The most important health care issue in the United States today is whether our current method of creating medical knowledge realizes the full potential of medical science to improve our health, and whether this knowledge is then best applied to clinical practice and communicated effectively to the public. By these standards, American medicine is clearly failing to fulfil its promise.

He also was concerned about the massive, increasing cost being imposed on society for little if any benefit:

I wasn't sure what I was going to find when I turned my full attention to these issues. But it was becoming clear that American medicine was like a runaway train, picking up speed, fuelled by the commercially generated belief that ever-increasing medical spending is necessary to achieve good health.

Dr Abramson's research led him to conclude that radical reform was needed to enable Americans to improve their health:

The bottom line is this: There has been a virtual takeover of medical knowledge in the United States, leaving doctors and patients little opportunity to know the truth about good medical care and no safe alternative but to pay up and go along. The ugliest truth of all is that these enormous costs do not come close to producing commensurate improvements in our health—the health of Americans is actually losing ground to that of the citizens in other industrialized countries, which are spending far less and at the same time providing health care to all of their citizens. [119]

Ray Strand, M.D. believes that following Congress's passing of the Prescription Drug User Fee Act (PDUFA) in 1992, it created a 'deadly partnership', between the FDA and the pharmaceutical companies that it was supposed to regulate:

Since Congress passed the PDUFA legislation in 1992, the FDA no longer plays an adversarial role against the pharmaceutical companies. Instead, the legislation made them partners. "User fees" make up approximately 50 percent of the FDA's budget and have allowed pharmaceutical companies to place certain demands on the FDA. Congress has placed the FDA under tough production guidelines, so that it must work together with the pharmaceutical industry to approve as many drugs as possible.[120]

The problem created by this 'deadly partnership' is that it has created the position where the FDA has 1400 employees for approving new drugs and only 65 full-time employees for monitoring more than 8,000 drugs, with fewer than ten of them with a PhD or M.D. degree.[121] If you add the situation whereby all drugs that the FDA approves are now based on trials lasting, at most, a few weeks and the data is being supplied by the industry itself—this leaves us open to a whole host of problems. The data that is used for this application is not available to independent scrutiny, and any unwanted side effects are easily hidden from superficial analysis even by the FDA. It has generally, only been through litigation that the extent of the deceit and falsification of data by the industry comes to light. Even when found out, however, the fines doled out to pharmaceutical companies that may be making billions per year off a drug are so pathetically small they could be considered an actual inducement to be unscrupulous—which according to available records—all the pharmaceutical companies are.

Falsehoods, Lies and Missing Data

One of the major complaints against the pharmaceutical industry is the complete lack of transparency in the trials and the data that they provide. Dr Ben Goldacre, writing in his book *Bad Pharma—How Medicine is Broken, and How We Can Fix*

It, cites numerous examples of how the pharmaceutical industry hides data that does not show its drugs in a positive light. He gives the example of a group of researchers who decided to review trials on antidepressants that came to the market between 1987 and 2004 that were reported to the FDA—no mean task. The researchers eventually assembled seventy-four studies in total, representing 12,500 patients. Thirty-eight of these trials had positive results, and found that the new drug worked; thirty-six were negative. All but one of the positive trials were published with great accompanying fanfare, but only three of the negative trials were published. Twenty-two were simply lost to history, buried in the archives of the FDA.[122]

Dr Goldacre cites another example (he devotes an entire chapter to missing data), that of the company GlaxoSmithKline who were applying for a marketing authorisation for their drug paroxetine for the use on children, in which he says 'an extraordinary situation came to light, triggering the longest investigation in the history of UK drugs regulation.' The investigation, which was published in 2008, had found that the company had withheld important data about the safety and effectiveness of this drug—effectively preventing doctors and patients from understanding the nature of the risk of taking it. He comments:

> It turned out that what the company had done—withholding important data about safety and effectiveness that doctors and patients clearly needed to see—was plainly unethical, and put children around the world at risk; but our laws are so weak that GSK could not be charged with any crime.

He cites how between 1994 and 2002 GSK conducted nine trials of paroxetine in children.[123] The first two apparently failed to show any benefit, and he mentions that the company made no attempt to inform anyone of this due—

according to a secret internal memo—to not wishing to 'undermine the profile of paroxetine'. Apparently, in the year after this secret memo, 32,000 prescriptions were issued to children for paroxetine in the UK alone. He further explains: 'More trials were conducted over the coming years—nine in total—and none showed that the drug was effective at treating depression in children.' He complains about the complete lack of care or accountability expressed by GSK's actions:

> It gets much worse than that. These children weren't simply receiving a drug the company knew to be ineffective for them: they were also being exposed to side effects…nobody knew how bad the side effects were because the company didn't tell doctors, or patients, or even the regulator about the worrying safety data from its trials. This was because of a loophole…you only had to tell the regulator about side effects reported in studies looking at *the specific uses for which the drug has a marketing authorisation*. Because the use of paroxetine was 'off-label', GSK had no legal obligation at the time to tell anyone about what it had found.[124]

What about moral obligation? Are we to accept that these companies can make massive profits at our children's expense, and also at our expense, with no moral obligation of any sort? Dr Peter C Gøtzsche, already mentioned, has campaigned for transparency, full disclosure, and accessibility to all trial data for independent analysis. One example he cites to show how deceit and complete indifference to harm dominate the pharmaceutical industry concerns Eli Lilly. This company, he explains 'continued its aggressive marketing of its NSAID, benoxaprofen (Opren or Oraflex), undisturbed by the terrible harms they knew their drug caused.' He explains:

The company touted that, based on laboratory experiments, the drug was different from other NSAIDS in having an effect on the disease process, but this wasn't true. Lilly presented a series of 39 patients that experienced a worsening of their joint damage, but the company concluded exactly the opposite.

Lilly ignored or trivialised the harms and failed to inform the authorities of liver failure and deaths, which a subsequent court case described as 'standard practice in the industry'. Lilly published a paper in the BMJ that claimed that no cases of jaundice or deaths had been reported, but this wasn't true. Furthermore, benoxaprofen causes other horrible harms, e.g. photosensitivity in 10% of patients and loosening of the nails from the nailbed in 10%...When independent researchers found that benoxaprofen accumulated in the elderly, Lilly tried to prevent the study from being published and, as always, the UK drug regulator's action was grossly inadequate and allowed Lilly to trivialise the problem. These omissions proved fatal for some elderly patients and the drug was withdrawn after only 2 years on the market.[125]

Dr Gøtzsche also cites the example of Cisapride (Propulsid from Johnson & Johnson) which was supposed to promote gastric emptying but was found to cause cardiac arrhythmias that led to numerous deaths. In 1998, the FDA warned about the contraindications for the drug through additions to the black box label, and practitioners were further warned through a dear doctor letter sent by the manufacturer. The warnings barely had any effect. Johnson & Johnson sold the drug for more than a billion dollars each year according to Gøtzsche the drug should never have been approved. When the FDA called for a public meeting in 2000, a company executive admitted that they had not even been able to show that the drug worked. [126] Dr Strand informs us that many children died using the drug Propulsid. Whilst more than three-quarters of all drugs on the market are not labelled for use in children, many are prescribed for children. He informs us that only five of the eighty most frequently used drugs in newborns and infants have pediatric use instructions—meaning only 5% have been tested in pediatric trials. He cites the case of Sarah, a young mother who gave birth to a daughter that was born four weeks earlier than planned. She mentioned to her paediatrician at her two-month well-baby checkup that the baby had a slight problem with the tendency to spit up some of her feeds, but was otherwise perfectly healthy. A month later she mentioned that the tendency persisted. The pediatrician suggested giving the baby a new drug, Propulsid, that was supposed to be effective in controlling acid reflux in young children. As the FDA had not approved Propulsid for use in children, this was considered off-label use. One survey revealed that of fifty-eight thousand premature babies, 20 percent received Propulsid. Dr Andre Dubois, an FDA medical officer who had reviewed a premarket clinical trial involving nearly 2,000 patients, discovered that 48 of the patients experienced heart problems as a direct result of Propulsid prolonging the QT interval [this in the heartbeat interval; this would be a cause for concern]. The FDA received reports of patients experiencing heart irregularities and even deaths due to cardiac arrest. The pharmaceutical company strongly denied that any of the deaths were due to the medication. Sarah's baby died, however, and, as the coroner had no idea that Propulsid played any role in the baby's death classified the death as SIDS (Sudden Infant Death Syndrome). Hundreds of deaths were reported to the FDA over the seven years and five label changes were made as the drug was on the market. Finally, Propulsid was removed from the market in July 2000.[127]

The story does not end with Propulsid, however, as other manufacturers have come up with their own version of what are commonly referred to as proton pump inhibitors. This class of drugs, however, can cause numerous side effects that range from minor to serious, ranging from problems like constipation, stomach pain, headache, diarrhea and vomiting to kidney disease, heart attacks, cancers, and bone fractures. Long-term use is not recommended. A 2016 study in the Journal of American Nephrology found long-term users were 28 percent more likely to suffer from chronic kidney disease They were also 95% more likely to experience kidney failure, also called end-stage renal disease. Several studies are also linked to bone fractures, and the FDA has required all proton pump inhibitors (PPIs) to carry a warning about the risk of bone fractures of the spine, wrist, and hip. The FDA found that the risk was greatest for people taking high doses for long periods of time. A 2017 study published in the journal *Gut* found that taking PPIs could double the risk of getting gastric cancer. The risk went up five-fold for people taking the medicines for a year. The risk went up more than eight times after taking the drugs for three years. This provoked the FDA to require gastric malignancy warnings for these drug labels in 2017. The researcher Terry Turner, writing in *Drugwatch* reviews many more problems associated with this class of drugs; he mentions, for example, a 2017 study in the journal *Pediatrics* that looked at children whose mothers took PPIs during pregnancy. It found their children faced a 30% higher risk for asthma.[128]

Thousands of people have sued the companies that make Nexium, Prilosec and other PPIs in one of the largest mass litigations in the United States. Proton pump inhibitor lawsuits claim that the drugs used to treat heartburn and acid reflux caused serious kidney problems in people who took them.

The lawsuits argue that manufacturers failed to warn people of the drugs' dangers. Lawsuits involving Prilosec, for example, claim AstraZeneca knew of kidney risks as early as 2004, but the company did not warn patients about them for another 10 years. By August 2019, there were over 13,000 PPI lawsuits pending in federal court. The claimants alleged that AstraZeneca, Takeda, and Pfizer, along with others involved in the manufacturing of the drugs, failed to adequately warn about the risk of kidney injuries related to the use of Prilosec, Nexium, Prevacid, and other PPIs. Hundreds of consumers also filed lawsuits against AstraZeneca, alleging Nexium caused bone deterioration, leading to loss of bone density and bone fractures. AstraZeneca, in 2015, had previously agreed to pay the US government $7.9 million to resolve kickback allegations involving Nexium. The government claimed AstraZeneca worked with another company to boost sales. Also in the same year (2015), AstraZeneca agreed to pay the US government and several states $26.7 million, plus interest, to settle claims that the pharmaceutical company underpaid rebates owed under the Medicaid Drug Rebate Program, according to the U.S. Justice Department.[129]

The only thing that you can predict about the outcome of the lawsuits for certain is that the fines will be paltry, and the pharmaceutical companies involved will try to hide information as best they can. Sales of Nexium in 2007 were in excess of $5.2 billion; whilst sales are lower now ($1.7 billion in 2018),[130] a few million to settle lawsuits will not affect the share price of AstraZeneca or the incentive to keep bringing new patents to market for them or any of the large pharmaceutical companies. All they have to do is play down and ignore any drug side effects, hope that they will not be too severe, or if they are, suggest the cause is not the drug. With the current regulatory practice, it will most likely take a number of years before the adverse effects come to light: as most drugs are only tested for a few weeks, the people that take the newly available drugs, in effect, become the guinea pigs in longer-term human trials.

When Merck was forced to recall its drug Vioxx, its nonsteroidal anti-inflammatory (NSAID) used for the treatment of arthritis, in September 2004, FDA official Dr David Graham estimated that Vioxx has probably caused 60,000 deaths. A vigilant researcher, Ron Unz, was drawn to the report of a huge drop in the death rate, which was reported in the media in April 2005. He noticed that it followed a large spike in the death rate that had occurred in 1999 the year Vioxx was introduced. He poses the question as to how many people really died due to Vioxx. The spike and eventual drop when Vioxx was recalled reflected 100,000 deaths a year. He conjectured that as many as 500,000 deaths could be attributed to the drug but admitted we may never know the true figure. What we do know for sure was that Merck knew the drug was dangerous and covered up the health risks and deaths. Twenty million Americans are understood to have taken Vioxx which was a big money-maker for Merck, generating about $2.5 billion in yearly sales.[131]

Disturbing Epidemic

Of all the areas of medicine the one with the most controversy, and, some argue, the greatest danger lies with the psychiatric drugs, in particular with their use in children and young people. It is also argued that this is an excessive over-medicalization, with profound and disturbing implications.

David Brodwin believes that absurdly high health care costs are undermining America:

> One of the greatest threats to the U.S. economy in the long term is the absurdly high cost of U.S. health care. We spend nearly 18 percent of GDP on it, whereas the rest of the developed world spends around 11 percent and gets about the same results.
>
> One of the major drivers of health care cost is mental illness. Spending on mental health care rarely makes headlines because it isn't dramatic. It doesn't grab attention like cancer and hepatitis drugs that cost over $100,000 per round of treatment. But the numbers add up because so many people are affected: In any given year about 20 percent of Americans are diagnosed with a mental health problem severe enough to

interfere with daily functioning. About 270 million prescriptions are filled each year for anti-depressants alone. And because mental illness affects people in their prime earning years (whereas most diseases primarily affect older people) mental illness has a catastrophic effect on people's earning power. The total earnings lost by Americans with mental illness – nearly $200 billion -- is nearly twice as high as the costs of drugs and psychotherapy used to treat them.[132]

According to the American Psychological Association, the larger proportion of this population is in the white non-Hispanic population, and they suggest that women are twice as likely to take antidepressant medication as men. This represents 16.5% of white Americans.[133] Alan Schwarz, writing in the *New York Times,* informs us more than 10,000 American toddlers 2 or 3 years old are being medicated for attention deficit hyperactivity disorder outside established pediatric guidelines, according to the Centers for Disease Control and Prevention. He further suggests this report "was the latest to raise concerns about A.D.H.D. diagnoses and medications for American children beyond what many experts consider medically justified. Last year, a nationwide C.D.C. survey found that 11% of children aged 4 to 17 have received a diagnosis of the disorder, and that about one in five boys will get one during childhood." [134]

What does this indicate to us all: is the USA afflicted with such a severely mentally disturbed population that it begins at such an early age as two years old and then necessitates continuing medication throughout life? Dr Peter Gøtzsche in, *Deadly Psychiatry and Organised Denial,* suggests that we might not all be so nuts after all: 'It is psychiatry that has become insane, not our children. Some child psychiatrists brag that they can make an initial assessment of a child and write a prescription in less than 20 minutes, and for some pediatricians, it takes only five minutes.'

Harvesting Sickness

Is that the true value of a child's life—that they are only worth five minutes of a doctor's time before what many consider to be mind-altering chemicals—are thrown at them? Gøtzsche brings up the name of a prominent child psychiatrist, Joseph Biederman, who he suggests has done more than anybody else to overdose our children with antipsychotics through the invention of juvenile bipolar disorder. Gøtzche accuses him of behaving in a 'God-like manner.' Biedermann was allegedly asked in court by an attorney about his rank at Harvard Medical School, to which he replied "full professor." The attorney asked, "What's above that?" To which Biedermann replied, "God."[135]

According to the *New York Times,* this was the same psychiatrist who was paid more than $1.6 million in consulting fees from drug makers which he failed to report to his university, violating federal research rules, according to documents provided to Congressional investigators. Fellow psychiatrists at the Harvard Medical School's psychiatry department Dr Timothy Wilens reportedly earned $1.6million and Dr Thomas Spencer reportedly earned at least $1million. None of them declared their incomes, as they were supposed to. According to the report, the Harvard group's consulting arrangements with drug makers were already controversial because of the researchers' advocacy of unapproved uses of psychiatric medicines in children. This is all the more troubling as Dr Biederman is considered one of the most influential researchers in child psychiatry and is widely known for focusing the field's attention on its most troubled young patients. Although many of his studies are small and often financed by drug makers, his work helped to fuel a controversial 40-fold increase from 1994 to 2003 in the diagnosis of pediatric bipolar disorder, which is characterized by severe mood swings, and led to a rapid rise in the use of antipsychotic medicines in children. [136]

As regards to the huge medication of children, Gøtzsche expresses concern that 'children of up to only four years of age are on psychotropic drugs, although the first three years of life are a period of rapid neural development, and about a quarter of the children in American summer camps are medicated for ADHD, mood disorder or other mental health problems.'[137]

So what is going on here? Either these children are clinically damaged and in need of powerful antipsychotic medication or not: surely it's a purely scientific question? Sadly, the evidence suggests this is not the case and that avarice, not science, once again plays a leading role. Let's turn to another source, this time to an executive from inside the pharmaceutical industry no-less: John Virapen, who worked for Eli Lilly in Sweden and was instrumental in obtaining approval for fluoxetine, marketed as Prozac in the USA. He discusses the *Diagnostic and Statistical Manual of Mental Disorders* (DSM) that many refer to as the bible of psychiatrists, he explains that all the members on the committee for mood disorders and schizophrenia and other psychotic disorders had contact with pharmaceutical companies, the leading categories of 'contact' being via research grants (42%), consultation (22%) and the spokesman's office. What he feels is interesting is how, for example, there were a hundred different manifestations of depression in the 1950s, which has increased three-fold since then, on which he comments: 'And that is the actual trick. You increase the profile, making it less clear, smooth out the boundaries between what is classed as healthy and what is classed as ill. You just make the whole catalog thicker. Add all possible states to the phenomenon of depression and you get an ever increasing number of people who fit into this category.' He discusses how marketing to children was extended: 'As of this year, Prozac can also be prescribed for children in Germany, where I live (the trade name for Prozac in Germany is Fluctin). It's what is called a *line extension* in marketing jargon: If a market segment has reached its upper limit, you start looking for a new market segment. Children are a new market segment. Now, it's their turn to swallow Prozac—a medicine that can make you aggressive and even tired of living.' It is obvious that he lost faith in the pharmaceutical industry, as his next comment demonstrates:

> Don't get me wrong: There's nothing wrong with maximization of turnover…but here we are dealing with the physical and mental well-being of people, whose destruction is deliberately accepted by the pharmaceutical industry, in order to make money and even more money. Hidden and unnoticed death. [138]

Dr Peter Breggin, a senior Harvard School of Medicine graduate and psychiatrist, and author of numerous books and scientific papers quotes physician Larry Brown: 'The practice of drugging children has no sound basis in law, medicine, or social policy. As such, it represents an ominous step along the Orwellian continuum of social control through psychotechnology'.

The practice of drugging children has no sound basis in law, medicine, or social policy. As such, it represents an ominous step along the Orwellian continuum of social control through psychotechnology.

He further writes [in 1993]:

> An estimated 180,000 to 300,000 young people a year are locked up in private psychiatric hospitals, and the numbers are increasing rapidly. Over one million more children are being prescribed drugs to control their behaviour in school and at home. Carving out this largely

involuntary consumer group has vastly increased the income, power, and influence of modern psychiatry. It has also greatly increased the psychiatric menace to children.

He makes an interesting comment about the background to this situation:

> Health insurers play a largely unexplored role in reinforcing the psychopharmaceutical complex. They tend to reimburse well for drugs, electroshock, and psychiatric hospitalization. On the other hand, they pay relatively little or nothing for psychotherapy and other forms of social rehabilitation, such a halfway houses, crisis centers, and residential homes, which ultimately can be more effective and less costly.

He makes a further point about the pharmaceutical complex; 'much of it also remains largely hidden from scrutiny, including the amounts of money paid by drug companies to the APA [American Psychiatric Association] and to leading psychiatrists.' He adds another dimension to the way the industry influences its market: 'One way to increase the overall size of the market is to convince the government, society, and individual citizens that its services are needed. From this motivation grows "official estimates" of the "prevalence of mental illness" that the media latch onto in their stories about the need for psychiatric treatment.[139]

Doctor Breggin mentions that decades ago when he was an intern and resident in psychiatry (1962-1966) they rarely saw or diagnosed manic depressive (bipolar) disorder. Currently, he suggests:

> Today, bipolar is so commonplace that most psychiatrists are treating many patients with that diagnosis in their practice at any one time. What has changed?... I am seeing children diagnosed with bipolar disorder because they have temper tantrums or seem excessively irritable,

when in reality their parents have not learned how to discipline them properly. Especially in regard to children, drug advocates have openly campaigned to increase the rate of diagnosing bipolar disorder in order to unleash powerful, adult medications on children.

This deluge of children diagnosed with bipolar disorder is quite extraordinary. I never saw a single case of childhood bipolar disorder during my psychiatric training and none that I can recall from the early years of my practice through the late 1980s, but nowadays I see many cases each year.

He mentions a 2007 study in the *Archives of General Psychiatry*, where the researchers found a fortyfold increase in children being diagnosed and treated for bipolar disorder:

Ninety percent of these children were being treated with medication. More than 47 percent were being treated with antipsychotic drugs, none of which were approved for children. Thirty-four percent were being treated with antidepressants, which can cause or exacerbate maniclike episodes, and 36 percent were being treated with stimulants, which also increase the risk of mania.

Well, does this mean that we are driving our children nuts or perhaps that, with the fantastical level of knowledge and expertise we now have, are better able to diagnose what must be a seriously screwed up society? Dr Breggin asks the obvious question:

What's the cause of the increased rates of severe cases of mania? Antidepressant medications, and to a lesser extent stimulants and tranquilizers, especially Xanax, are causing the upsurge of manic episodes. In almost all the adult cases that I have evaluated in the last decade, and in *every* child and teenage case I have seen in my office, the manic symptoms had begun after starting antidepressants and, more occasionally, stimulants or Xanax.

In his book *Medicating Madness—The Role of Psychiatric Drugs in Cases of Violence, Suicide, and Crime,* he suggests that none of the cases of children and their parents, and none of the adults who were driven into mania by prescription drugs, were told by the treating doctors that they had a medication-induced disorder. He further reveals: When occasionally the drug was implicated in any way, it was portrayed as a benign agent that happened to "unmask" a preexisting, underlying bipolar disorder—a theory based not on science but on the physician's impulse to avoid blame for the disaster.

When occasionally the drug was implicated in any way, it was portrayed as a benign agent that happened to "unmask" a preexisting, underlying bipolar disorder—a theory based not on science but on the physician's impulse to avoid blame for the disaster. [140]

Dr Peter Gøtzsche quotes Marcia Angell, former editor of the *New England Journal of Medicine,* giving some further credence to our concerns about the dangers and the overuse of psychiatric drugs:

> I have spent most of my professional life evaluating the quality of clinical research, and I believe it is especially poor in psychiatry. The industry-sponsored studies … are selectively published, tend to be short-term, designed to favor the drug, and show benefits so small that they are unlikely to outweigh the long-term harms.

Dr Gøtzsche expresses his own concerns about the industry:

Harvesting Sickness

Psychiatry is the drug industry's paradise as definitions of psychiatric disorders are vague and easy to manipulate. Leading psychiatrists are therefore at high risk of corruption and, indeed, psychiatrists collect more money from drug makers than doctors in any other speciality. *Those who take the most money tend to prescribe antipsychotics to children most often* [my emphasis]. Psychiatrists are also 'educated' with industry's hospitality more often than any other speciality.

This has dire consequences for the patients. The *Diagnostic and Statistical Manual of Mental Disorders* (DSM) from the American Psychiatric Association (APA) has become infamous. It is now so bad that Allen Frances, who chaired the task force for DSM-IV (which lists 374 different ways to be mentally ill; up from 297 in DSM-III) believes the responsibility for defining psychiatric conditions need to be taken away from the APA.

Gøtzsche notes that the DSM-IV has already created three false epidemics because the diagnostic criteria were too wide: attention deficit hyperactivity disorder (ADHD), autism and childhood bipolar disorder. [141] His concerns are shared by other researchers. Ray Moynihan and fellow researchers in their *BMJ* paper titled "Medicalisation—Preventing overdiagnosis: how to stop harming the healthy", wrote:

Medicine's much hailed ability to help the sick is fast being challenged by its propensity to harm the healthy. A burgeoning scientific literature is fuelling public concerns that too many people are being overdosed, overtreated, and overdiagnosed. Screening programmes are detecting early cancers that will never cause symptoms or death, sensitive diagnostic technologies identify "abnormalities" so tiny they will remain benign, while widening disease definitions mean people at ever lower risks receive permanent medical labels and lifelong treatments that will fail to benefit many of them. With estimates that more than $200bn (£128bn;

€160bn) may be wasted on unnecessary treatment every year in the United States, the cumulative burden from overdiagnosis poses a significant threat to human health.

They also shared the particular worry regarding the overdiagnosis in children, and give a salient example of how significant the problem is:

> One focus of concern is the possible overdiagnosis of children, who have no say in the appropriateness of a label that can permanently change their lives. This is particularly salient with attention deficit hyperactivity disorder. A recent study of almost a million Canadian children found boys born in December (typically the youngest in their year) had a 30% higher chance of diagnosis and 40% higher chance of receiving medication than those born in January, with the authors concluding their findings "raise concerns about the potential harms of overdiagnosis and overprescribing." [142]

You may be forgiven for thinking that this is some small problem, some overlooked and easily rectifiable issue. The more you look into the issue, however, the more concerns are raised. The pharmaceutical insider John Virapen, whom we have previously referred to, introduces his book with a few points that suggest again that avarice plays an essential role:

- Did you know that more than 75% of the leading scientists in medicine are paid by the pharmaceutical industry?
- Did you know that there are drugs on the market where bribery played a role in the approval process?
- Did you know that the pharmaceutical industry invents illnesses and promotes them with targeted marketing campaigns to increase the market for their products?
- Did you know that the pharmaceutical industry increasingly has its sights on children?

Virapen makes the following observations regarding the introduction of fluoxetine (Prozac), a drug that he was intimately connected with, and how it was marketed to become a blockbuster. It was essential to broaden the scope of the drug market beyond 'sick people': 'sick people represent a relatively small market. Imagine if you could talk those who aren't ill into taking pills. Then you would reach a new dimension of marketing. That is the new quality of a blockbuster. And that was exactly the role fluoxetine was supposed to play.'

In his book, *Side Effects: Death—Confessions of a Pharma-Insider,* Virapen reveals how he bribed the psychiatrist that would evaluate fluoxetine as an independent expert for the regulatory authority. He believed that it would be the only way to get approval due to the appalling side effects of the drug. His director, after discussions with his Eli Lilly superiors in Geneva, called Virapen regarding using bribery and said: "John, do whatever you think is necessary. We won't put any obstacles in your way." Apparently, after accepting the offer of the bribe, the investigating psychiatrist additionally demanded that he and his colleagues receive a research assignment from Lilly for fluoxetine. Virapen commented that it 'would earn him and his colleagues a lot of money, for years to come. A whole department could live off this one contract alone.'

The result was he had to send him one of his colleagues to prepare the existing data in such a way that the regulatory authority wouldn't need to ask any awkward questions. Files were 'newly arranged and shuffled like the cards in a game of poker. Statistics—playing with figures. Deaths disappeared in footnotes … And already, that awful word suicide is no longer to be found.' On top of it, the investigating psychiatrist placed his own personal letter of recommendation. How sweet is that? Virapen had also to get the right price, which he was able to successfully negotiate. But his comments add a sour note, writing at this time: 'The price I negotiated for an incompletely tested, faulty product, which drove and still drives a lot of people crazy or to their death, was the basis for gaining approval, throughout the world.'

Virapen mentions that the director of the review board, who was a recognized expert, had reported from her own clinical studies that, with as little as a quarter of the dose, i.e. 5mg, there had been difficulties and patients had tried to commit suicide. The drug was marketed as a 'mood lifter' and advanced as a 'lifestyle drug', and supposedly 'conveyed a positive attitude to life.'[143]

The Eli Lilly marketing machine went into overdrive: in less than two years Prozac was outselling all other antidepressants. In March 1990, the green-and-white Prozac capsule appeared on the cover of *Newsweek* under the banner "The Promise of Prozac," where it was described as a medical 'breakthrough' it said, "even healthy people have started asking for it." *New York* magazine called it a "wonder drug." Peter Kramer's influential book, *Listening to Prozac,* gave glowing reports of the drug and said that the drug made people feel "better than well". Prozac became the number two best-selling drug, with more than 60 million prescriptions written for it in 1998. Half a million children were prescribed it, which became one of the fastest-growing markets, even though repeated studies have shown antidepressant drugs are no more effective in children than placebos.[144]

Prozac became the most successful antidepressant: according to Dr Ann Tracy, it was handed out like candy for depression, yeast infections, post-surgical pain, PMS, chronic fatigue syndrome, flu, acne, hormonal imbalances, hypoglycemia, etc. However, the adverse side effects by October 1993 had amounted to more than 28,000 reports to the FDA. This included 1,885 suicide attempts and 1,349 deaths. According to the FDA, this generally represents anywhere from 1% to 10% of actual figures. Nevertheless, this represented more adverse reactions than any other drug in its history. Not to be put off by a few adverse reports, in April 1998, the American Psychiatric Association and the American Academy of Pediatric Psychiatrists asked the FDA to consider serotonergic antidepressants for use in children *as young as two years old,* and drugs for anxiety, aggression, and manic depression in *one-month-old babies*! Talk about insanity! Am I missing something here? Why don't they put it in the water supply and have done with it? In case you think I am just having a go at Prozac, Dr Tracy informs us the use of Ritalin (a stimulant) increased in children age six and *under* by 23% between 1995 and 1999, although the use of the Prozac family of drugs increased in the same age group by a staggering 580%—even though the drugs are not approved for children under 18. Dr Tracy expresses her concern about this use: 'Even more alarming to learn that Ritalin and Prozac are being prescribed *together* [my emphasis] for at least 30% of those given an SSRI antidepressant. Considering both are serotonergic agents, that combination is very dangerous and can easily lead to serotonin syndrome.'

Tracy gives some examples of the effects of serotonin syndrome:

> Three cases come to mind where an adolescent was given Prozac and Ritalin together or back to back and suffered violent reactions from the combination. One is that of Kip Kinkle in Springfield, OR who killed his parents and then went to school where he killed two classmates. The other case was in Huntsville, AL where Jeff Franklin used a sledgehammer, hatchet, butcher knife and pointed mechanic's file to kill his parents as they returned home from work and then attacked his younger brother and sister. The other in Amarillo, TX was a young man who burned down a church and the pastor's home after his medication was changed to a prescription of Prozac and Ritalin combined with yet another antidepressant on top of that! How can children be expected to

handle such powerful drugs and then the combinations of such drugs besides?!¹⁴⁵

Dr Tracy in her book, *Prozac—Panacea or Pandora,* documents many, many cases of violent suicides and homicides that were attributed to antidepressant use, especially SSRIs. I discuss a few more in the next section.

Robert Whitaker, in his book, *Anatomy of an Epidemic,* reports on some chilling facts regarding the creation of the psychiatric epidemic we have fabricated and the untold damage done to people's lives due to this misuse. He reports that in 1995 a Harvard psychiatrist determined that 25% of children and adolescents diagnosed with depression convert to bipolar within 2-4 years. Another researcher, Washington University's Barbara Geller, extended the follow-up period to ten years, and in her study, nearly half of prepubertal children treated for depression ended up bipolar. Whitaker suggests that we can make a reasonable guess as to the number of people who will be more than likely permanently damaged by antidepressants: 'These findings give us our second mathematical equation for solving the bipolar epidemic. If 2 million children and adolescents are treated with SSRIs for depression, this practice will create 500,000 to 1 million bipolar youth.' He further adds that children in the USA consume 3 times the quantity of stimulants consumed by the rest of the world, which can only add to the disaster befalling America's children. He mentions that the US Government Accountability Office reported in 2008 that 1 in every 15 young adults (18-26 years old) is now found to be seriously mentally ill, 680,000 with bipolar and another 800,000 ill with major depression. Whitaker comments:

> Twenty years ago, our society began regularly prescribing psychiatric drugs to children and adolescents, and now one out of every fifteen Americans enters adulthood with a "serious mental illness." That

is proof of the most tragic sort that our drug-based paradigm of care is doing a great deal more harm than good. The medicating of children and youth became commonplace only a short time ago, and already it has put millions onto a path of lifelong illness.[146]

Peter Breggin expresses the problem facing us with the over-prescribing of drugs: 'A huge proportion of the general population accepts that psychiatric drugs are the answer to everyday problems from fatigue and a broken heart to conflicts in the family between parents and their children. The drugging of children has become an epidemic of medical child abuse leading me to call for a halt to giving psychoactive substances to children for the control of their minds and behaviour.' Breggin, in my view, is one of the more clued-up psychiatrists, who actually engages people in conversation and therapy that does not automatically involve taking medication. He does not mince his words when he discusses the nature of mind-altering drugs: 'All drugs that impact on the brain and mind "work" by partially disabling the brain and mind. No psychoactive substance corrects biochemical imbalances or any other real and presumed defects, deficits or disorders of the brain and mind, and none improve the function of the brain and mind. The so-called therapeutic effect is always a disability'.

All drugs that impact on the brain and mind "work" by partially disabling the brain and mind. No psychoactive substance corrects biochemical imbalances or any other real and presumed defects, deficits or disorders of the brain and mind, and none improve the function of the brain and mind. The so-called therapeutic effect is always a disability.

If these drugs disable the brain why you may ask, are they prescribed so much? Breggin again gives his understanding, based on his many years of observation and experience:

> The shared or common capacity of all psychiatric drugs to compromise brain and mind function helps to account for the current practice of using psychiatric drugs off label and combining multiple drugs into "cocktails." It is a matter of increasing the disability of the brain and mind until the required effect is achieved, such as docility and passivity, indifference to self and others, emotional numbness or anesthesia, robotic behavior, or reticence about emotional distress.

Aside from the mind-numbing and disabling effects that are deemed useful and worth the risk in some circumstances with a severely disturbed individual, Breggin informs us of some of the less-discussed side effects: 'These drugs suppress both sexuality and love, often without full recovery when the drugs are stopped.'[147]

Not-So-Hidden Violent Reactions with Antidepressants

One of the favoured myths created by the pharmaceutical industry is that the drug you are taking is correcting an imbalance in the brain, as with the Serotonin Reuptake Inhibitors—their very name implies that their action on serotonin is addressing a serotonin imbalance. Their effects on people, however, do not create favourable outcomes after what may be perceived as an initial positive response. Sarah Bosely, writing on Prozac in the *Guardian* in 1999, says: 'Disturbing evidence has now emerged, showing that, after the initial relief and euphoria of the first dose, Prozac can push some patients into so agitated a state of mind that they are a danger not only to themselves, but to others, too.' She reports on the spate of 'disturbing accounts of violence and suicide committed by people prescribed the drug by their doctors.' At the time of her report, a number of victims filed claims against Eli Lilly:

> Some 200 cases have come to court in the US. Victims and families of killers have sued the multi-national Eli Lilly, manufacturers of the world's most commercially successful drug. Until recently, not one case reached a verdict. Either it was dropped, or Lilly settled out of court, sometimes for millions of dollars - Lilly's defence has always been the same: blame the disease, not the drug. Depressed people get put on Prozac. Depressed people are often suicidal. Keep on taking the tablets.

She also reports on Dr David Healy, a leading UK psychiatrist and author of numerous books, who became involved in litigation against some of the drug companies who came to the conclusion that Lilly was guilty of failing to warn doctors and the public of some of the terrible consequences for some people taking Prozac that they knew about. She reports Healy's discoveries: "Based on published data and on Lilly's internal documents, the only reasonable estimate for the number of people who have worldwide, because of Prozac, tried to kill themselves since it was introduced would be a quarter of a million - around 25,000 will have actually succeeded," says Healy.

> Terrifying things happen to a number of people within the first few weeks of taking the drug, says Healy. They become agitated, restless and anxious. Out of the blue, and completely out of character, they may try to kill themselves in extremely violent ways, and they may try to take others with them.

Bosely also informs us how Lilly's own internal documents as early as 1978 identified a fairly large number of reports of adverse reactions that included patients developing psychosis, restlessness and akathisia. Some patients converted from severe depression to agitation within a few days, and in one case the agitation was so marked that they were taken off the drug. She also informs us that the documents further state that: "in future studies the use of benzodiazepines to control the agitation will be permitted". She points out that from that point on, 'Lilly's trial subjects would be put on tranquillizers to get them over the akathisia experienced by some in the early days on the drug. Yet once Prozac was on the market, there was no warning to doctors that such action might be necessary.' [148]

One trial case, that was made public, is worth bringing to your attention, because of the revelations of the underhand and despicable actions of, in this case, Eli Lilly, as reported by Doctor David Healy, in his book, *Let Them Eat Prozac.* This was the case involving Joseph Wesbecker, who one day walked into the Louisville printing plant where he worked, armed with an AK-47 and some handguns and went on the rampage shooting twenty fellow workers, killing eight of them, before turning his weapons on and killing himself. One month prior to the shooting Wesbeker had been put on Prozac after being diagnosed with depression by his physician. Apparently, Wesbeker stopped the medication after two days, claiming it didn't suit him. He went on disability in the spring of 1989, and when his disability payments were cut he was faced with returning to work which he was not keen to do. On August 10, his doctor suggested that he try Prozac again. When his doctor saw him a month later he found him much more agitated and more volatile. He suggested that Wesbeker discontinue the Prozac, but Wesbeker refused. On September 14 he went on his rampage. The case eventually came to trial in September 1994, and one of the expert witnesses, Nancy Lord, who had previously worked in the pharmaceutical industry was able to make a number of important points in court on record that were highly revealing:

When I looked at the Lilly data, I didn't find it was adequate to study this drug. The data was flawed for a number of reasons. First of all the protocols were not well designed...Not only did they permit the use of concomitant medications, but they permitted the use of psychotropic concomitant medicines.

It looked like they did everything possible to kind of tone down the problems with the drug rather than give them a rigorous, systematic and comprehensive evaluation to define what the problems were and then put it in the package insert so the doctors could be warned not to use the drug in certain types of patients, or to use it more carefully.

In my opinion, this drug has not been approved. It's been approved with sedatives, but taking fluoxetine all by itself has never been studied.

When the case came to trial, Judge John Potter had ruled that evidence on another Lilly trial was inadmissible. This was the trial regarding Oraflex, the brand name for benoxaprofen (Opren in Britain), a new pain killer which had been released in mid-1982 in the US. It was considered an expensive aspirin that was found to produce some serious side effects such as liver and kidney problems, rashes, peeling fingernails, and a number of deaths. Lilly denied that the drug was causing these side effects. An independent laboratory, however, was able to show there was a dangerous accumulation of the drug in older people. Oraflex was withdrawn and Lilly was prosecuted for failing to report to the FDA the full details of its clinical trials program and the reports of toxicity. Healey reports that over one hundred deaths were attributed to Oraflex in Britain, and over four thousand people suffered serious side effects. In the USA forty-nine deaths were attributed to it, and in one case the jury awarded $6 million to one of the claimants. During the proceedings in the Prozac case, one of Lilly's experts made comments about having confidence in any drug that the FDA had given approval for, the claimant's counsel claimed that this had opened up the opportunity to detailed questioning on its standards for conducting clinical trials. The lawyers asked for permission to introduce the Oraflex material and Judge Potter agreed. However, Lilly's lawyers asked for a short adjournment. When the court re-adjourned, the claimant's lawyers did not ask to admit the evidence from the Oraflex case and offered no further evidence. The jury came back with a nine to three majority in favour Lilly.

For Lilly this was a great opportunity for discouraging future litigation. Chief Executive Randall Tobias was reported as saying that "the jury after hearing the scientific and medical facts…came to the only logical conclusion— that Prozac had nothing to do with Joseph Wesbecker's actions." Judge Potter smelled a rat and was apparently informed by one of the plaintiffs that a deal had been made in the corridor outside the courtroom. Potter subsequently filed a motion to have the not-guilty verdict quashed and replaced with "dismissed with prejudice as settled." The case went to the Kentucky Supreme Court, which found that "there may have been deception, bad faith conduct, abuse of the judicial process or perhaps even fraud."[149]

Circuit Judge John Potter, believed that Lilly bribed plaintiffs and their lawyers before the jury verdict. He uncovered evidence of bribery, and fought Eli Lilly for years but failed to obtain proof of the terms of the deal. Jon Rappoport reports that "Lilly succeeded in keeping its criminal action from a judicial proceeding. As is Eli Lilly's norm and practice; it trashed the judge for his pursuit of the truth." He reveals that Lilly secretly paid the victims $20 million (in 1994) to help ensure a verdict exonerating the drug company. He reports "Indianapolis-based Eli Lilly vigorously shielded the payment for more than two decades, defying a Louisville judge who fought to reveal it because he said it swayed the jury's verdict."[150]

Harvesting Sickness

This is just one example of one company pursuing its goal of maximizing returns and its profits by any and all means at its disposal. It would be wrong to treat this example as just 'one bad apple', a term often used to make us believe that these practices are not endemic and universal in the pharmaceutical industry. I could fill this book with many more examples of dishonest and criminal actions by the pharmaceutical industry that have been used to promote dangerous drugs that produced violence, suicide, or appalling and disabling symptoms and even death in their victims. I do not wish to over-indulge you with this a whole lot further. I know some people, who may have been harmed by antidepressants, for example, feel that the human side of the story can be missing. I agree that this helps to bring the story of this type of tragedy to life. Dr Ann Tracy's book is full of such stories; here is one further example: that of Maria Malakoff and her husband Gary, both Florida pharmacists, who got sucked into taking Prozac, something that would change their lives forever. After a few months of taking Prozac she impulsively attempted suicide: part of her, however, suspected she was reacting to the drug, and she avoided harming herself and immediately stopped taking the drug. She then tried to warn her husband as to what had happened to her and her suspicion that it was provoked by Prozac. He, however, said that he felt fine on it. He did finally stop taking the drug the day he put a gun in his mouth and blew his brains out in front of his wife and four children. Her pharmacy was one of the first to remove Prozac from its shelves. Dr Tracy warns: "The day is not far off that every family in this country will be affected in some way by Prozac." Her book cites many examples where people who, before trying to kill themselves said they felt so agitated that they felt desperately like "jumping out of their skin."[151]

What I feel is useful about this story, played out over time, are the revelations that through litigation, and further scientific scrutiny, it provides us with the obvious conclusion that is shared by many—that the pharmaceutical industry has become a pathologically dangerous entity. This will be discussed further in the next chapters, but suffice it to say at this juncture, that it would be a mistake just to focus on one drug or one pharmaceutical company. There will always be a new 'wonder drug', but it will only be, with the passage of time, that the drug's side effects and ability to cause damage will come to light. In some cases, as with the great cholesterol con and the statin scam, that can lead to damage to its victims spread slowly over long periods of time, so-much-so that many may not understand that they are victims of damage until it is too late. The same could be said in some respects with the antidepressant crisis, due to what Dr Breggin refers to as the 'spellbinding effect', where the damage to a person's brain is such that their awareness is so dulled they are no longer aware that they are not the same person they were. It is often only the people around them who see the change in personality, mood swings, lack of interest, lack of care, lack of passion, lack of love, and abandoned sex life and notice the damage that was done but the drugged individual may not. We now know that these antidepressants are extremely hard to stop taking in many cases, and the withdrawal symptoms can be appalling. We know the industry consistently denied that their drugs were the cause of these symptoms and that they have insisted that these effects are due to the illness of the person taking the drug: that these symptoms were simply masked before taking the drug. According to Dr Breggin, this is utter rubbish. Once off the drugs, if people have not been on them too long most people will make a full recovery.

We only know this through the passage of time, when people like Dr Breggin were able to get their clients successfully off these types of drugs, and in many cases enable their patients to get their own selves back that this information even came to light. None of this hazard is ever going to surface with a poorly regulated six-week trial for a drug overseen by a regulator that is openly regarded as working for the pharmaceutical industry.

Peter Gøtzsche informs us that there are over 5,000 media stories of massacres, homicides, suicides, and school and college shootings dating back to 1966 that involve antidepressants and ADHD drugs, in some cases detailing the drugs and legal defences. He comments: 'Psychiatric drugs are so harmful that they kill more than half a million people every year among those aged 65 and over in the US and in Europe. This makes psychiatric drugs the third leading cause of death, after heart disease.' He further explains the way these drugs are dishonestly marketed: More than half the patients believe their mental disorder is caused by a chemical imbalance in the brain. They have this misperception from their doctors, which means more than half the psychiatrists lie to their patients … I have come to the conclusion that psychiatric research is predominantly pseudoscience, and…reliable research constantly tells us a very different story to the fairytale that leading psychiatrists want us to believe in.'[152]

To illustrate the idea that this pathological system will continue to create the same so-called "wonder drugs", that will continue to exploit sales in markets that will be addictive or lead to huge sales—the blockbuster mentality with no real regard to the human consequences—let us jump forward in time to the current epidemic and briefly review the current opioid crisis that is taking such a toll on America—a toll that threatens to engulf the world. For those of you who would like further information on any of the topics so far discussed, there is much more information to be found in the cited works and my previous book *Unhealthy Betrayal—How the Manipulation of Science and Politics By Corporate Interests Destroys Health and Threatens the Future of Humanity.*[153]

Prescription Addiction

Chris McGreal, the reporter and author of *American Overdose—The Opioid Tragedy in Three Acts,* asks the question "How was the greatest drug epidemic in American history allowed to grow virtually unchecked for nearly two decades with no end in sight?" He estimates that opioids have claimed more than 400,000 American lives since 1999 and that drug overdoses now kill more people in the United States each year than all the American soldiers who died in the Vietnam War. He claims that overdoses are the leading killer of people under the age of fifty and are dragging down life expectancy in the USA. He suggests that by the time the opioid epidemic has run its course, the number of deaths may well have doubled, compounded by a second wave of heroin and synthetic opioids such as fentanyl. McGreal quotes a former head of the FDA describing the mass prescribing of narcotic painkillers as "one of the greatest mistakes of modern medicine," but he claims that "It is neither a mistake nor the kind of catastrophe born of some ghastly accident. It is a tragedy forged by the capture of medical policy by corporations and the failure of American institutions to protect the public."

"…one of the greatest mistakes of modern medicine," but "It is neither a mistake nor the kind of catastrophe born of some ghastly accident. It is a tragedy forged by the capture of medical policy by corporations and the failure of American institutions to protect the public."

One of the significant players in the whole epidemic was a company called Purdue, who developed OxyContin, a pure narcotic that was marketed as having "delayed absorption" and believed to "reduce the abuse liability of the drug". McGreal tells us how Purdue launched OxyContin, touting it as a "New hope for millions of Americans," 'positioning the drug as a valuable weapon in the war on untreated pain'. They suggested that millions of people lived in agony due to "unwarranted fears of uncontrollable side effects and/or addiction by physicians and patients alike," which the company claimed was largely exaggerated and unfounded. Purdue, the company responsible for the sale of the opioid, OxyContin, was formed by the Sackler family, who had already achieved great economic success previously persuading Americans that they had far too much stress in their lives and what they needed was a good tranquillizer such as Valium. It was offered as a way to treat sleep problems, stomach upset, worry about exams, heartburn and even "psychic tension." With such a pedigree, the next generation of Sacklers unleashed a marketing program for their new drug, OxyContin, that included the distribution of fifteen thousand copies of a CD, *Get in the Swing with OxyContin,* that they distributed to doctors without the approval of the FDA. That led the Drug Enforcement Administration to comment that they 'had never seen anything like it in promoting a narcotic.'

McGreal reviews the story of the opioid crisis: the way Purdue was able to avoid conducting a clinical trial of a standard addiction and overdose test in animals, and how the FDA official who oversaw the approval process, Curtis Wright, sided with the company enabling the company to avoid this action. Wright approved OxcyContin for wide use as an appropriate remedy for moderate to severe pain. He was well rewarded for his work with a job working for Purdue within a couple of years of leaving the FDA. [154]

In October 2017, US President Donald Trump declared opioid addiction a public health emergency, and federal research funding to control opioid misuse and pain management reached US$1.1 billion. Deaths due to drug overdoses were estimated at 70,000 in the United States in 2017, and of those—more than two-thirds were caused by opioids which, by now, included prescription pain killers, the synthetic opioid fentanyl and its analogues, and heroin. According to Judith Feinberg, writing in *Nature* in September 2019, this opioid crisis is an epidemic that is a symptom 'of the fraying of the socio-economic fabric of the rural United States. The epidemic arose in the 1990s in areas that had experienced economic decline, a brain drain and population loss over decades.' She relates it to the loss of key industries such as coal mining and aggressive marketing by the pharmaceutical industry. She cites the example of Kermit, West Virginia, a coal town with about 400 inhabitants, with a local family-run pharmacy that received 9 million pain pills in a space of two years.[155]

People related the rise of the opioid epidemic to numerous reasons, such as the massive advertising campaigns by the pharmaceutical industry, who were spending more than $5 billion a year pushing their products on television following the FDA's loosening of the advertising regulations which allowed them to directly advertise their drugs to the general public—the USA being the only country in the world other than New Zealand where this is allowed. Chris McGreal cites numerous events, such as Purdue Pharma's David Haddox and the American Pain Society writing a policy document reassuring doctors that they would not face disciplinary action for prescribing narcotics, even in large quantities. He also cites the Pain Care Forum that spent close to three-quarters of a billion dollars over a decade (up to 2015), on pushing policies, writing legislation, and funding elected officials in Washington DC and across the country to 'promote opioids and oppose curbs on prescribing.' Its members included the American Pain Foundation (APF), the American Pain Society, and the American Academy of Pain Medicine. As is predictable with many seemingly independent organizations that support the industry view, he suggests, 'But peel back the covers, and the forum was a web of interwoven corporate interests and specialists in their pay.' McGreal reveals how the APF was very quick to the defence of doctors who were accused of illegally prescribing opioids, and that they claimed the arrests and curbs on prescribing were driven by "opiophobia." He mentions how the foundation spent considerable sums on "educational guides" promoting prescription narcotics, and that Purdue Pharma gave it $150,000 to promote the Institute of Medicine's report that suggested that 100 million Americans were living with chronic pain. He also points out that, in the year that the Pain Care Forum was founded and was pushing its report on pain, that suggested approximately 11,000 people were killed by overdosing on prescription opioids, and by 2011 the death toll had reached an unbelievable number of 17,000 victims a year. Over this same period, Purdue's income from OxyContin rose by a billion to more than $3 billion a year.[156]

Purdue Pharma, was, however, only one player in the opioid epidemic this epidemic would see even the great pharmaceutical behemoth, Johnson & Johnson facing numerous lawsuits over its role in the opioid crisis. In August 2019, an Oklahoma judge ruled that the company had blood on its hands, after it had tried to shift responsibility for the biggest drug epidemic in America's history, that has claimed more than 400,000 lives as a "drug abuse crisis", shifting blame onto the victims as Big Pharma so often likes to do. Judge Thad Balkman, however, after listening to two months of evidence suggested the company's "false, misleading, and dangerous marketing campaigns have caused exponentially increasing rates of addiction, overdose deaths". He accused Johnson & Johnson of lying about the science in training sales reps to tell doctors its high-strength narcotic painkillers were safe and effective when they were addictive and had a limited impact on pain. Oklahoma's attorney general, Mike Hunter described the marketing strategy as "a cynical, deceitful multimillion-dollar brainwashing campaign" to pressure doctors into prescribing large numbers of narcotic painkillers even as the death rate was increasing. Balkman also implicated Johnson & Johnson as being part of the much wider collaboration by opioid makers to subvert medical policy, particularly in America, by fostering the illusion of an epidemic of untreated pain to which they suggested narcotic drugs were the only solution.[157] From 2000 through 2011, members of Johnson & Johnson's sales staff made some 150,000 visits to Oklahoma doctors, focusing in particular on high-volume prescribers, the state said. In addition, the pharmaceutical giant supplied most of the nation's opioid material to other drug manufacturers, refined by one of its companies from a variety of poppy that Johnson & Johnson developed and grew in Tasmania. The state said that the company aggressively promoted the safety of opioids generally, through campaigns tailored for women, teenagers, and veterans. It said the company engaged with "front groups" of pain patients and pain medicine specialists, who insisted the drugs were effective for quotidian pain and minimized the risk of addiction. Oklahoma has suffered mightily from opioids. According to Mr Hunter, between 2015 and 2018, 18 million opioid prescriptions were written in a state with a population of 3.9 million. Since 2000, his office reported, about 6,000 Oklahomans have died from opioid overdoses, with thousands more struggling with addiction. "Judge Balkman has affirmed our position that Johnson & Johnson maliciously and diabolically created the opioid epidemic in our state," Hunter said.[158]

This trial followed from earlier bad news for Johnson & Johnson when they were ordered to pay $8 billion when a jury upheld the claim that young men were not warned of breast growth linked to their drug Risperdal used to treat psychiatric disorders. They were ordered to pay punitive damages to Nicholas Murray. This verdict came after they were previously ordered to pay $2.5 million in another associated case, which claimed the drug caused an autistic child to grow large breasts from when he was eight years old—growth that cannot be reversed. The plaintiffs claimed that Risperdal caused gynaecomastia, or swelling of the breasts in men, which was considered due to the activation of the hormone prolactin. The plaintiffs also claimed that the company pushed Risperdal to be used "off label" in children.[159] "The company has cultivated this reputation as this family-friendly, public-minded company, but these cases suggest otherwise," said Carl Tobias, a law professor at the University of Richmond. "So there's a huge public relations problem." He also points out that there are 14,000 other cases involved with Risperdal, as well as 15,000 talc cases, 25,000 pelvic mesh cases, and possibly thousands of opioid-related lawsuits to follow. In addition to selling Duragesic fentanyl patches through a subsidiary, Johnson & Johnson had earned richly as a leading supplier of opioid from its poppy fields in Tasmania.[160]

Sales of Purdue's OxyContin peaked in 2011 when sales of all opioids peaked, and between 2007 and 2016 the most widely prescribed opioids were hydrocodone (Vicodin) and oxycodone (Percocet). It has been suggested that the Sackler family responded to this fall in sales by investing in a global network, which included Mundipharma in order to expand sales of OxyContin. Opioid sales are now rising in many other countries. Former USFDA Commissioner David A. Kessler has called the failure to recognize the dangers of painkillers one of the biggest mistakes in modern medicine. Speaking of Mundipharma's push into foreign markets, he said, "It's right out of the playbook of Big Tobacco. As the United States takes steps to limit sales here, the company goes abroad." The spectacular success of OxyContin has generated nearly $35 billion in revenue over the last two decades and made the Sacklers one of the nation's wealthiest families. Three generations of the family now help oversee Purdue and the Mundipharma-associated foreign corporations. Mundipharma is not alone in seeking new markets for opioids outside American borders. Mundipharma expanded first in Asia, then Latin America, and then the Middle East and Africa, ultimately having a presence in 122 developing markets. The head of Mundipharma Emerging Markets, Raman Singh, has overseen 800% sales growth in the developing world. Since 2011, Mundipharma has hired more than a thousand employees, most of them sales representatives, and now has a presence in 300 cities. Many companies are looking to increase sales in other countries, following the drop in sales in the USA; in the last year, two other manufacturers, Teva and Grunenthal, each bought drug companies in Mexico.[161]

Former USFDA Commissioner David A. Kessler has called the failure to recognize the dangers of painkillers one of the biggest mistakes in modern medicine.

At its peak, America was dealing with 211million opioid prescriptions in a year and in 2016 a fifth of all deaths among Americans aged 24 to 35 were due to opioids. Between 2006 and 2012 US drug companies saturated America with 76 billion oxycodone and hydrocodone pills alone.[162]

It was announced that Purdue Pharma had made an offer to make a comprehensive settlement involving thousands of claims against it for its role in the crisis. The settlement does not, however, include an admission of wrongdoing and involves plaintiffs in nearly 2,300 lawsuits, including numerous municipal governments nationwide and nearly two dozen states. Not all the attorney generals, however, agree with the settlement terms. Maura Healey, the Massachusetts attorney general, who was one of the first to sue members of the Sackler family, said in a statement, "It's critical that all the facts come out about what this company and its executives and directors did, that they apologize for the harm they caused and that no one profits from breaking the law."[163] The chances are not high that this is likely to occur if past experience is anything to go on. The American legal system has been shown to be loath to criminally convict pharmaceutical executives and put them in jail. Apologizing could be seen as an admission of guilt and culpability. As far as the law goes, the pharmaceutical industry has demonstrably marketed dangerous drugs that they knew would cause death, time and time again: is legalized genocide too strong a wording for us to describe this behaviour?

Chris McGreal informs us that in May 2019, a jury for the first time actually convicted the head of an opioid manufacturer for a criminal offence over the epidemic. He tells us prosecutors used the racketeering laws that were written to pursue organized crime to charge the billionaire founder of Insys Therapeutics, John Kapoor, and four of his executives for bribing doctors to prescribe their powerful spray, Subsys, which contained fentanyl, to patients who did not need it. Insys paid more than a million in bribes to doctors to prescribe high doses of Subsys, and watched sales rise from $14 million in 2012 when Insys came on the market, to nearly half a billion dollars five years later. The mayor of the West Virginian city of Huntington, Steve Williams, had watched the opioid epidemic wreck his city's social fabric; he voiced what many considered to be an increasingly widely held view that likened pharma executives to "drug dealers in Amani suits." He posed the question "Just because this person is working on a street corner selling drugs and this other person is working in the executive suite fifty stories up, is there really a difference? Just because you are in the executive suite doesn't mean that you are immune from the results of the corporate decisions that you make. Just because you have billions of dollars at your disposal doesn't mean that you shouldn't be held accountable." Insys subsequently filed for bankruptcy after pleading guilty to fraud and agreed to pay a penalty of $225 million. [164]

How To Survive in the 21ˢᵗ Century

New York State Attorney General Letitia James, who has sued Purdue and the core multibillionaire members of the Sackler family, said: "While our country continues to recover from the carnage left by the Sacklers' greed, this family is now attempting to evade responsibility and lowball the millions of victims of the opioid crisis." She continued in a statement: "A deal that doesn't account for the depth of pain and destruction caused by Purdue and the Sacklers is an insult, plain and simple. As attorney general, I will continue to seek justice for victims and fight to hold bad actors accountable, no matter how powerful they may be." [165]

Purdue Pharma filed for bankruptcy Sunday evening, September 15, 2019, in a move to shield itself and its owners from the lawsuits. The filing itself came scarcely 48 hours after an announcement late on the Friday afternoon by the New York attorney general, Letitia James, that her office had uncovered almost a billion dollars in previously undisclosed wire transfers from Purdue to private accounts held by one of the Sacklers. The discovery came from just one of 33 subpoenas that the state had recently issued to financial institutions and advisers that had done business with the Sacklers. It was suggested that these conveyances amounted to "fraudulent conveyance," that some states have claimed may pierce the bankruptcy shield against litigation. Following the revelations by New York attorney general's office about the money transfers by members of the Sackler family, they also added: "any deal that cheats Americans out of billions of dollars, allows the Sacklers to evade responsibility, and lets this family continue peddling their drugs to the world is a bad one."[166]

Sick Industry

The opioid crisis in America is set to infect much of the world, few countries will likely be unaffected by it. It is a story of corporate and human greed with little care for the consequences to human life. Why is it that organizations that were previously perceived as supporting the health of a country, the medical industry and the pharmaceutical industry—are now so easily revealed as the main threat to our health? This is a useful question but does not have a simple answer.

The pharmaceutical industry has grown increasingly powerful and as previously revealed has been enabled to escape any real scrutiny, and been able to achieve massive wealth and profitability. How this has been possible is worth examining. One of the most significant factors is the way in America, for example, drug companies can charge whatever they like for their drugs. In 2003 Congress passed a law that was written by the industry to prevent what just about every other government does in the developed world, that is, negotiate prices for drugs. Congressman Billy Tauzin, chair of the Energy and Commerce Committee, shepherded the legislation limiting price negotiations into law. He was rewarded for his endeavours—after giving up his seat in Congress, he took up a $2 million a year post as head of the drug manufacturer's trade group PhRMA. McGreal informs us that Tauzin became the highest-paid industry lobbyist in the country earning more than $11 million a year. This is at a time when drug makers were pouring close to $2.5 billion into lobbying and funding members of Congress over the decade to 2016. Following are some examples of drug pricing that help illustrate how this law enables unbridled returns to the pharmaceutical industry: the UK National Health Service pays $70 for the drug EpiPen, a drug antidote for allergic reactions, in America it is charged at $600.[167] During the 2016 election in California, according to figures released by the non-profit organization MapLight, the pharmaceutical industry invested $70 million in an effort to fight Proposition 61, which would have limited the prices state agencies pay for prescription drugs. Bay area reporter Tracy Seipel commented: "Some observers are predicting drug company contributions will top $100 million by Election Day".[168]

How To Survive in the 21st Century

Having the freedom to set whatever prices you feel like sets a dangerous precedent and attracts the wrong kind of people to the industry. The biotech investor Martin Shkreli, described as the "most hated man in America", was responsible for hiking the price of Darapim by $5,000, a drug that was considered very effective for treating toxoplasmosis in patients with compromised immune systems, such as cancer patients. According to market reporter Barbara Kollmeyer, Shkreli, the former chief executive officer of Turing who was facing civil and criminal securities fraud charges 'drew particular scorn from the committee [the House Committee on Oversight and Government Reform] after the price of Daraprim soared to $750 from $13.50 per pill overnight.' Shkreli purchased the drug for $55 million with the expectation that he would be able to increase the drug's revenues from the previous $10 million a year to several hundred million dollars a year. In one of his emails, he is quoted as saying: "I think it will be huge. We raised the price from $1,700 per bottle to $75,000…So 5,000 paying bottles at the new price is $375,000,000—almost all of it is profit and I think we will get 3 years of that or more. Should be a very handsome investment for all of us. Let's all cross our fingers that the estimates are accurate." Another email reported: "Martin [Shkreli] did say that he had to maximize profit for investors and that was why price is high. He did not say it was for research primarily that it was a high price. He called that the 'dirty secret' of pharma." Another company, Valeant Pharmaceuticals was in the spotlight for raising the prices of two of its heart drugs—Isuprel by 525% and Nitropress by 212%. [169] Just in case you think that these are isolated examples, here are a couple more revelations of how pharmaceutical companies seek to maximize returns: Cycloserine, a drug used to treat dangerous multidrug-resistant tuberculosis, was just increased in price to $10,800 for 30 pills up from $500 after its acquisition by Rodelis Therapeutics. Doxycycline, an antibiotic, went from $20 a bottle in October 2013 to $1,849 by April 2014. [170]

Harvesting Sickness

So all we have to do to make a mint is to buy up the rights on a drug and up its price, or even take over a company and then up its price, particularly when it's a very useful drug. Is this really a sensible way to behave? Professor's Leslie Sekerka and Lauren Benishek in their review of the pharmaceutical industry looking at it from the regulatory point of view and specifically at the advertising side noted that spending on advertising for television by pharmaceutical companies more than doubled in four years, which represented a 65% increase from 2012, investing $6.4 billion in US advertising in 2016. They inform us that in 2016, 80 prescription drug advertisements were televised every hour, totalling 1,920 drug ads directed at American viewers per day. They make the useful comment: 'All this advertising can increase the cost of prescription drugs. Ironically, these ads actually serve as tax deductions for pharmaceutical firms.' They made the further observation regarding the success of their advertising, that it is no surprise that, in the two countries in the world that allow direct-to-consumer-advertising, USA and New Zealand, citizens 'take an average of more than two prescription medications regularly.' They also comment: 'To understand what drives these ads, it is necessary to examine the trillion-dollar pharmaceutical industry known as Big Pharma.' National health expenditures are projected to reach growth forecasts of 4.8% in 2019, up from 4.4% growth in 2018, and to reach $3.8 trillion. Growth forecasts averaging 5.7% leading up to 2027 predict expenditure to reach nearly $6 trillion. [171]

If you create a situation where there is little real regulatory control of an industry connected with healthcare, one that is generating such vast profits, and allow them to cause significant injury and even death without any real incentive to adhere to any moral compass or social norms, simply allowing them to focus on making money—the tendency would lead to developments that are not going to create real health in society. Not only is this not going to lead to health-creation, it will actively subvert health—and actively develop a more pathological

171

business model that is fed by self-interest and motivated by greed—particularly if similar conditions exist in other sectors of that economy. In *Hijacked—How the Banking Industry, Finance, and Corporate Interests Have Hijacked Our Economy and Corrupted Democracy,* we have already revealed how the economy has been subverted into what I referred to as "casino capitalism", which developed from its feudal roots following modernization and significant deregulation. Such a situation, particularly following the inevitable crises that such a malfunctioning economic system produces, leads to 'investors' chasing whatever returns they can get. It creates a self-perpetuating parasitic situation, where the medical industry—dominated by pharmaceutical interests—not just fails to generate health, but actively destroys it and feeds off that destruction.

Creating Sickness

There are many ways that the pharmaceutical industry undermines our health. We have already discussed the way that the industry created the so-called "mental health crisis", the "epidemic of ADHD" leading to the bipolar epidemic. We would be mistaken to believe that this is the only area of health that the industry has subverted. You don't have to look very far to find that far from being an isolated example, creating illness has, in fact, become its major method of expanding its markets and thus its profits.

The US healthcare system has been the most easily-exploited market due to the ability to use direct-to-consumer-advertising. Ray Moynihan, Iona Heath, and David Henry, in their report, "Selling sickness: the pharmaceutical industry and disease mongering", explain their findings:

> There's a lot of money to be made from telling healthy people they're sick. Some forms of medicalising ordinary life may now be better

described as disease mongering: widening the boundaries of treatable illness in order to expand markets for those who sell and deliver.

In their article published in the British Medical Journal in 2002, they describe the way the industry operates to extend their markets:

> Within many disease categories, informal alliances have emerged, comprising drug company staff, doctors, and consumer groups. Ostensibly engaged in raising public awareness about underdiagnosed and undertreated problems, these alliances tend to promote a view of their particular condition as widespread, serious, and treatable. Because these "disease awareness" campaigns are commonly linked to companies' marketing strategies, they operate to expand markets for new pharmaceutical products.

They cite a number of examples, irritable bowel syndrome being one that has long been considered as common functional disorder, associated with poor dietary choices. They suggest it is currently experiencing something of a global "makeover," following the arrival of new drugs which: 'has seen manufacturers seek to change the way the world thinks about irritable bowel syndrome'. They obtained information from a leaked industry document that revealed the way science is manipulated:

> A confidential draft document leaked from a medical communications company, In Vivo Communications, describes a three year "medical education programme" to create a new perception of irritable bowel syndrome as a "credible, common and concrete disease." The proposed 2001-3 education programme is part of the marketing strategy for GlaxoSmithKline's drug Lotronex (alosetron hydrochloride)...
>
> According to the documents, the education programme's key aim is this: "IBS [irritable bowel syndrome] must be established in the

minds of doctors **as a significant and discrete disease state.**" Patients also "need to be convinced that IBS is a common and recognised medical disorder." The other main messages are about promoting the new "clinically proven therapy"—Lotronex.

They describe how the first step 'is to set up an "Advisory Board" comprising one KOL [key opinion leader]', in this case, from each state in Australia, with its chief role 'to provide advice to the corporate sponsors on current opinion in gastroenterology' and on "opportunities for reshaping it". They go into details of different marketing strategies and groups to be targeted with promotional material, such as pharmacists, nurses, patients, and a 'medical foundation described as already having a "close relationship" with In Vivo.' They describe further initiatives but inform us:

> Although billed as a medical education plan, the document is clearly part of the Lotronex marketing strategy. One clause explicitly stipulates that all publications and manuscripts must be approved by the drug company's marketing, medical, and legal departments. The document also makes clear the media's role in changing public perceptions about irritable bowel syndrome, stating that "PR [public relations] and media activities are crucial to a well-rounded campaign—particularly in the area of consumer awareness."

They mention that the campaign was halted following the withdrawal of Lotronex from the market, after reports to the FDA of serious adverse reactions which included fatalities. The article also examines other examples, such as medicalising baldness, extending the conception of what constitutes osteoporosis, and making the menopause a form of pathological illness that has to be treated by drugs. They inform us that their key concern with the examples they discuss: 'is the invisible and unregulated attempts to change public perceptions about health and illness to widen markets for new drugs.'[172]

Melody Petersen, *New York Times* investigative reporter, in her excellent volume *Our Daily Meds,* discusses the many tactics that the pharmaceutical industry use to get people to unnecessarily take their drugs. She cites how they created National Depression Screening Day and invited students to take their test for 'mental illness.' She reports of the 190 students who took the test almost half had a score that indicated "diagnosis likely, further evaluation needed." Of these students, two-thirds were said to have depression and 58% were categorised as having "generalized anxiety disorder" which was further defined as "excessive worrying." More than 25% of them, as a result, started taking antidepressants. She also cited industry experts who revealed the secret of creating drug sales suggested the "ultimate goal" was for the drug companies to "sell the consumer a message or product without the consumer even being aware that a 'sell' is taking place'. She reveals how the industry created a market for their drugs by cleverly targeted campaigns, such as one that supposedly revealed a 'disorder said to be destroying the lives of millions of Americans' with 'a potentially humiliating problem' that of 'overactive bladders.' Nevermind, the drug companies have come to the rescue—the solution was at hand with their nice drug Detrol. It was suggested that taking a drug such as Detrol made people feel better when they went out and this type of product was a market that was growing at 30% a year. Apparently, they considered if you went to the bathroom more than eight times in 24 hours you were a candidate for their drugs. Well, you might want to consider how big a problem this is when one of the side effects from taking these drugs was according to Petersen, associated with the onset of dementia, and in those with Alzheimer's already, the disease significantly worsened.[173] Most nutritionists would advise drinking a minimum of 2 ½ litres of water a day, which would involve more visits than 8 a day to the bathroom. I recommend Petersen's book for anyone who would like a more in-depth review of the pharmaceutical industry.

To illustrate the all-pervasive nature of the way the pharmaceutical industry operates, take the example of blood pressure medication. This example is cited in a series of articles by *Seattle Times* staff reporters Susan Kelleher and Duff Wilson, who interviewed more than 160 doctors, patients, medical analysts, regulatory officials and other experts for "Suddenly Sick." They travelled to Europe, Canada, and around the country, obtaining records and interviews with patients, officials with the World Health Organization, and doctors attending medical conferences. These articles state that the series also relied on thousands of pages of medical-journal articles and a lot more information. They begin their series with this question: 'A woman is healthy one day, but the next day she has a life-threatening disease. Nothing in her physical condition has changed. How can this be?' They state that: 'The answer to this riddle involves billions of dollars in health-care costs and likely touches the lives of everyone reading this newspaper.' They reveal:

> Pharmaceutical firms have commandeered the process by which diseases are defined. Many decision makers at the World Health Organization, the U.S. National Institutes of Health and some of America's most prestigious medical societies take money from the drug companies and then promote the industry's agenda.

They reveal how their research has led them to understand that, 'Some diseases have been radically redefined without a strong basis in medical evidence,' and further that:

> The drug industry has bolstered its position by marketing directly to the health-conscious consumer, leading younger and healthier people to consider themselves at risk and to start taking medications.

Harvesting Sickness

Every time the boundary of a disease is expanded— the hypertension threshold is lowered by 10 blood-pressure points, the guideline for obesity is lowered by 5 pounds— the market for drugs expands by millions of consumers and billions of dollars.

The result? Skyrocketing sales of prescription drugs. Soaring health-care costs. Escalating patient anxiety. Worst of all, millions of people taking drugs that may carry a greater risk than the underlying condition. The treatment, in fact, may make them sick or even kill them.

They reveal information they uncovered from the prestigious Dartmouth Medical School:

Dartmouth Medical School researchers estimate that during the 1990s, tens of millions more Americans were classified as having hypertension, high cholesterol, diabetes or obesity simply because the definitions of those diseases were changed. Today, three of every four Americans technically have at least one of those diseases. But millions of them are not truly sick and may never be, even without medication.

They report that in 1998 the WHO task force that agreed to guidelines affirming that anti-hypertensive drugs should be used as the first form of treatment was chaired by Dr Albert Zanchetti, an Italian cardiologist. Zanchetti, a professor of medicine at the University of Milan and, founder of the European Society of Hypertension, had numerous ties to the drug industry, such as Italy's largest drug company, Recordati where he was paid to consult and give speeches. He also took grants or consulting fees from 18 other drug companies including most of the world's largest, but WHO did not require that he disclose how much money he was paid by the drug companies. As well, he also appointed the 17 other members of the committee, and all but one of them had close financial ties to drug firms. The committee proposed 80 as the ideal number for diastolic pressure, claiming anything higher was unhealthy and recommended that as the first course of treatment doctors choose from any of the five classes of hypertension drugs. Despite a protest signed by 888 doctors, pharmacists and scientists from 58 countries claiming the committee had misrepresented medical evidence WHO supported the guidelines.

The US National Institutes of Health's own panel recommended broader use of hypertension drugs at new lower blood pressures, and the Seattle Times article informs us that nine of the eleven authors of their guidelines had ties to the drug companies, the details of which they disclose in their article. They also refer to the largest hypertension study undertaken, that was funded by the federal government, the Antihypertensive and Lipid-lowering Treatment to Prevent Heart Attack Trial (ALLHAT trial) that concluded that the newer blood pressure drugs were less safe and no more effective than the much cheaper and older diuretics: 'The study found that Lisinopril and Amlodipine…were no more effective than water pills in preventing deaths. On the other hand, Lisinopril was linked to 60 percent higher frequency of strokes. Amlodipine…was linked to 38 percent more heart attacks and increased rates of suicide and depression.'[174]

In February 1999, WHO announces that half-a-billion people worldwide needed hypertension treatment. By defining hypertension as over 140/90, "normal" as 130/85 and "optimal" as 120/80, the recommendations would classify 45% of people of all ages, and nearly 60% of elderly people, as hypertensive. In May 2003 – A new U.S. guideline says 45 million Americans have "prehypertension," defined as systolic pressure from 120 to 139, or diastolic from 80 to 89. It also recommends that doctors add one or more different blood-pressure drugs if diuretics did not lower patients' blood pressure below 140/90.

More people visit doctors for hypertension than for any condition other than the common cold. And no wonder, as the threshold for hypertension has dropped from160/100 to140/90 and now, with pre-hypertension, to 120/80. More than 50 million Americans are considered hypertensive, meaning blood pressure of 140/90 or higher. Additionally, 45 million US adults are said to have prehypertension—a level of 120-139 (top number) or 80-89 (bottom number).

Kelleher and Duff in a following article in their series reported on the way the goalposts were moved on obesity turning it into a disease in its own right:

> In making obesity a disease, these experts helped create a billion-dollar market for the drugs that maimed… killed hundreds and damaged the hearts and lungs of tens of thousands. The story of obesity shows how it became acceptable for doctors to risk killing or injuring people on the premise that it would save them from illnesses they might never get.[175]

They discuss the disaster caused by the use of Phen-Fen and Redux (sold as weight-loss drugs) and the fatal side effects of these drugs and others that were touted as drugs that would save lives, but in reality, took so many lives they were recalled. I reported on this tragedy in a previous volume, *Unhealthy Betrayal.*[176] It is clear that the pharmaceutical industry is able to move the goalposts and capture a larger market for their drugs as long as they can maintain the idea that taking drugs is the only way to obtain health or to achieve respite from the onslaught of criticism that can be directed to an overweight person, or someone who is informed they have a cholesterol problem or they have high blood pressure.

Leslie E. Sekerka, and Lauren Benishek in their review titled "Thick as Thieves? Big Pharma Wields its Power with the Help of Government Regulation," inform us:

How To Survive in the 21ˢᵗ Century

Americans are barraged by an endless flow of ads that claim to remedy medical maladies with prescribed drugs. The commercials depict productive and happy lives, with suggestive associations that human flourishing can be achieved via pharmaceutical intervention. The appeals are accompanied by an exhaustive inventory of potentially negative life-altering side effects. As ads end with this depiction of relational bliss through drug use, viewers hear a fast-paced listing of monotone non-segmented disclaimers, which can range from modest impacts (e.g., slight weight gain) to very serious implications (e.g., suicidal ideations).

It is obvious that this advertising works. They cite an example: 'in 2011 Boehringer Ingelheim spent $464 million advertising its blood thinner Pradaxa. The investment appears to have paid off: the drug passed the $1 billion sales mark the following year.' Pfizer's cholesterol drug Lipitor was heavily promoted and became the best-selling drug of all time, with $125 billion in sales over 15 years. They inform us how vast the market for prescription drugs has become: 'Americans spent $325 billion in 2015 (equating to 1.8% of GDP and 10% of total national health expenditures) on retail prescriptions alone (not including drugs administered directly by healthcare providers).

Their research raises some disturbing implications: 'If, for instance, a consumer suffers a psychiatric or neurological illness that can impair their decision making capacity, they may be at risk of undue influence from these ads. Yet, one study found that 18% of the 50 drugs advertised most assiduously in the U.S. were medications used to treat these kinds of disorders.' They mention that Allen Frances, chair of the DSM-IV Task Force, 'warns that the gradual mislabeling of everyday problems as illness has toxic implications for individuals and society: stigmatizing people, introducing them to potentially harmful medications, misallocating medical resources, and draining the budgets of families and the nation.'[177]

Roxanne Nelson echoes these thoughts when she comments 'Many consumer advocates and health care professionals believe that direct-to-consumer advertising should be prohibited or, at the very least, more closely regulated.' In testimony before the Senate Special Committee on Aging in 2005, Peter Lurie, MD, deputy director of Public Citizen's Health Research Group, called direct-to-consumer advertising "nothing less than an end-run around the doctor–patient relationship—an attempt to turn patients into the agents of pharmaceutical companies as they pressure physicians for medications they may not need." Research confirms that when doctors are directly asked for a particular drug by their patients they generally oblige with prescribing what is requested, even when they believe the drug is no better than tried and tested older drugs. Invariably the drug is much more expensive than the older drug. [178]

Sekerka and Benishek, come to the conclusion about the pharmaceutical industry that reflects the problem we face: How this industry moves forward presents one of the biggest ethical challenges of the 21st century, seeking a balance between capitalism and the corporation's duty to its share and stakeholder constituents.[179]

One of the challenges facing most people today is the conflicting information that they are exposed to. How do you navigate your way through all this information and make any sense out of it and determine what to do with it? How do we protect ourselves and our loved ones? In the next chapter, I hope to give you some tools that will enable you to make a better-informed choice to decide how to respond to much of this information.

Chapter Seven

Surviving the Carnage

What does it take to survive in the 21st century with such an invasion of man-made chemicals? And it's not just the chemical onslaught, but also dealing with all the mixed messages from the media, from supposed 'experts', from doctors, professors and such authorities who we have been led to believe have our best interests at heart. It would probably be useful to address the issue of so much misinformation and the reasons we are faced with so many mixed messages, just to clear the air.

We have already discussed how the wealth of the pharmaceutical industry has enabled it to buy the influence of many opinion leaders, to promote their agenda. The same approach can be said for the food industry, the agriculture industry, the chemical industry, and realistically, just about any business that is wealthy enough to buy 'experts'. Marion Nestle, in her book *Food Politics—How the Food Industry Influences Nutrition and Health,* discusses the many ways that industry subverts scientists, academics and public opinion, fairly comprehensively. Some examples of how opinion is manipulated can help us take a more sceptical approach to some of the ways corporations seek to influence us.

It would probably be useful to use an example of a major institution that everyone assumes is honestly supporting our health. Take, the American Heart Association (AHA). Nestle discusses how the AHA brings in a lot of revenue by allowing food companies to use their heart logo symbol on food products so that they could claim that their products were heart-healthy. Apparently, even food companies complained that the program was "an extortion racket", so they revised their fees and introduced a new pricing policy. By October 1997, 55 companies were participating, with over 643 products certified.[180]

I took a look at what their requirements were for inclusion in their scheme, to get an idea of what foods could be passed as heart-healthy. According to their website, in the section Heart-Check Food Certification Program Nutrition Requirements, they list a number of items worth commenting on: Yoghurt: 20g or less total sugar per standard 6 oz serving; Snacks: 5 grams or less added sugar per serving; Smoothies 2 teaspoons (8g) or less added sugar per serving, Total Fat: Less than 5 g (also per 100g); Saturated Fat: Less than 2 g (also per 100g); Cholesterol; Less than 95 mg (also per 100g). Liquid Vegetable oils: Total fat: no limit.[181]

We discussed vegetable oils in chapter two, and as expected, the AHA does not discuss the harmful nature of these fats and are happy to put no limit on their consumption. I can only reiterate my position, that in an unadulterated state, they are a great benefit but are very susceptible to damage, and when processed are easily degraded, producing unhealthy free radicals which will attack the body.

I also listed some items which included sugar, such as, Yoghurt: 20g or less total sugar per standard 6 oz serving. The food industry uses sugar far too much to sell their products and make them seem more palatable. In my view, sugar should never be added to yoghurt which is still allowed to be called 'yoghurt'. Yoghurt traditionally was simply cultured milk, mostly cultured with bacteria such as Lactobacillus acidophilus, which is considered one of the useful bacteria that contribute to the health of what people like to refer to as our 'gut biome'. In this form, particularly if the milk is organic and free of contaminants and pesticides, and has not been processed in any other unhelpful way, it is considered a useful and beneficial food. This is assuming that the recipient is not lactose intolerant or suffering from a general milk intolerance or allergy. I mention the intolerance because it is quite prevalent in Western culture. Many western countries homogenize milk, a process that forces the milk through high-pressure filters (usually 10 microns in diameter), which breaks the fat nodules into much smaller particles. This size reduction whilst enhancing shelf-life in a supermarket creates the situation where drinking this milk, which contains molecules that are smaller than human cells in diameter, can pass into the body without going through the normal digestive process. Swill around the milk in your mouth and the milk can enter the bloodstream without even being swallowed. This can create antibodies to the foreign invader and lead to a dairy food intolerance. Adding the sugar in the yoghurt during the manufacturing process, along with sugar-laden fruit, discourages the survival of Lactobacillus acidophilus (assuming that it is even used in the creation of such products) and encourages pathogens instead.

Whilst on the subject of sugar indexed in the AHA site (and highlighted by me), I would have to comment that I suspect the sugar interests had to be accommodated. In my view, sugar is not a food: it is a poison, much as Professor Yudkin discovered in his early work. Whilst I would be the first to admit that its sweetness is something we all find very pleasing, it nevertheless does not contribute to health in any way. It is not something that should be recommended in *any* degree, particularly to children, who are so easily seduced by the taste and are in the process of developing an intestinal microbiome that is forming part of their immune system that will be an essential part of their life-long protection against illness, particularly food-borne pathogens.

As regards to the items on total amounts of fat, saturated fat and cholesterol, I can only reiterate, that low-fat diets are not going to produce health. It is much more important to look at the *quality* than the quantity, though a diet lacking in fats, particularly the essential fatty acids is going to create significant health issues.

We introduced the example of the AHA to illustrate the power and influence that invested economic interests are able to bring to bear to affect the agenda of such a public body. We have previously revealed much criticism of the FDA and the EPA: again these organizations are integral to protecting our health and wellbeing. Being able to subvert these organisations and the political institution of government is something that big money and powerful interests are able to do.

However, let us explore how we can navigate our way through the situation that we find ourselves in, living in the twenty-first century, and navigate a way through what many may consider a challenging and confusing situation.

Fundamental Nutrition

A useful point to address is a simple fact: we are all unique beings. There is no one-size-fits-all with nutrition and therefore there is no one diet that will suit everybody. There are many factors that can affect the choice of food, that could be due to blood type, the person's location, such as living in a hot climate compared to a colder climate, food availability, current health status, financial status etc. Nevertheless, there are some basic principles that we can utilize to guide our food choices, that are useful to discuss.

I was influenced by the writings of Dr Paavo Airola, writing back in 1971, in his book *Are You Confused,* where he addressed some of the confusion that was reigning at that time about diet. He would address the question "Is milk good for you?" by questioning what you might mean by the word "milk?" He would—and I am just pulling this out my memory and not quoting his work directly—he would likely ask whether you had a cow running around out back grazing on free-range pasture that you just milked ready for consuming, or whether you were referring to supermarket pasteurized or even homogenized milk that invariably contained pus from mastitis, pesticides, antibiotics, and other residues? The result of consuming either of these different kinds of 'milk' would not be expected to confer the same benefits. If you asked whether wheat was good for you, he would invariably question what "wheat" was being referred to. Do you have a supply of the ancient variety of wheat our ancestors, grew on free-range pasture, or are you referring to the modern hybrid that was developed after the war? This modern plant that is grown in large volumes in the USA and Canada, is the short-stemmed hi-gliadin and hi-gluten-content variety, treated with man-made chemical fertilizers and grown on deficient soils, chemically sprayed with herbicide throughout its growth cycle, and even sprayed to be killed so that it can be harvested at the same time. Obviously consuming these products is going to create a different experience, a different metabolic experience, leaving aside taste.

How To Survive in the 21ˢᵗ Century

I feel it is useful to use the same kind of questions with regard to any food source. Take meat as another food source, and the example of beef. It is obvious you will not have free-range cattle on your doorstep: the majority of people obtain their food from supermarkets. In the USA, most beef is fattened on food lots on grain, miles from the nearest farm or fields of grass where they can freely roam and graze. The resultant beef is raised with hormones and antibiotics and will have a different fatty acid profile than grass-fed animals. This meat will come with a much higher omega 6 content compared to grass-fed animals, which would be higher in omega 3. As I previously mentioned omega 3 fatty acids are anti-inflammatory and therefore much more beneficial; the omega-six are considered more inflammatory. This is more of an issue in the USA, as the common American diet is already much too high in omega-six fats found in corn and vegetable oils used in so much American food. Web MD informs us that too much omega 6 can raise blood pressure, lead to blood clots that can cause heart attack and stroke, and cause your body to retain water. Conversely, they agree we don't eat nearly enough omega-3, which can reduce our risk for heart disease and cancer. Omega-3 is found in fish oil, all green leafy vegetables, flaxseed, hempseed, chia seeds, and walnuts (walnuts are also high in omega 6). [182] The lack of grass, of course, is only one aspect of the cattle's diet: what are the levels of pesticides, antibiotics, genetically modified products etc. that these animals are raised on, and do we assume all the food comes from degraded soils that are fed by artificial chemicals?

You can see how the question "is it good to eat meat?" is not likely to get a yes or no answer from me. Obviously, if you wished to consume beef, the better source would be grass-fed beef. Better still would be grass-fed beef organically reared, on really rich, fertile soil. Some of you may have heard of Joe Salatin, the owner of Polyface farm, North Virginia and author of *Folks This Ain't Normal—A Farmer's Advice for Happier Hens, Happier People and a Better World.* I was first inspired by this great farmer waxing lyrical about the 'grass' his cattle ate, a veritable food palette of herbs and different grasses, he was identifying and praising the characteristics and use of each plant that his cattle actively searched out at various times to adjust their health—something he learned by watching his animals year after year. Now if you were fortunate enough to be a recipient of any food from this farmer, either animal or vegetable, you would be receiving as good a nutritional status as could be expected in 21st century America. America needs more farmers like him, who are actually creating more fertility in their soils.

I am sure, for some of you, what I am saying might sound a little idealistic, especially to those on lower incomes, people saddled with more debt than they would otherwise wish, or others who simply feel that the money issue is too insurmountable. The money issue, of course, is significant but it is not, in my view, insurmountable. I personally, do not believe that chemical pollution is insurmountable either, nor just about any other problem that, we have created. I am not trying to be superficial here, it is just that I believe humanity has the creative capacity, and the creative talent to meet and deal with just about any challenge that human ignorance and actions based on greed have created. This topic will be further dealt with in the next chapter.

Good Fats and Bad Fats

We briefly discussed fatty acids and vegetable oils in the previous paragraphs, and in chapter two. It is a topic that I feel is important to get to grips with, as there is so much ignorance about this subject, even amongst nutritionists and academics of all kinds. We can use the same basic approach that we used with regards to milk and beef in the previous paragraphs with regards to fats and oils. There is a rich source of fats and oils to be obtained from seeds and nuts, fatty fish and animals. If you are a vegetarian or a vegan seeds and nuts should play a large role in your diet, preferably organic and in as natural a state as possible. It is important to understand that fats and oils can react to heat, light and exposure to oxygen. The rate they react is important for your health. Flax seeds, which are an excellent source of omega 3 essential fatty acids, are vulnerable to oxidation by heat, light, and oxygen. For this reason, you do not want to heat and cook with them. They should be consumed raw. I consume them mixed with raw oats (I grind them up in a coffee grinder and soak them in water), mostly with berries in the summer (berries are high in antioxidants and polyphenols). If you use flax oil, it is important to obtain an organic supply if possible, but it is more critical that you get a source that cold processes the seeds, preferably in an air-evacuated environment. The oil should be packed in a dark or opaque container, preferably nitrogen-flushed, and once processed it should be refrigerated. All these precautions limit heat, light and oxygen causing rancidity. This does not lend itself to mass-production, nor does it come cheaply, as it is time-consuming and it takes a lot of care. The final product should be refrigerated, and if sold in a store the same rule applies. The final product should not taste bitter: if it does, that would suggest it is rancid, due either to using old seed, or lack of care in extraction or storage. If you have obtained a good quality product, your body will be able to use this fantastic reactivity to heat light and oxygen *inside* your body to create the myriad reactions, creating phospholipids, hormones, cell walls etc. that the omega 3s are renowned for.

Similar principles apply to other sources of oils such as nuts. Once you remove the shell of an almond, for example, air has access. How you choose to store nuts affects how long they can be kept and how quickly they begin to spoil. I buy my nuts in bulk and store them in the fridge, as I do with all seeds. They get used quite quickly. I rarely heat them: I occasionally make a nut roast inside a hollowed-out squash. The squash protects the nut roast from getting over-exposed to heat, but by the time the squash is cooked the resultant nut roast is very satisfying.

Many of the pesticides and herbicides used are fat-soluble and are very persistent in biological systems, for this reason, wherever possible, I would recommend choosing organic nuts, seeds, and oils. This of course also applies to animal fats as well.

As regards to oils for cooking, coconut oil, which has a saturated fat component, withstands heating much like animal fats, such as lard or beef dripping. Animal fats have been used for centuries, and withstand destruction much better than most vegetable oils. Olive oil—strictly speaking, a fruit oil—cannot stand high heating as well as the saturated fats, so it is best to heat it sparingly it is much better used raw and makes an excellent dressing for salads. Sesame oil is a more resilient oil when heated but again is better used raw. The other vegetable oils, are all high in omega 6 and are too reactive when heated to recommend. The mass-produced vegetable oils sold in supermarkets are not kept refrigerated as most of them are so destroyed there would be no point in going to this expense. Revisit the section on the hazards of vegetable oils in chapter two, for a more complete picture of this issue.

I previously quoted the WebMD article by John Casey here is what he wrote in 2003:

How To Survive in the 21ˢᵗ Century

To make the switch to heart-healthy fats, start by avoiding the truly unhealthy fats—trans fatty acids. These trans fats come from vegetable oils that were chemically modified so they are solid like butter. Because these oils don't spoil as quickly as butter, they are used in most packaged cookies, chips, crackers and other baked goods sold in the supermarket, as well as in margarines.

The solidifying process—called hydrogenation—extends the shelf life of food, but it also turns polyunsaturated oils into a kind of man-made cholesterol. Trans fats can increase your level of "bad" LDL cholesterol, and may increase your risk of heart disease. What's more, these man-made fats are taken up by the body much easier than are omega-3s. So trans fatty acids not only harm your health, they also block the absorption of healthy fats. [183]

In 2005, the Dietary Guidelines for Americans advised the public for the first time to limit trans fat to less than one % of calories (U.S. Department of Health and Human Services & U.S. Department of Agriculture 2005). This followed on from the reports issued by the Institute of Medicine (2003/2005), the WHO/FAO expert consultation of 2003 and the European Food Safety Authority in 2004. Following these recommendations and the stream of negative reports, from Mary Enig and others, the food industry reduced the levels of trans fats in food products, including margarine. Following the FDA determination in June 2015 that partially hydrogenated oils are not able to be supported by the designation as generally recognised as safe (GRAS status) a further reduction of trans-fats from partially hydrogenated oils is expected over the next three years in the food supply including spreads.[184]

It is to be welcomed that trans fats are being phased out. They still exist: many margarines still contain partially hydrogenated oils. Unfortunately, whilst the unfounded persecution of saturated fats persists, which is supported by pharmaceutical interests to support their massive sales of statins, vegetable oils will still be predominantly used in the food industry. This will add to the disease burden. They, of course, are particularly problematic and the wrong choice for deep fat fried food, where they will degrade to ever more harmful products such as aldehydes which, as I have previously mentioned, have been linked to illnesses including cancer, heart disease, and dementia.[185]

Twenty-first Century Food Choices

Surviving in the toxic world that we live in, and maintaining a good degree of health is challenging for many people. There are a great number of factors that can tip the balance as far as our health is concerned; sometimes it is just due to simple good fortune or perhaps better genes that we are able to stay healthy where others may succumb to disease in one form or another. However, there are measures that we can take to stack the cards more in our favour.

One of the most obvious measures we can take is simply to restrict our exposure as much as we can to some of the manmade chemicals in our food, air, water, and the environment we live in. For many, this easier said than done. One of the biggest problems is identifying the source of our exposure, as oftentimes we may not be aware that we are being exposed. The food supply is a classic case. Whilst we may all appreciate that, for example, by choosing organic produce we are limiting our exposure to numerous chemicals, such as herbicides, pesticides, and fungicides, this only works if we choose to purchase fresh produce, or perhaps even grow our own food, and then make our own freshly prepared meals instead of buying pre-prepared meals. For some people, this is not an easy option for a number of reasons.

The food industry is no more interested in creating health than the pharmaceutical industry. All their research and technology is devoted to making money out of supplying, not exactly food, but products—"why buy ingredients when you can buy solutions?" These are the new buzzwords according to Joanna Blythman, who wrote a book called *Swallow This—Serving Up the Food Industry's Darkest Secrets.* The industry remains almost completely opaque to outsiders: she nevertheless obtained access to some of the inner secrets of the food industry in the UK, where they manufacture over 12,000 different chilled food recipes, earning more than £10 billion a year in sales. In 2012, the UK ate its way through 3 billion ready meals. Blythman found that much of the industry speaks a pretty impenetrable language, talking of 'flavour technology systems' and 'flavour delivery systems'. She went to a food industry event, where there was little real food of any kind to be found. She came to the conclusion as she walked around the exhibition that the main point of the food ingredients was to sell food manufacturers wonder products which allowed them to reduce their spending on more costly real ingredients. She mentioned her disappointment when she eventually found something that looked like real food, a fruit salad, and was told that the salad was treated with NatureSeal, and which was able to add 21 days to the shelf life of the product without any discolouration, leaving the fruit 'appearing fresh and natural'.

In 2013, just 25 major chilled food companies operated from 100 highly streamlined production sites, employing around 60,000 people supplying all the major supermarkets in the UK. The executives did not talk about food, but 'product' and 'food ingredient technology'. The technology is constantly changing to meet the different demands of the food technologists. Currently, they are trying to develop product that does not have to appear on any label, as consumers are becoming increasingly aware of the ingredients list and have become more averse to purchasing foods with E-numbers and additives with long and unfamiliar chemical names. Blythman informs us that a ready meals manufacturing facility can be churning out as many as 250,000 servings a day made up of 60 or 70 different products, with one manufacturer boasting making 2.5 million meals a week. [186]

Eric Schlosser, writing back in 2001, in *Fast Food Nation—What the All-American Meal is Doing to the World,* informs us how the American consumption of fast food grew from a mere $6 billion in 1970 to more than $110 billion by 2000, with people spending more on this than higher education, fast cars or computers and software (in 2109 it was estimated to be in excess of $208 billion). He also reveals that the American flavour industry had revenues of $1.4 billion and was churning out ten thousand new processed food products every year in the USA. [187] By 2018 its market had grown to $13.31 billion and is projected to reach $19.72 billion by 2026.[188] The flavour industry has evolved and professes to be able to create virtually any taste requirement, however, the full list of ingredients might prove a little daunting. Schlosser's list of the ingredients that go towards strawberry flavour runs to approximately fifty components, with just a few mentioned here: benzyl isobutyrate, ethyl butyrate, dipropyl ketone, ethyl heptanoate, ethyl methylphenylglycidate, hydroxyphrenyl-2-butanone, 4-methylacetophenone, methyl anthranilate, neryl isobutyrate etc. [189] Tasty huh?

One of the problems we face is that we really have little idea of what actually is in processed food. We are aware of some of the more obvious issues with processed food, from writers such as Michael Moss, who informed us how the food industry worked out the "bliss point", that magical mixture of sugar, salt and fat that captured the consumer's tastebuds, and how they developed the "mouthfeel" by playing with the distribution size and shape of fat globules, and that they found that the size and shape of the salt molecules also affected a swifter and more powerful impact on our tastebuds. He makes the comment:

How To Survive in the 21st Century

Inevitably, the manufacturers of processed food argue that they have allowed us to become the people we want to be, fast and busy, no longer slaves to the stove. But in their hands, the salt, sugar, and fat they have used to propel this social transformation are not nutrients as much as weapons—weapons they deploy, certainly to defeat their competitors but also to keep us coming back for more.

The industry discovered that children's bliss point for sugar was much higher than adults which is why they have been targeted through sweet products, that the industry knows will get them hooked. In 1977, twelve thousand health professionals signed a petition asking the Federal Trade Commission to ban the advertising of sugary foods on children's television shows. It was known that the typical American child in 1979 would watch more than 20,000 commercials between the ages of two and eleven—and more than half of them were promoting sweetened, cereals, candies, snacks and drinks. Sugar was promoted as many as seven times per half hour. The industry, however, successfully fought back against any person or organization that would dare to confront its right to make vast profits at our children's or our expense. They were, however, unable to prevent the rising obesity epidemic in children and in adults, and the rising levels of diabetes. In 1990, a Yale study made headlines for revealing that children's behaviour was affected just by eating two cupcakes. They suffered a tenfold increase in adrenaline and exhibited abnormal behaviour. The WHO proposed changing the recommended daily level of sugar to 10% of a person's calorific intake, citing numerous links between sugar and diabetes, cardiovascular disease, and obesity. In 2011 an independent group from the University of California at Davis reported the finding that those drinking high-fructose corn syrup beverages experienced a 25% jump in their triglycerides, LDL cholesterol, and a fat-binding protein—all markers for heart disease. Moss mentions in his book the work of Anthony Scalafini who discovered how addictive sugar was in a study on rats when he fed them cookies, candies, and sweetened cereals, and found they grew quickly obese. When the sugary food was withdrawn the animals showed signs of withdrawal such as chattering teeth.[190]

Some have responded to the warnings about sugar and highly processed food, and the weight gain associated with this type of diet by cutting down on sugar and choosing low-calorie sweeteners the so-called diet-sodas, that use compounds like aspartame as a sweetener which do not add calories but gives the sweetness. It is known that 36% of people who use sweeteners are obese and, 23% overweight, however, which reveals that there are problems with this approach for people who wish to lose weight. There are a number of studies that do not show weight-decline: in fact, the opposite—they actually show weight gain using alternative sweeteners. Studies show children on diet sodas, for example, gain weight, particularly in boys. Saccharin use in the Nurses' Health Study, that assessed long-term health factors, conducted in the 1970s, was associated with an eight-year weight gain in 31,940 women. Animal studies show a similar response. The current understanding is that artificial sweeteners can make you feel hungry and actually eat more.

Lead researcher Associate Professor Greg Neely from the University of Sydney's Faculty of Science explained their findings: 'After chronic exposure to a diet that contained the artificial sweetener sucralose, we saw that animals began eating a lot more. It was found that in one study fruit flies that were exposed to a diet laced with artificial sweetener for prolonged periods (more than five days) were found to consume 30 percent more calories when they were then given naturally sweetened food.' Neely found that 'chronic consumption of this artificial sweetener actually increases the sweet intensity of real nutritive sugar, and this then increases the animal's overall motivation to eat more food.' They found that there was a significant response to the sweetener in the brain:

'Through systematic investigation of this effect, we found that inside the brain's reward centres, sweet sensation is integrated with energy content. When sweetness versus energy is out of balance for a period of time, the brain recalibrates and increases total calories consumed.'[191] This will not be good news for the manufacturers of these products: no doubt they will fund studies that 'prove' this is not the case, or at least muddy the waters to leave some 'doubt' as they have done in so many other instances.

Obesity is considered to be a global epidemic. In the United States, 30% of adults are classed as obese and 50% of children are considered as being overweight. This creates health problems that increase medical expenses, which are $147 billion annually in the United States and $81 billion in the European Union. The official guidelines recommend reducing calories to lose weight, but the current evidence shows using artificial sweeteners to lose weight is not working. It also introduces further problems. Sucralose, when heated becomes chemically unstable and releases chlorinated aromatic polycyclic hydrocarbons (Cl-PAHs) which are toxic compounds that can accumulate in the body and are associated with various cancers in humans. Another study published in 2018 by Thiago Magalhães Cabral et al, in an international collaboration, came to the same conclusions as the previous studies and further suggested: 'artificial sweeteners, precisely because they are sweet, stimulate the preference for the taste, the desire and the dependence for sweet foods, favoring an increase in the consumption and consequently, weight gain.' They, however, were concerned about the changes such artificial sweeteners were having on the gut flora or the gut microbiome. This is worth reviewing, as it is my belief that if you take care of your gut biome, you will have a much better chance of living a healthy life. It is your direct connection to health: its importance cannot be overstated. Here is their view of the microbiome:

The gut microbiota is a complex environment and influences many functions such as nutrition, energy homeostasis and body control. The microbiota and its metabolites are involved in intestinal permeability, in the mucosal immune function, in intestinal motility and even in the enteric nervous system.

They looked at different populations and found some useful observations:

The main trigger for changes in the flora is the type of food ingested. For example, African children who used to eat grains and large amounts of fiber had microbiota colonies with gram-negative bacteria, to improve the absorption of macronutrients. However, the same children exposed to a diet high in sugar and fat showed a significant change in their microbiota, increasing the Firmicutes and decreasing Bacteroides. With this change, not only did they gain weight, but also presented decreased glucose tolerance. The same change in microbiota is seen with the use of saccharin in animal and human models and in patients with diabetes.

They mention that it is already known that the high-fat, high-carbohydrate diet that we regard as the typical Western diet alters the microbiota. They found that artificial sweeteners also change the flora in the gut, but the changes varied and affected different locations. For example, the metabolism of sucralose happens in the large intestine, whereas the metabolism of aspartame occurs in the small intestine, and each alters the flora in different ways. Their findings should give us some pause for concern, as their model flora using saccharin 'looks like the model flora of diabetes, and the model flora using sucralose looks like the model of autoimmune diseases, with less commensal bacteria, less mucous and more pathogens.' The problem, however, is that many of us will not know whether we are ingesting additives such as sucralose because 'they are intrinsic in foods and not described in labels.'

How To Survive in the 21ˢᵗ Century

They discovered that the gut biome was critically linked to weight gain which, in my view, can help explain why so many people have problems with trying to lose weight:

> The microbiota is important for weight maintenance, as shown by an experimental bypass model that proved that surgically transplanting the flora of thin people would result in lower intake and, consequently, weight loss. Other examples are a study with rats given antibiotics and subsequent use of sweeteners, leading to dysbiosis and insulin resistance, the SUEZ study or even epigenetics of SGA [Small-for-Gestational-Age] newborns with sparing phenotype being more susceptible to obesity. All corroborate the importance of the microbiota and its impact on weight.

The SUEZ study that they refer to was remarkable in its revelations regarding the impact the three main sweeteners; saccharin, sucralose and aspartame on glycemic metabolism, in that they produced a worsening of the glucose tolerance curves, associated with increased insulin resistance and impaired β-cell function, which is the beginning of metabolic syndrome. The feces of, in this case, rats with their altered biota were sampled and transferred to healthy rats without any prior intolerance. What was found, is that these animals began to exhibit the same glycemic changes as their flora donors. Here is what they inferred:

> In this way, it shows that the impact was directly related to the flora. At the end of the study, it elevates the animal-to-human model by placing the glucose-tolerant human microbiota in germ-free mice, and these mice begin to respond poorly to glucose. Leading to the belief that the metabolic pathways used in rats and humans are the same.

This is remarkable and would confirm why oftentimes targeting the gut biome by dealing with any dysbiosis and, introducing a different dietary regime to improve the flora composition, sometimes aided by fasting, is able to turn around our health status and defeat both diabetes and obesity. They tell us that saccharin and aspartame raise the production of butyrate in the body and that has led to an increase in the number of Bacteroidetes in the gut. It is these bacteria that 'are directly associated with weight gain'. They also inform us that 'sweeteners such as sucralose and saccharin do not stimulate the hypothalamic area. They have other reward areas'. Which could contribute to the brain's response to increasing the feeling of hunger. Finally, these products 'lead to a typical inflammation of obesity, and worsening response to sugar intake'.[192]

Gut Biome and Health

There is much more interest in discussing what is now commonly being referred to as "the microbiome": this is being recognized as having a much more important role in our health than was previously thought. This is an area of study I have been interested in for some time. When I studied nutrition, Dr Jensen's book *Tissue Cleansing Through Bowel Management* was required reading, and *Probiotics—How 'Friendly Bacteria' Can Restore Health and Vitality*, by Leon Chaitow, written in 1990, was already a familiar read. Whilst the former volume may not have a rivetingly exciting title, the contents had a lasting impression. I particularly remember the images accompanying the story of a woman who was heading for a foot amputation due to the ulcerations on her foot and lower leg were failing to heal and turning gangrenous. This woman desperately, not wishing to lose her foot and lower leg, sought help from Dr Jensen. She was given colonic irrigation, and pictures were taken of her foot over a period of a few weeks as it slowly healed. Pictures were also taken of the results of colonic irrigation, which produced long lengths of dark fetid material that had previously impacted along the length of her intestine, not just the colon—all due to excessive ingestion of over-processed white flour products. [193]

Discussion of anything to do with bowels is normally considered taboo. People just don't like to talk about this subject. As a nutritionist, however, trained old-school, it is a topic that is important to discuss with any patient, as are energy levels and general health. Leon Chaitow's book introduced the reader to the benefits of real yoghurt, typically cultured with Lactobacillus bulgaricus, and Streptococcus thermophiles. Whilst not considered big-time residents of the human GI tract, they were considered helpful bacteria. Both, for example, were shown to have powerful anti-tumour activity. The intestinal flora is known to be helpful in many different ways. One way is the ability to manufacture B vitamins, such as biotin, niacin (B3), pyridoxine (B6), B12, and folic acid. Many of the beneficial flora are known to play a role in protecting against the negative effects of radiation and toxic pollutants, aside from enhancing the immune function. Certain strains of the Lactobacillus acidophilus are able to produce antibiotic substances such as acidophilin, lactolin, and acidolin, which help protect us from unfriendly invading pathogens, such as some of the Salmonella bacteria. By producing acids, the Lactobacilli inhibit potentially dangerous pathogens such as E.coli and Streptococci.[194]

Interest in the microbiome by mainstream science is to be welcomed. When you consider that the bacteria in our gut outnumber our cells by estimates that vary from ten to one to one hundred to one, it raises the question of just how human are we? Yet this relationship with bacteria is ancient. Estimates for human cells vary from 30-100 trillion: this represents more than 300-3000 trillion microbes, representing approximately 5,000 different species, and weighing roughly a kilo in the gut. We cannot exist without these bacteria. That is why using antibiotics should be considered very seriously before taking them, loss of the microbiome leads to diarrhea, rapid weight loss, dehydration, and death if the bacterial colonies are destroyed. The evidence of microbes in meconium, and the fact that when babies are born (in natural deliveries) they adopt their mother's flora suggests an intricate and historic relationship. This suggests that our evolution is alongside a co-existence with the world of bacteria (and also viruses and fungi), a symbiotic relationship stretching back to the beginning of human life.

Researchers from Emory University, Atlanta, Georgia, found that gut microbiota differ in obese individuals versus lean individuals, and differs again between healthy individuals and those with atherosclerosis, diabetes, and metabolic syndrome. They mention that when fecal microbiota are transplanted from lean, healthy donors, it was found to improve insulin sensitivity in men with metabolic syndrome. They found that atherosclerosis is associated with specific gut microbiota and may be fueled by the intake of specific dietary components that the gut microbiota synthesize into trimethylamine-N-oxide (TMAO) which is associated with increased risk of major cardiovascular events. They also found that individuals with type 2 diabetes had distinctive gut microbiome makeup that had fewer anti-inflammatory properties. They concluded that diversity was key to health:

> A wide diversity of gut microbiota is currently thought to be the healthier composition than having only a select few bugs. This diversity is affected by a varied diet rich in plants, vegetables and fruit, so those who have a limited diet also have a low diversity of microbiota. Aging is associated with decreasing microbial diversity and the reduced diversity correlates with nutritional status, increased inflammation and frailty.[195]

Interest is such that researchers are examining gut flora all over the world, and finding a very wide diversity, much wider compared to that found in the Western countries which is linked to processed food and extensive use of antibiotics. Michael Pollan became interested in the microbiome and reiterated the importance of the gut biota's role in vitamin manufacturing, such as the B vitamins and vitamin K, but also neurotransmitters such as serotonin, short-chain fatty acids, and amino acids. In an article titled "Some of My Best Friends are Germs," he mentions research that shows how the gut epithelium is supported by certain bacteria, such as the Bifidobacteria and Lactobacillus planetarium which are common in fermented vegetables. They actually feed the epithelium layer of the gut by producing short-chain fatty acids which maintain the structural integrity of this layer. When the epithelium is not well nourished, it is known to become permeable which can allow endotoxins from pathogens and even proteins from foods like gluten can gain passageway directly into the blood system, creating low-grade inflammation, and provoking an immune response. This can lead to food intolerances, allergies, infection, and chronic disease.

Pollan refers to a study by Patrice Cani that found when a junk food diet was fed to mice their gut flora changed and they also developed a more permeable gut barrier which allowed endotoxins to leak into their bloodstream. This led to a low-grade infection and eventually to metabolic syndrome. Pollan believes that if this suggests that inflammation in the gut may be the cause of metabolic syndrome, which it seems to imply, and not just in animals but humans, 'then medical science may be on the trail of a Grand Unified Theory of Chronic Disease, at the very heart of which we will find the gut microbiome.'[196]

Sayer Ji, the founder of GreenMed Info, adds to the mystique of the microbiome by adding a few useful detoxifying properties of some microbes, such as Bifidobacterium breve and Lactobacillus casei. They have been found to help the body detoxify Bisphenol A, the ubiquitous plastic toxicant. Lactobacillus bacteria have also been found to attach themselves to heavy metals in the gut which allows them to be safely excreted. They also are able to safely break down heterocyclic aromatic amines, the compounds that can be produced when meat is cooked at high temperatures, compounds which are extremely mutagenic. He also reports on the ability of the probiotic strains of kimchi, a traditional Korean dish of fermented cabbage to degrade organophosphorous pesticide compounds. Bifdobacterium bifidum, which is found in breast milk has been found to degrade the toxin perchlorate, an ingredient in jet fuel that is also a ubiquitous toxin, This was linked to the discovery that babies that are breast-fed have much lower levels of this toxicant than bottle-fed babies.[197]

No doubt we will hear more about the marvellous gut biome. Suffice it to say here that I believe if you nurture your gut biome, it will nurture you. If you choose to treat it like a sewer and eat a lot of highly processed food, fast foods and drinks that are laced with unknown chemicals and sweeteners, including sugar, the chances are not good that it will support your gut biome and your health in the long term.

Foods that actively support healthier intestinal flora supply plant fibre, much of it from inulin, a fibre known to promote gut bacteria, reduce constipation and help break down fat. Foods like chicory root, dandelion greens, and the onion family, including staple onions, garlic, and leeks all promote a healthy gut but also supply antioxidants, anti-inflammatory compounds, anti-cancer compounds, and antimicrobial effects. Garlic and onions also contain another prebiotic called fructooligosaccharides (FOS) that feed the beneficial bacteria. Asparagus, oats, apples, and flaxseed are all great prebiotics; they each provide additional benefits with antioxidants, anti-inflammatory and anti-cancer properties. Flaxseeds also help regulate blood sugar levels and supply omega-3 essential fatty acids. Seaweed also is a potent prebiotic, it is rich in antioxidants and supplies a useful source of minerals. However, is rarely used in Western countries. Jerusalem artichokes are also high in inulin, so are very beneficial, and also have the added benefit of high levels of thiamine and potassium.[198]

Toxic Food

We briefly mentioned aspartame. Used as an artificial sweetener, it has been labelled as an excitotoxin as has Monosodium glutamate (MSG). In the early 1950s, a neuroscientist by the name of Dr T Hayaski found that when MSG was injected into the grey matter of a dog's brain, the dog would fall down in his cage and begin to convulse wildly. He concluded that glutamate was causing the dog's brain cells to become overexcited and fire uncontrollably. Despite the importance of this discovery, he was mostly ignored. Other researchers found a similar effect with another amino acid, aspartate. Eventually, they discovered over seventy such excitatory amino acids. Meanwhile, the food industry found that these products so enhanced the taste of their bland foods, they were being used in more and more products and being disguised. MSG and its related toxins were disguised as "hydrolysed vegetable protein", "natural flavourings" and "spices" In 1974, Dr John W Olney demonstrated that MSG fed to pregnant rats would cause brain damage to their offspring. He also found that the amount of MSG in commercially available soup was high enough to raise the blood glutamate level in children that predictably caused brain damage in immature animals. He found that humans concentrate glutamate in their blood to a greater degree than other animal species, and he was well aware that a child's brain is four times more sensitive to excitotoxins than an adult's. Neurosurgeon Dr Russell Blaylock, in his book, *Excitotoxins—The Taste That Kills,* informs us how neurons exposed to high amounts of MSG swell up and then die within an hour with low doses, however, they don't swell they just suddenly die two hours later. This is something he finds is characteristic of MSG, aspartate and other excitotoxins.

What troubles him is that he believes the typical American diet can contain anywhere from 10-20 grams of excitotoxin a day. The foods he has listed that contain MSG include plant protein extract, yeast extract, textured protein, hydrolysed flour, and sodium caseinate, amongst others. He further lists other additives that frequently contain MSG: malt extract, malt flavouring, bouillon, broth, stock, natural flavouring, natural beef or chicken flavouring, and seasoning. This is by no means an exhaustive list.[199] As regards to health symptoms, Dr Janet Starr Hull, in her book *Sweet Poison—How the World's Most Popular Artificial Sweetener Is Killing Us My Story*, lists 92 negative health effects.[200] Obviously, a lot more could be said about this, but this is beyond the scope of this volume. Those who wish further information on any of the topics I raise are advised to further explore the sources provided.

Joanna Blythman, already mentioned, has looked into the components of the food industry a little deeper than most and what she has discovered might give us pause for concern. Just picking a random page and she is discussing plastic food packaging and how they are treated with a microscopic layer of chemicals, such as alkyl mono- and disulfonic acids, aluminium borate and N,N-bis(2-hydroxyethyl) dodecanamide. Apparently, they are there to provide an 'anti-fog' effect, by stopping the build-up of dewy moisture in the container. She reports that the Food Packaging Forum, a not-for-profit, independent foundation recently warned that 175 dangerous chemicals are found in food packaging, 'Chemicals of Concern', linked to cancer, reduced fertility, genital malformations, and hormone disruption. Apparently, because it is associated with packaging the food, the industry can use whatever chemicals they feel disposed to and do not have to declare their use. She also mentions the use of nanoparticles, an emerging technology that uses particles so small (about one tenthousandth the width of a human hair) that they can end up in places in the human body that larger cells would not be able to reach. She cites the example of nanoscale zinc oxide, which has been found to cause lesions in the liver, pancreas, heart, and stomach in animals. Nanoparticles of titanium dioxide have been found to damage DNA, disrupt cell function and interfere with the immune system. Apparently, 400-500 nano packaging products are estimated to be in use currently, and are expected to account for 25% of all food packaging by 2020. Nanosized titanium dioxide is apparently already in use in coffee creamer, cookies, cream cheese, turkey gravy, lemonade and chocolate. Nanoparticles may even be in the coating on your 'fresh' fruit and vegetables, to extend shelf life.[201]

Novel Enzymes

Brief mention can be made of the use of enzymes in the food industry, as nearly all commercially prepared foods contain at least one ingredient that has been made with one of the 150 enzymes believed to be in use in the food industry. Regulators have classified enzymes as processing aids and as such, under European law, they do not have to be labelled, even if they are genetically modified, which many of them are. Blythman expresses concern about enzymes that survive heat in the production process and leave us with fungal alpha-amylase, where 20% of its allergenicity can survive in the crusts of bread. She also mentions transglutaminase, an elasticizer used in bread, pastries and low-quality meat products, that has been found to generate the epitope [part of a molecule] responsible for coeliac disease. She believes that the proteases, enzymes that are effective as detergents but are commonly used in baking, as being 'the most likely to cause allergies and sensitivities because they have the easiest access to the bloodstream and soft tissues.[202]

There are about 3000 known enzymes produced by all animals, green plants, fungi, and bacteria that catalyze about 4000 biochemical reactions. A number of them have been known to play an important role in the food manufacturing industries. Genetically modified recombinant microorganisms have been used to synthesize enzymes for further application in food. The rDNA techniques have been available since the 1970s. Using genetic engineering has enabled increased production processes. There are numerous microorganisms that have been genetically modified to produce a variety of enzymes, which are said to contribute to their role in industries such as baking, beverages, cheese, dairy, egg-based products, and so forth. One important GMO-derived enzyme used in the dairy industry is chymosin (a microbially produced rennet-like enzyme) employed for cheese-making. In 1990, this chymosin obtained from GMO technology was granted generally regarded as safe status by the FDA in the United States and approximately 90% of the cheese produced in the United States is made using fermentation-produced chymosin. Two enzymes, lipase and GO, are often produced with the help of GMMs that are normally added in order to preserve and maintain egg powder along with its colour. Another enzyme manufactured by GMOs, such as pectinase for fruit-and beverage-processing has been in use for more than 15 years.[203]

Acrylamide

In 2002, the discovery that acrylamide, a chemical used in the manufacture of plastics and in water treatment, was found in a large number of foods sounded alarm bells, as it was known to be genotoxic and a carcinogen. The discovery was made by Swedish researchers undertaking blood tests in men following a tunnel accident. It sparked research that showed many foodstuffs, predominantly starch-based products were the source. Jenni Russell, writing in *The Guardian* in 2002, revealed that foods such as crispbreads were found to contain from 330-2,300 micrograms per kilogram of acrylamide, oven chips from 301-1,104 (the over-cooked ones scoring the higher reading), breakfast cereals from 340-1,400. This raised concerns particularly for children who were seen as more likely to consume many of the products tested. Leif Busk, the head of research at

Sweden's National Food Administration, suggested that children were more likely to be damaged by it because their cells are dividing more rapidly and acrylamide is known to affect dividing cells. He also indicated that he believed acrylamide is 1,000 times more dangerous than the majority of carcinogens in food.[204]

Acrylamide is one of the by-products created by what is known as the Maillard reaction, one of the most common and most complex reactions that takes place mainly in foods. The Maillard reaction occurs on heating or during prolonged storage and is one of the deteriorative processes that take place in stored foods. It is one on the non-enzymatic browning reactions. One of the most common being the reaction of carbonyl compounds, especially reducing sugars, with compounds which contain a free amino group, such as amino acids, amines and proteins.[205]

Research shows that even the youngest of our offspring are affected by the industrialized food system, with powdered infant formulas found to contain significant levels of acrylamide. A group of Brazilian scientists found that during prolonged heating or storage of the powdered infant formula, a wide variety of reactive compounds are formed, which can then polymerize with protein residues and form dark pigments or melanoidins. This is following the manufacturing process that includes: pasteurization, homogenization, concentration in a vacuum evaporator, and drying in spray dryer, processes that incorporate 'a large number of thermal processes, the formulas' that 'are subject to a series of reactions that can negatively impact their quality, among them the Maillard reaction'. They mention that the Maillard reaction also contributes to other volatile compound formation, primarily aldehydes and aminoketones. The melanoidins, however, have metal chelating properties, which means they bind to metals that according to the researchers 'may be undesirable when they affect nutritionally essential minerals (Ca, Mg, Cu, Zn, Fe) and subsequently impede metabolism and mineral absorption.' The researchers also point out that the final products resulting from the Maillard reaction are advanced glycated end products (AGEs), which we introduced in chapter three, in the section on metabolic syndrome. They point out 'A large number of AGEs have been identified in vivo' which all 'contribute to AGES accumulation in the body'.[206]

They also inform us that AGEs can cause tissue damage generated by structure and protein changes; inter- or intramolecular cross-linking; free radical formation, and inflammation due to the interaction of these compounds with specific receptors. They suggest as a result, 'excess AGE accumulation in body tissue seems to contribute to the development of chronic disorders such as diabetes, weight gain, cardiovascular diseases and neurodegenerative diseases, i.e., Alzheimer's, Parkinson's, and schizophrenia. In addition, AGEs may contribute to the development of arthritis, bone mass loss, and disorders involving the function and/or structure of DNA and RNA molecules'.[207]

This is a brief review of some aspects of food production that may or may not affect your food choices. It is not my intent to scare everyone to death and make people paranoid about what they eat. It is my hope that this information may actually bring about a real change of thinking. Many people may feel that they have little choice as to what they can eat, perhaps due to financial circumstance, some perhaps due to where they live—perhaps they live in an area with poor shopping facilities. I do, however, believe that having the capacity for a more-informed choice should enable us to not just live healthier lives but also create a better world.

How To Survive in the 21ˢᵗ Century

We have reviewed some fundamental principles in nutrition that have hopefully enabled people to have a clearer picture of what can constitute "healthy food". Understanding about the fats and oils will hopefully be seen as important and useful and will, in itself, lead to a better health outlook. Introducing the importance of the gut biome will hopefully enable more people to develop a better and more respectful relationship with their own body and its *real* needs. The information about the food industry should help inform us how to make better food choices and realize that reliance on their products creates serious challenges for our bodies. Radical change is required if we truly wish to create a world than nurtures health and protects our children and their future. In the next chapter, we can look at some further strategies that will help create more survivors and fewer casualties of the industrialized food and agricultural system.

Chapter Eight

Primary Ingredients of Life

There are some ingredients that are fundamentally important to life. Getting them in the right format and in the right amount, without unnecessary adulteration, is very important for plant health, animal health, and for our health. In this chapter, we will look at this idea briefly, and give some examples of what this really means for our health.

The issue of health has fostered massive media coverage, including numerous books, articles, podcasts, interviews etc. I didn't want this volume to be just another 'health' book: I wanted it to reflect where my research was taking me, and offer a different perspective and examine some of the deeper issues involved. Whether it is immediately obvious or not, much of the information on health is trying to sell you something. It is not enough to say simply "follow the money" and look for the financial ties behind the information you are being asked to believe. Most of the time, the information you are being asked to swallow may be coming from an eminent authority, no doubt with expert credentials, and often their ties to corporate interests are not easily discovered. One thing I have discovered, however, is how to dig, how to uncover, and how to tell the difference between someone selling the corporate agenda, and true science—of which I feel there is far too little.

How To Survive in the 21st Century

One of the ways corporations seek to manipulate us is to make things complicated and seem difficult to understand. If they can numb your mind and put you off enquiring too deeply, they can exploit this to their advantage—just look at the statin or antidepressant or opioid explosions as an example—a classic miss-selling of drugs that we don't need, and health consequences that we are still unravelling. Whilst I will engage you with some science, underlying this will be a simple principle or objective—basically that human beings to maintain health need basic nutrients that are essential to support life, and that whatever prevents this from occurring needs to be addressed.

One idea that is presented here is how there has been a huge reluctance, particularly by the medical fraternity, to acknowledge the true nutritional value of food. This can be illustrated by some of the stories that I share with you below that illustrate how it took decades for doctors to accept the importance of B vitamins, for example, and to take this information on board—though some, it could be argued, still have not taken on board. It has been suggested that the medical profession felt threatened by the world of nutrition because it was a subject they had never really studied, and today this is still considered to be the case for a great majority of doctors. Nevertheless, the basic principles and ideas of nutrition are fundamental to health and relatively easy to understand, and at least with a few examples of the story of their discovery are worth sharing with you.

Take water, for example, something that is absolutely essential to life—yet access to something so fundamental as water that is fit to drink is not as easy as it should be.

Primary Ingredients of Life

Water for Life

Water is the basis of all life. The human body is composed of more than 60% water. Our brains have an even higher requirement for water, being approximately 73% water. Supplying our requirement for water in the 21st century is challenging, not so much for its lack of availability (though for many this is an important consideration) but more due to the quality. In industrialized countries, the challenge is to be able get access to water that is fit to drink and not encumbered with numerous contaminants that are either hazardous to our health or make the water taste so poor that many choose not to drink it and instead choose beverages that seem more appealing—which unfortunately is far too often the case.

It is important to establish a good source of drinkable water. This may not be as easy as you might think. In my previous volume *Unhealthy Betrayal*, I reported on the contamination from pesticides and herbicides, such as atrazine which affects much of the groundwater in numerous American and European states. Agricultural pollution, however, is not the only source of water contamination: much contamination comes from industrial production, and from some unsuspecting sources. In 2016 the German Environment Agency undertook a review of human and veterinary pharmaceutical substances that reported worldwide on surface water, groundwater, tap/drinking water, and the environment generally. They found 631 different pharmaceuticals. They found the anti-inflammatory drug diclofenac in the environment of 50 countries, and in several locations at 'ecotoxicologically relevant concentrations'. The non-steroid anti-inflammatory drug diclofenac is believed to have caused the near-extinction of vultures on the Indian subcontinent due to the birds feeding on the carcasses of cattle treated with the drug. It is also believed to be responsible for damaging the inner organs of rainbow trout. More than 100 different pharmaceutical substances have been found in several European countries and the USA. The most commonly found therapeutic substances are antibiotics, analgesics, and hormones. The study concluded that 'pharmaceuticals in the environment are a global challenge calling for a multi-stakeholder and multi-sector approach to prevent, reduce, and manage pharmaceuticals entering the environment.'[208]

I wrote more about the industrial contaminants in *Unhealthy Betrayal,* about DDT, PCBs, dioxin contamination, and the various sources etc. Due to limited space, all I intend here is to discuss how the water treatment plants in most countries rely on simple filtration systems that minimally filter the water, and generally treat the water with chlorine to control the pathogenic content. Filtering out the many manmade chemicals is highly costly so is generally not undertaken. This is problematical, as it leaves us with an unknown array of chemicals, depending on our respective water sources and suppliers, and the chlorine treatment which in itself is a hazard.

Chlorine chemistry can be compared to entering a minefield, or according to Professor Joe Thornton: "Chlorine chemistry is a Pandora's box, opened less than 100 years ago and still spewing its demons into the environment." He reports that the German government's Council of Environmental Advisors concluded in 1991, "The dynamic growth of chlorine chemistry during the 50s and 60s represents a decisive mistake in twentieth century industrial development, which would not have occurred had our present knowledge as to environmental damage and health risks due to chlorine chemistry then been available." Chlorine is a highly reactive chemical, being a large atom with two electrons in its inner shell, eight in its middle shell and seven in its outer shell—which leaves it unbalanced and needing another electron to give it stability. Sodium, on the other hand, has a single electron in its outer shell, which it will happily part with, and which will readily react with chlorine, combining violently, to produce sodium chloride—which then becomes a more stable compound. We know this as our common table salt. Chlorine, being so highly reactive, particularly with organic matter (carbon-based molecular compounds) gives rise to a huge range of what are referred to as 'organochlorines'. The trouble with them is they can be highly toxic to biological systems, and there are more than 11,000 of them. The organochlorines tend to persist and accumulate in biological systems, particularly the fat-soluble ones. Because historically we were never exposed to such manmade chemicals, we have not evolved the enzymes in our bodies to break them down. The infamous 2,3,7,8-tetrachlorodibenzo-p-dioxin (TCDD), is not just one of the most toxic products, created in numerous chemical processes by man, it is also one of the most persistent, and will most likely exist indefinitely. This is why Professor Thornton suggests we should abandon the use of chlorine and replace it with less dangerous products. Here is what he has to say about us opening Pandora's box: 'While governments, cheered on by those who benefit from the open box, try to chase down each and every tiny demon that escapes, we miss the simplest and most obvious solution: close the lid.'[209]

The issue we are faced with, due to engaging with so many products that use chlorine in their chemical manufacture is that so many harmful by-products are being continuously created by many industries, such as the paper pulp industry, pesticide industry, plastics and PVC industry, wood preservative industry etc. It would greatly serve the interests of mankind if the love affair with chlorine would end. The PVC industry also incorporates in excess of 4 million tons of phthalates and more than 124,000 tons of lead in its worldwide production. Combusting PVC will lead to the serious release of these products aside from the notorious dioxin TCDD. In the USA thousands of tons of PVC are sent to incinerators (estimated in 2000 at between 200,000 to 300,000 tons).

It should be obvious that we need to find a better way of purifying our water than methods currently employed that rely on adding a poison like chlorine. Yes, it will kill microorganisms that might otherwise cause us problems, but it does so with an added threat, that is to permit this highly-reactive molecule to react with many other chemicals in the water, forming more dangerous and hazardous products and further enabling the chlorine to react with the contents of our bodies creating yet more hazardous products. Among the by-products created by water chlorination are the trihalomethanes, including chloroform, and dichlorobromomethane, which are produced in relatively large amounts and are known to be carcinogenic. Studies on water and birth outcomes have shown chlorinated water to be associated with various birth defects including reduced birthweight, malformations of the heart, oral cleft, and nervous system.[210]

Reducing personal exposure can be aided by simple filtration systems. Avoiding water consumption due to the taste or concerns about the problems raised here are not recommended, as we can limit our exposure by simple filtration remedies. Turning to other drinks does not necessarily mean that these drinks do not contain chlorinated water and even more hazardous products, although perhaps masked by other tastes. Drinking water has to be a pleasure and aid us in staying healthy: it is the basis of life itself.

Maintaining Sanity

How do we keep our mental balance when surrounded by so many things that seem to pose a threat to our health and greater wellbeing? The explosion of the use of antidepressants and opiates, and the alarming increase in dementia and

Alzheimer's disease, suggest that a significant portion of the population might be having difficulty with keeping mind, body, and soul together.

Mental health is a subject that has interested me greatly: it is an area of study that I have pursued for many years. There is now emerging a much greater interest in the metabolic status of people and the effect of various diets on our health status. Even within this development, however, there is still much confusion. I add this discussion because it can play a hugely significant part in someone's life. In my view, some doctors are far too quick at prescribing antidepressants that can add more problems to a person's life. Most people are resilient and, with emotional support and perhaps some therapeutic guidance will meet the challenge of their depression, overcome their anxiety, and learn how deal with what life is throwing at them, actually learning something valuable about themselves in the process. Unfortunately, in the USA their health insurance does not cover the alternative approaches, whereas it does cover medication that can harm them.

Dr Carl Pfeiffer was influential in highlighting how a number of simple nutrient deficiencies were found to be responsible for problematic mental conditions. Working as the director of the non-profit Brain Bio Center in Princetown, New Jersey, with a team of thirty-five, including seven other scientists, they published more than 300 scientific research papers in leading journals throughout the world. One of the discoveries he reported on was the finding that many depressed and mentally ill people were deficient in vitamin B_6 and zinc, and that it was no ordinary deficiency, but caused by the abnormal production of pyrroles. They found that approximately 30% of schizophrenics suffered from "pyroluria", and 11% of normal people suffered from it as well. They also found that 50% of schizophrenics had low blood levels of histamine.

This imbalance was found to be linked to too much copper in the body, which was linked to lack of vitamin C and exposure to copper. Both vitamin C and vitamin B$_3$ were used to great effect to counter this imbalance. The source of this problem varied: in some people, it was caused by contraception (both birth control pills and copper IUDs), in others, from copper pipes. As regards to schizophrenia, he found five principal causes:

1. Histapenia—low blood histamine with excess copper (50% of schizophrenics).
2. Histadelia—high blood histamine with low copper (20% of schizophrenics).
3. Pyroluria—a familial double deficiency of zinc and vitamin B$_6$ (30% of schizophrenics).
4. Cerebral allergy—includes wheat-gluten allergy (10% of schizophrenics).
5. Nutritional hypoglycaemia--20% of schizophrenics. [211]

These percentages do not add up to 100% due to the fact that some of the patients suffered from more than one of these symptoms. Hypoglycemia refers to low blood sugar whilst this is not a disease, it nevertheless is a situation that can affect our ability to adequately function. People on highly processed carbohydrates and high sugar diets can experience real highs and lows in blood sugar levels that affect cognitive functioning in measurable ways.

The use of niacin (vitamin B$_3$) for the treatment for schizophrenia was associated with Dr Abram Hoffer (M.D., PhD), a Canadian biochemist, physician and psychiatrist, who pioneered the use of megavitamin therapy and other nutritional interventions for the treatment of schizophrenia, which developed to become known as Orthomolecular Medicine.

Primary Ingredients of Life

Niacin is such an important vitamin, it is worth diverging here to inform you about its discovery and its significance to your health. It is worth repeating that niacin raises the HDL cholesterol level (the "good" cholesterol) more than any known pharmaceutical, whilst simultaneously lowering total cholesterol, triglycerides and LDL cholesterol, the supposed "bad" cholesterol. Niacin is transformed in the cells into nicotinamide adenine dinucleotide (NAD) and is used in more than 450 biochemical reactions, more than any other vitamin-derived co-factor. Many nutritionists believe the story of how niacin was discovered should be taught in schools: I offer a brief version here.

In 1914, pellagra had reached epidemic proportions in the American South Doctors were convinced it was contagious. Whole areas of South Carolina, Georgia and Mississippi were swept with the strange flame-red skin rash 100,000 people died from pellagra. No doctors could be persuaded to go and discover the cause. Eventually, Dr Joseph Goldberger, an excellent bacteriologist from New York and an expert on tropical diseases volunteered to deal with the outbreak. He went straight to the hospitals and insane asylums at the centre of the outbreaks and quickly discovered that it was not a contagious disease. He became convinced that it was diet-related. He found the disease was more pronounced in the less wealthy members of the population, and all were eating a lot of highly processed and sugary foods: cornmeal mush, hominy grits, and cane sugar syrup. Goldberger changed the diets in two of the orphanages in the affected area by removing the sugar and over-reliance on the processed corn—in the face of considerable scepticism—as few doctors believed the disease could be related to diet. He, nevertheless, succeeded in restoring health in the two orphanages. Still faced with disbelief in the medical profession, he instituted a trial with some male prison volunteers to go on a diet on the best white bread, corn pone, hominy grits, sweet potatoes, salt pork, cane syrup, cabbage and coffee. Eventually, the diet produced the tell-tale signs of pellagra, the red rash. Doctors confirmed it was indeed pellagra. William Dufty, who reported on this story, in his excellent book *Sugar Blues,* suggested that Goldberger was totally unappreciated for what he did. 'Was Goldberger awarded a Nobel Prize that year or any year? Did he receive a Congressional Medal of Honor or a medal from the AMA? A few of the best minds in medicine accepted his findings. The vocal majority landed on Goldberger like a ton of bricks. They challenged his findings, they vilified him.' He made the fatal error of promoting the importance of the role of nutrition and diet in health, which was perceived even then as threatening to the pharmaceutical industry and to doctors with no training in nutrition. It took until the 1940s before the US government mandated the addition of niacinamide to flour: they also mandated the addition of thiamine (B_1) and riboflavin (vitamin B_2).[212]

It is hard to over-emphasize the importance of B vitamins, particularly when mental impairment is concerned. Check out this list of symptoms:

- Irritability
- Apathy
- Sleeplessness
- Suspiciousness and paranoia
- Depression (including postpartum depression)
- Memory loss
- Dementia, intellectual deterioration
- Hallucinations
- Violent behavior
- Development delay and autism in children
- Decreased vision, loss of vision
- Tremor paralysis

- Weakness, chronic fatigue

This is just a partial list of symptoms for B_{12} deficiency, part of the symptom list provided by Dr Jeffrey Stuart and his fellow author Sally Pacholok, in their excellent volume *Could It Be B12?—An Epidemic of Misdiagnoses.* They wrote their book after Sally self-diagnosed B_{12} deficiency in herself which led them to discover that, 'An epidemic is raging and virtually undetected by medical professionals,' and that epidemic was B_{12} deficiency.

This epidemic is caused by a number of factors in different populations. The older section of society is already considered a vulnerable population due to a lowering of their ability to produce intrinsic factor which is essential for the absorption and use of B_{12}. Added to this problem can be a number issues involving the use of medications, such as proton pump inhibitors, H2 blockers for heartburn or ulcers, antacids, and biguanides for diabetes (which is just a selection, not a full list of antagonists that affect B_{12} uptake). Another source can be pernicious anemia, in which an autoimmune process destroys the cells that produce the intrinsic factor. Birth control pills are another common culprit as a B_{12} antagonist, and so is the use of nitrous oxide as an anesthetic.

One source of deficiency has been found among mothers on vegetable-based diets, such as vegans and vegetarians, due to the main source for B_{12} being animal protein. There is a much higher demand for nutrients when producing a baby and following delivery to, sustain a baby's health via breastfeeding. Stuart and Pacholok report a 2000 study finding that 24% of vegetarians and 78% of vegans were found to be deficient in B_{12}. Mothers with lower levels risk compromising the health of their child and, if not rectified, it can cause permanent impairment. They recommend not using a microwave for heating milk formula, milk or meat, as it destroys B_{12}. They suggest that giving autistic children supplemental B_{12} via injections, reduces hyperactivity and gives improvements in speech. They believe that normal plasma levels of B_{12} should be higher than 550pg/ml. For brain and nervous system health and prevention of disease in older adults, serum B_{12} levels should be maintained near or above 1,000 pg/ml. There is a lot more that could be said on the topic of B_{12}, as its effect on the brain and nervous system is so critical and deficiencies left too long, particularly in young, growing children, can lead to permanent impairment. Stuart and Pacholok also believe that older people in retirement homes should be routinely tested for B_{12} levels.[213]

Before leaving our discussion of some of the B vitamins, another anecdote is worth repeating that illustrates how our over-refining of food can cause serious problems for us. Our story takes place in Java in the 1890s and concerned the outbreak of beriberi disease. Top German doctors were sent to discover what caused beriberi, most of them died or were sent home on stretchers. One doctor who survived decided to undertake a return visit and worked in a small hospital for beriberi victims. His name was Dr Christian Eijkman. His interest was aroused by the behaviour of some of the chickens, who at one point seemed to be suffering from the same symptoms but then seemed to recover. This happened when the supply of rice was changed. They apparently had a shortage of the white refined rice and so fed the chickens on brown unrefined rice. He discovered that the native population did not suffer from beriberi, nor did their chickens. The natives refused to eat the diet of white bread, jams, and sweet deserts, and white rice of the colonial population. As the chickens had improved on the diet of brown rice he concluded that there was something on the outside of the rice grain that protected the animals from getting beriberi. He made his report to the authorities in 1893. He was, however, totally ignored. It wasn't until 1911 that a Polish chemist by the name of Dr Casimir Funk decided to look into Eijkman's theory that the truth was discovered. Funk spent months grinding rice until he had enough of the polishings, the rice bran, to make into a solution. He fed a sample to a pigeon paralyzed by beriberi. It recovered within a few hours. He believed that a vital substance for health was removed by the refining of rice, and he decided to call it a vitamin, from the Latin word vita for life, and the word amine from amino acids, the components of protoplasm. It wasn't until 1936, when Dr Robert R Williams finally was able to produce crystals from a whole ton of rice polishings and discover its molecular makeup that he was able to say that thiamine or vitamin B_1 had been truly discovered and Eijkman's theory proved.[214] I reported this story in my first volume, *Unhealthy Betrayal,* as with the pellagra story because I feel they are both important stories and very little known. And have we learned anything from them? It would appear not if the sales of white rice and its use in the restaurant trade are anything to go by. Am I wrong?

The Wonders of Vitamin C

It is beyond the scope of this volume to delve into the world of supplement use to any great depth. Vitamin C, however, is too important not to discuss. If for some reason I was going to restrict myself to taking only take one supplement, vitamin C would be my obvious choice. Personally, with such an impoverished food supply, even with a good intake of fruit and vegetables, I believe it would be difficult to obtain adequate nutrients to produce optimum health and maintain it in the face of so much pollution. It would be hard not to suggest taking some supplements, at least a multivitamin and mineral supplement would be my minimum recommendation with the addition of vitamin C.

Vitamin C is useful in so many ways, it has been suggested as the single most threatening substance to the pharmaceutical industry's profits that exists. It is well known that they funded innumerable studies on vitamin C using such low levels therapeutically that they showed little or no benefit, simply so they could then say that 'there are innumerable studies that show vitamin C as ineffective in treating'…. whatever health issue they wish to promote their drug use over. For many of you what I reveal here about vitamin C will no doubt be news to you, which in many ways is a shame: it shouldn't be hidden information. However, I hope to reveal some of vitamin C's secrets and use here and give you some sources to get further information if you so wish.

Dr Abram Hoffer, who we have already discussed, used to use vitamin C alongside his use of B$_3$ to decrease the oxidation of adrenaline into psychosis causing adrenochrome. He found schizophrenia 'one of the severest oxidative stress conditions.' What he discovered was that some of his schizophrenic patients who also had cancer began to respond to the large doses of vitamin C. He found that sarcomas were particularly responsive to large doses of vitamin C. One of his patients with cancer was taking 40,000 milligrams each day; six months later her tumor was no longer visible on the CT scan. Hoffer was so astounded that he worked with more cancer patients treating more than 1500 patients and found, 'The results of my treatment have been generally good, much better than the results of surgery, radiation, and chemotherapy, used alone or in combination.'[215]

Dr Thomas Levy, writing in his volume, *Curing the Incurable-Vitamin C, Infectious Diseases, and Toxins,* discussed the work of numerous pioneers such as Dr Frederick R Klenner who cured polio and hepatitis with vitamin C. Levy maintains that 'Vitamin C actually has been documented to have readily and consistently cured both acute polio and acute hepatitis, two viral diseases still considered incurable'. He maintains that Klenner demonstrated repeatedly that vitamin C appears to be the most ideal agent for killing any infecting virus. Not just was it able to kill the virus but vitamin C was able to help eliminate any toxic chemical or substance capable of poisoning the body, including the toxins associated with several infectious diseases. What Levy makes abundantly clear is that for vitamin C to work therapeutically that it was important to meet strict criteria:

1. That vitamin C be given in the right form.
2. That it is administered with the proper technique.
3. Given in frequent enough doses.
4. That it be administered in high enough doses.
5. That it be administered along with certain additional agents in some cases.
6. That it be administered for a long enough period of time.

As an example, when Dr Klenner treated polio as he did in the 1947 epidemic, he cured it within 72 hours using frequent injections of large doses of vitamin C of between 6,000 – 20,000 mg in a twenty-four hour period. He would also add thiamine (vitamin B_1) to help nervous tissue recovery. None of his patients would have any lingering symptoms or paralysis. The epidemic was stopped in its tracks in his town. Levy discusses most of the infectious diseases, mumps, scarlet fever, measles, diphtheria, pertussis (whooping cough), smallpox… (the list goes on). He makes the point, 'Yes, many viral infectious diseases have been cured and can continue to be cured by the proper administration of vitamin C. Yes the vaccinations for these treatable infectious diseases are completely unnecessary when one has access to proper treatment with vitamin C.' Well, here is a serious reason that the pharmaceutical industry does not want you to know about how useful vitamin C really is—vaccinations are one of their most profitable products. They don't need advertising or marketing, most governments just promote their use for free, and better, even make it compulsory in some cases. In my view, Levy's book should be required reading for all health professionals. He says, 'To date, no viral infection has been demonstrated to be resistant to the proper dosing of vitamin C' [my emphasis]. He further adds, 'Even today, modern medicine does not have a single effective and non-toxic virus-killing drug.'

Dr Klenner treated people with viral encephalitis, and in some cases where the patient was already comatose and near death. Klenner termed the response that he repeatedly witnessed as "dramatic," yet even with the possibility of sudden death, he never failed to see a full recovery. He also reported excellent results with chickenpox, shingles, and herpes simplex. Levy reports that where the severe pain associated with shingles can sometimes persist for weeks, it was usually resolved within two hours with adequate vitamin C. Levy also reports that vitamin C is useful for the treatment for exposure to ionizing radiation. He suggests the associated symptoms will generally be consistent with a large increase of free radicals and oxidative stress in the affected tissues. He says, 'A potent antioxidant like vitamin C is ideally suited for coping with the onslaught of oxidant stress unleashed by a significant exposure.' He mentions that Klenner asserted that vitamin C will "prevent radiation burns." Levy suggests that vitamin C 'has been shown to be the ideal agent for helping in the destruction of most bacteria, fungi, and other microbial agents that continue to afflict mankind.' [216]

Anybody who uses vitamin C successfully will no doubt tell you that the RDA (recognised daily allowance) for vitamin C has been set too low, and our impoverished diets based on too many over-processed carbohydrates and too much sugar are causing irreparable harm to our bodies. Philip Washko and Mark

Primary Ingredients of Life

Levine showed how glucose interfered with vitamin C transport around the body and disrupted uptake by neutrophils (white blood cells) so that vitamin C levels were seriously compromised when there were high levels of glucose in the blood.[217] This can seriously compromise the immune system. Vitamin C supports the immune response in numerous ways.

Andrew Saul PhD., and Steve Hickey PhD., in their book *Vitamin C: The Real Story,* discuss how vitamin C protects against atherosclerosis, and how the loss or lack of vitamin C affects the levels of nitric oxide in the blood vessels that keep the vessels smooth and blood flowing well. Vitamin C also maintains the elasticity of the vessels and is important in collagen formation and maintenance. Saul and Hickey quote the work of the American pharmacologist Louis J. Ignarro, PhD., who received the Nobel Prize in Physiology for his work on nitric oxide signalling in the cardiovascular system. He proposed that the use of vitamin C with other antioxidants (vitamin E and alpha-lipoic acid) together with the amino acid L-arginine would prevent blood vessel inflammation and subsequent damage. [218]

There is actually more interest in vitamin C in mainstream medicine currently, which is inevitable as the benefits of vitamin C use are extensive. A recent positive development has been reported by Sander Rozemeijer et al., who were looking at new technology that could check vitamin C status by the bedside of critically ill patients. The researchers note that, 'Vitamin C deficiency is common in critically ill patients. Vitamin C, the most important antioxidant, is likely consumed during oxidative stress and deficiency is associated with organ dysfunction and mortality.' They report on the use of a point-of-care device that can measure the 'static oxidation-reduction potential (sORP) which reflects the level of oxidative stress, and antioxidant capacity (AOC).' They note: 'Vitamin

C deficiency is common in critically ill patients with severe sepsis, trauma or ischemia/reperfusion injury and is associated with endothelial damage, cellular injury, organ dysfunction, and mortality.' Their study, however, involved giving their patients 10g of vitamin C per day, which, therapeutically speaking, is not considered a huge dose. Dr Cathcart could use 10 times that level of dose for treating a cold. Klenner would use ten times that amount in cases of acute toxicity.[219]

An international study in July 2018, by intensive care specialists, Aileen Hill and associates evaluated the use of vitamin C in cardiac surgery patients to improve outcomes following surgery. Unfortunately, the size of the doses was small, but the study was nevertheless encouraging and upbeat about its use. They cite some of the benefits:

> The pleiotropic biochemical and antioxidant functions of vitamin C have sparked recent interest in its application in intensive care. Vitamin C protects important organ systems (cardiovascular, neurologic and renal systems) during inflammation and oxidative stress. It also influences coagulation and inflammation; its application might prevent organ damage. The current evidence of vitamin C's effect on pathophysiological reactions during various acute stress events (such as sepsis, shock, trauma, burn and ischemia-reperfusion injury) questions whether the application of vitamin C might be especially beneficial for cardiac surgery patients who are routinely exposed to ischemia/reperfusion and subsequent inflammation, systematically affecting different organ systems.

They acknowledge that even after less invasive and elective surgery such as maxilla-facial surgery that higher doses of vitamin C (500-2000 mg/day, mean 1150 mg/day) were required to compensate for the losses observed from just this type of procedure. They suggested that a dosage of 3-4g/day was required in the case in patients with burns or sepsis or critically ill trauma patients. Compare the levels of vitamin C that Dr Klenner routinely used for the treatment of diphtheria where he would administer 700mg/kg body weight given intravenously through a twenty-gauge needle "as fast as the patient's cardiovascular system would allow." This would approximate to 50 grams per day. That's a big difference, and sepsis can become a serious threat quickly. The big difference is that, when vitamin C is used adequately, antibiotic use can be curtailed, so the immune system, instead of being compromised is actually supported. The researchers nevertheless point to the perceived benefits for its use:

> Any conclusive evidence of the benefits of vitamin C in cardiac surgery patients would lead to rapid implementation of this promising therapy for four reasons: (1) The overall safety profile of vitamin C may enable a broad use; (2) the feasibility of vitamin C administration without any dose adjustments; (3) familiarity for clinicians and patients as a therapy for cancer and in some burn units; (4) low costs to produce and administer.[220]

One of the ways that the pharmaceutical industry and the medical industry have been able to keep so many doctors oblivious to the benefits of not just vitamin C, but arguably the role of nutrition and the value of supplements in our health, has been to restrict access to important studies. They have successfully made sure that Medline and the PubMed national database of US National Library of Medicine, National Institutes of Health, leave out such important publishing resources as the *American Journal of Clinical Nutrition*, which was cited more than 6,500 times in 2018. Another journal about nutrition that is left out of these databases is the *Journal of Orthomolecular Nutrition*, started by Abram Hoffer which is another example of what can only be considered a form of censorship. In fact, you will find no journals of nutrition of any kind searching these databases. [221] The articles in the *Journal of Orthomolecular Nutrition* are also free.

Whilst on the subject of censorship, I would like to point out another way valuable information is effectively withheld. In the pharmaceutical industry, when a drug's patent expires other companies are allowed to produce this product, which invariably reduces its price. If I wished to get access to a journal article, even if it is more than ten years old, journals still demand full payment, even if the article is 20 or 30 years old. This is no benefit to true science, to true discovery. It should be mandatory that after 10 years the article becomes available in the public domain. If you also consider that the vast majority of the science that covers the pages of these journals was funded by public money, it makes it even more reprehensible when access is so restricted.

In spite of this kind of censorship, more medical professionals are beginning to discover the value of vitamin C. Despite the fact that for decades mainstream medicine has maintained vitamin C use is only required for the elimination of scurvy, there is overwhelming evidence that its role is essential in so many functions in our bodies. James May and Fiona Harrison in an article in 2013 on the role of vitamin C in the vascular endothelium reported: 'Beyond simply preventing scurvy, evidence is mounting that ascorbate is required for optimal function of many dioxygenase enzymes in addition to those involved in collagen synthesis.' They have recognised that 'many diseases and conditions have either systemic or localized cellular ascorbate deficiency as a cause for endothelial dysfunction, including early atherosclerosis, sepsis, smoking, and diabetes.' They report: 'Indeed, it may even require megadoses of the vitamin to replete the vitamin and improve endothelial function in some of these conditions.'[222]

Primary Ingredients of Life

Before we leave the subject of, in this case, the blood system, Frie et al., writing in the *Proceedings of the National Academy of Sciences* in 1989 described vitamin C as 'an outstanding antioxidant in human blood plasma.' They also acknowledged the error in the low level set for the RDA. 'In light of the well-known antioxidant properties of ascorbate, it is noteworthy that the US recommended daily allowance (RDA) for ascorbate is based exclusively on its function in collagen synthesis (its anti-scorbutic effect) and not on its antioxidant activity.' One of the important aspects of vitamin C's protection is the lipids in our body that are so vulnerable to oxidation, particularly from excess glucose, these researchers found, 'Our data demonstrate that ascorbate is the most effective aqueous-phase antioxidant in human blood plasma and suggest that in humans ascorbate is a physiological antioxidant of major importance for protection against diseases and degenerative processes caused by oxidant stress.' They were also able to 'show that it is indeed ascorbate that completely protects plasma lipids against detectable peroxidative damage induced by aqueous peroxyl radicals and that ascorbate is the only plasma antioxidant that can do so'.[223] I added this information to point out how important vitamin C is in protecting us, particularly when we are exposed to so many damaged fats and oils created by the industrial food supply. Levels of vitamin C are compromised in our bodies from so many sources: from infections of all kinds, from highly processed carbohydrates, such as sugar and white flour, from stress, injury, and numerous toxins—this leads to the situation whereby vitamin C levels can be severely depleted and unable to keep up with all the toxins that the body has to deal with—hence the reason for considering supplementation.

The highest concentrations of ascorbate (vitamin C) in the body are to be found in the brain and in the neuroendocrine tissues, such as the adrenal glands. This points to an important relationship. Researchers Harrison and May

How To Survive in the 21st Century

from the Department of Medicine, Vanderbilt University School of Medicine, Nashville, posit the importance that these facts suggest:

> Combined with regional asymmetry in ascorbate distribution within different brain areas, **these facts suggest an important role for ascorbate in the brain.** Ascorbate is proposed as a neuromodulator of glutamatergic, dopaminergic, cholinergic, and GABAergic transmission and related behaviors. Neurodegenerative diseases typically involve high levels of oxidative stress and thus ascorbate has been posited to have potential therapeutic roles against ischemic stroke, Alzheimer's disease, Parkinson's disease, and Huntington's disease.

They point out that James Lind in his Treatise on Scurvy of 1772 discovered that in sailors whose organs were severely ravaged by scurvy, the "brains of these poor people were always found to be sound and entire." Subsequent animal studies had found the same situation. Apparently, the brain holds onto its vitamin C even as the body becomes ravaged by scurvy. They also point to studies that show when vitamin C was removed from their diet, in one case guinea pigs that are, like humans, unable to make their own vitamin C—these animals developed a progressively ascending paralysis and died within 24 hours. It has to be said that this demise was also due to the withholding of vitamin E at the same time—effectively losing two important antioxidants. The animals did not, however, show signs of scurvy, but it was revealed they suffered widespread neuronal loss. These researchers mention other animal studies that were related to ischemic stroke which illustrated the value of vitamin C. They observe:

> Perhaps the most dramatic acute oxidant stress in the CNS is the ischemia-reperfusion injury that occurs with ischemic stroke. Ischemia initially depletes intracellular GSH [the antioxidant

glutathione] and ascorbate in the brain. If reperfusion with oxygen-rich blood occurs, the ROS [reactive oxygen species] generated due to abnormal mitochondrial metabolism will extend tissue damage to areas with decreased oxidant defences.

They cite the study that involved giving monkeys 1g/day of ascorbate for six days before experiencing 'middle cerebral artery occlusion' which is where blood supply is blocked. The result was 'brain infarct size was decreased by 50% in the ascorbate-treated group compared to the control group not treated with ascorbate.' Which basically showed that vitamin C limited the damage of a stroke by 50%, and that was just 1 gram a day. They also noted that Alzheimer's disease patients had lower plasma levels of vitamin C and that there was improvement with ascorbate supplementation, as well as reduced disease incidence. Regarding Parkinson's disease, they suggest, 'Oxidative injury is also thought to play a key role in the pathogenesis of the disease.' They also mention how ascorbate helped improve the bioavailability of levodopa which could be converted into the neurotransmitter dopamine in elderly Parkinson's disease patients with low levels. In their report they concluded:

> That ascorbate is important for neuronal maturation and function, as well as for protection of the brain against oxidant stress is well supported by the evidence presented in this review. The vitamin is maintained at high concentrations in brain and in neurons in particular relative to other organs. In addition, strong homeostatic mechanisms maintain brain and neuronal ascorbate concentrations within very tight limits.[224]

The study above used 1gram a day, which is a very small amount. I would like to see the effect of larger doses. I will leave you with a story that shows the human relevance of this information, by a great nutritionist, Andrew Saul

PhD, who we have already introduced. I read this excerpt posted as a review for the book *Ascorbate: The Science of Vitamin C* by his collaborator Steve Hickey PhD, which I have copied here. I am sure he won't mind, aside from being a great nutritionist (I can recommend his books) he has a great sense of humour, and he would be happy for me to support Steve Hickey's book. Here is what he has to say:

> What is it about a little left-handed molecule of six carbons, six oxygens, and eight hydrogens that ticks off so many in the medical community? Maybe it's cases like this one: Ray, a health professional I know, had an 11-month old son who was very sick for over a week. No one and I mean no one, in their family had had any sleep in a long time. They were up night after night with this child, who had a high fever, glazed watery eyes, tons of thick watery mucus and labored breathing. The child would not sleep, and did little else but cry. The baby was under the care of a pediatrician, who, in the infant's eleven months on earth, had already prescribed twelve rounds of some very serious antibiotics. That they clearly were not working was all too apparent to Ray, who out of desperation decided to try something he previously had been taught to not try: bowel tolerance quantities of oral ascorbate. Ray and his wife gave their baby some vitamin C about every 15 minutes. As a result, the baby was noticeably improved in a matter of hours, and slept through the night. With frequent doses continuing, the child was completely well in 48 hours. Ray calculated that the baby had received just over 2,000 mg vitamin C per kilogram body weight per day. This is even more than what Dr. Frederick Robert Klenner customarily ordered for sick patients. Remarkably, at 20,000 milligrams of vitamin C/day, that 20-pound baby never had diarrhea.

> With such a little body, you have to marvel at where all of it was going. Of course, it is the opinion of those who promulgate the US RDA and related nutritional mythology that almost all of that baby's vitamin C

went uselessly into the toilet. Ray and his wife would tell you differently. They would say that their sick child soaked it up like a sponge, and then promptly got better. [225]

Dr Thomas Levy reports on a great number of uses for vitamin C that many people will find interesting in another excellent volume on vitamin C, called *Primal Panacea*, which would be a useful book for most people. He reports on a case of swine flu where a patient was completely cured by the use of vitamin C. The patient was comatose at the time, and doctors were going to turn off the life support machine. The patient had also been diagnosed with whiteout pneumonia and "hairy cell" leukemia. The family insisted on trying vitamin C in Klenner-sized doses. According to Levy 'the clinical response was quick and stunning.' Almost at once, the patient's lungs began to clear and the patient recovered enough to be removed from life support. A few weeks later he walked out of the hospital. What was even more remarkable, was that his leukemia had also appeared to have resolved along with the swine flu. The only tragedy of the story, in this case, was the completely dismissive attitude of the doctors towards vitamin C: they suggested his recovery was a coincidence. [226]

I added this account to further illustrate how effective vitamin C is with viruses and bacteria. It is a shame that the medical profession lives in ignorance of such a great tool against such pathogens when they have so little else of such value.

Coronavirus Outbreak

As I write this we are in the grips of a worldwide epidemic of the coronavirus, covid-19. This outbreak has coincided with the publication of this volume and forced me to consider adding some further information. The book was at the final editing stage, but the events of the now declared pandemic have introduced a new dimension to consider. The previous section devoted to vitamin C which revealed its ability to destroy all known viruses now takes on a more imperative message.

Communication via the *Orthomolecular Medicine News Service* posted the following comment: 'No matter which hospital a coronavirus patient may seek help from, the question is, Will they be able to leave walking out the front door, or end up being wheeled out the basement backdoor? Prompt administration of intravenous vitamin C, in high doses, can make the difference.'[227] The following communication informed us that China was conducting a clinical trial of 24,000 mg/day of intravenous vitamin C to treat patients with coronavirus and severe respiratory complications at Zhongan Hospital of Wuhan University. They suggested that credit for making this happen should be given to Dr Zhiyong Peng, chief physician and professor at the hospital which they suggest was 'close to ground zero for coronavirus'.[228] This was encouraging: could it be that vitamin C treatment was actually going to have the opportunity to prove itself and get recognized for its true value at last? As the covid-19 issue unfolded we had further interesting developments from China. We were informed that the chief supplier of vitamin C in China is DSM Jiangshan Pharmaceutical, and it had shipped 50 tons, yes that's right, 50 tons of immunity-boosting vitamin C to the province of Hubei, of which Wuhan is the capital city. This was promising news, as with the polio epidemic in 1948 when the use of intravenous vitamin C enabled Dr Frederick Klenner to stop it in its tracks and cure all those infected within 72 hours, this has the potential to help a large number of people deal with Covid-19 infection.[229]

This covid-19 pandemic story is changing our world by the day. No doubt by the time this book hits the press the story will have significantly changed. As I write this, I have just completed a fifth article on the coronavirus and vitamin C's ability to deal with viruses on my website www.Fundamental-Health.com. One recent article was about the censorship of postings by people such as Andrew Saul PhD who we have already introduced. Saul had articles that were blacked out by Facebook. He had so many interfered with that he lost patience with Facebook and decided to move to another site (MeWe.com). I have posted his new location. Others experienced similar experiences. Saul mentioned how WHO met with internet providers such as Facebook, Google and Amazon, and were told the internet was "awash with misinformation." Vitamin C was singled out 'because of false reports that it can cure the coronavirus.' [230]

One of the victims of this censorship was Richard Cheng MD. PhD. a US board-certified specialist in anti-ageing medicine, and cardiologist with a PhD. in biochemistry. He was visiting China at the time of the covid-19 outbreak to spend time with his parents. As the outbreak became serious he decided to stay and help. He was able to communicate with colleagues in America, virtually, on a daily basis, many of them were in the *International Society for Orthomolecular Medicine,* and they issued a number of progress reports via the *Orthomolecular Medicine News Service.* Some of these reports were singled out for censorship and were blacked out by Facebook, and YouTube removed a presentation made by Dr Cheng. What seems to have been the reason in some cases was the claim that vitamin C can successfully treat and even cure covid-19.

For those of us that have studied vitamin C, and know the extensive history of numerous physicians that included doctors like Frederick Klenner, and later Dr Robert Cathcart who used high-dose vitamin C with great success to treat serious infections—successfully dealing with this outbreak is not a surprise. Cathcart treated more than 22,000 patients with vitamin C and advocated treating influenza with up to 150,000 mg a day (yes, that is 150 grams). He found the sicker the patient was, the more ascorbic acid they could take orally. He graded illness by the amount of vitamin C it took to cure it. A mild cold would be 30 to 60 grams, a bad cold would be 100 grams, flu would be 100 grams, and with mononucleosis and viral pneumonia, he would find 200 grams or more ascorbic acid could be tolerated without diarrhoea. He used to call it 'titrating to bowel tolerance.'[231] Apparently, even the medical pioneer, Dr Robert Cathcart III himself, is now being censored by Wikipedia, in this case, as they have decided to remove his page. Curiously, at this time, there is a concerted effort to bury information about the established benefit of high-dose vitamin C. The cynics amongst us might wonder whether it has anything to do with the plans that the pharmaceutical industry has in rolling out approximately 300 new vaccines. [232]

Dr Joseph Mercola published an article in February (2020), "Vitamin C works for Sepsis, Will it Work for Coronavirus?" Sepsis is known to be responsible for 1 in 5 deaths worldwide every year, killing 11 million people in 2017. Sepsis is one of the leading causes of influenza deaths. He reported on the work of Dr Paul Marik, Chief of Pulmonary and Critical Care Medicine, Eastern Virginia Medical School, USA, who had developed a protocol shown to dramatically improve the chances of survival in septic patients. His IV protocol for adults included 200 mg of thiamine every 12 hours, 1500 mg of ascorbic acid every six hours, and 50 mg of hydrocortisone every six hours for two days. It was found to reduce mortality from 40% to 8.5%.[233]

More recently, Dr Marik has been working with covid-19 patients, and has included a protocol that incorporates 3 grams of vitamin C every six hours and steroid treatment. Dr Marik is not alone using vitamin C in the USA for treating Covid-19 patients, he is part of a group of physicians called the Frontline

COVID-19 Critical Care Working Group that are achieving spectacular results with their protocol. One of his associates from Houston, Texas, Dr Joseph Varon, using a similar protocol reported, 'To date, we have 0% mortality at United Memorial Center. Zero percent. I know it's too good for people to believe in this but it's working.' The drug protocol is not new, he has been using a similar protocol for years for treating sepsis (as reported in the previous paragraph). Some physicians are reluctant to utilise large-dose vitamin C without seeing published studies, for these people Dr Varon emphasizes his priority: 'Yes there is need to do a study…But at this time, if I see that something is working I'm not going to let my patients die.' Their website has the comment, "Our MATH+ protocol saves lives. So why isn't the world using it?"[234] Why indeed?

Dr Pierre Kory, one of the members of the Critical Care Group, in testimony to a US Senate Committee hearing, discussed the group's frustration with trying to get the group's protocol to a wider audience as it saved lives. He explained that they had successfully treated 100 patients and had only two deaths, and that was of two patients in their eighties with 'advanced chronic medical conditions.' He explained that his group were dismayed that most of the treatment recommended was only for supportive care, which they found was of limited value. They also felt it was a 'tragic error in analysis of medical data, and that is the fact that all societies in the beginning of covid have advised against the use of corticosteroids in covid-19.' Their protocol which included methylprednisolone, a corticosteroid combined with high-dose vitamin C, which they believed worked very effectively together. They were able to get their protocol delivered to the White House, but at the time of the hearing had not had a response. Dr Kory, who had been working in New York for a couple of weeks was further dismayed that people who were sick with Covid-19 were not coming for treatment early enough. One critical aspect was getting the treatment early enough to be effective, and this was not being publicised.[235]

I reported on the situation in New York, where Andrew G Weber, a pulmonologist and critical care specialist, affiliated with the Northwell Health facilities based on Long Island. He informs us that his intensive-care patients with covid-19 immediately receive 1500 mg of intravenous vitamin C. They are given repeat doses 3 or 4 times a day. He explains that he found vitamin C levels in coronavirus patients drop dramatically when they suffer sepsis and that an inflammatory response occurs when their bodies overreact to the infection. He says, 'It makes all the sense in the world to try and maintain this level of vitamin C.'[236]

What can you do on a personal level to protect yourself and your family at times like this? It seems sensible to suggest beefing up your body's ability to resist infection when there are serious infections around. Whether you find yourself reading this book with the covid-19 infection still in full swing or at some time later, the following protocol should be of use to you:

Supplement protocol for boosting the body's ability to fight off attack:

- Vitamin C 3,000 milligrams (or more) spread over a number of doses per day.
- Vitamin D3, 5,000 IU for 2 weeks then reduce to 2,000 IU per day.
- Magnesium 400 mg per day (as citrate, malate or chloride).
- Zinc 20 mg daily.
- Selenium 100 mcg (micrograms) daily.

If you are confronted with an infection, increase the vitamin C with each dose until you reach bowel tolerance, then back off slightly. When the infection subsides gradually reduce the dose. If symptoms return increase the dose again. Once the infection clears reduce the dose to the maintenance dose. If the symptoms worsen and you are unable to increase oral dose of vitamin C and require hospitalization, inform the critical care team you have been taking oral vitamin C and request high-dose IV vitamin C (IVC) as a matter of urgency. High-dose IVC is safe and effective and can be used with other medications. Experience with covid-19 revealed by Dr Marik and Dr Cheng found that early application was critical.[237] The treatment protocols used by Doctor Marik and his cohorts can be found on my website accompanying the highlighted text by Dr Marik: **URGENT! Please circulate as widely as possible. It is crucial that every pulmonologist, every critical care doctor and nurse, every hospital administrator, every public health official receive this information immediately.** The protocol is updated regularly. [238] The April 20th update in the introductory page adds "If what you are doing ain't working, change what you are doing."

There is information on my site that explains some of the detailed science behind the reason vitamin C is essential to defeating this particular covid-19 pathogen, and preventing the damage that is precipitated by the cytokine storm that causes so much damage. It is just as Dr Thomas Levy suggests in his books, that vitamin C's crucial action here is not as a simple vitamin, but as an electron donor. Much of the damage caused by the virus is caused by the destruction of haemoglobin, and the subsequent release of free heme which is accompanied by the further release of its sequestered iron. In its free unbound form it is oxidised by the virus into its ferric form (Fe^{3+}) which is transformed into a highly reactive and destructive molecule in the lungs. On top of that the vitamin C levels by this stage unless added to in high doses render the immune system seriously crippled. Immune cells like macrophages, neutrophils, and lymphocytes all produce cytokines. Cytokine storms from immune cell dysfunctions lead to further collapse of the immune system that has found to be the ultimate cause of fatality in Covid-19. [239]

Immune Support

A lot more could be said about vitamin C, such as vitamin C deficiency being associated with every known heart disease risk factor. Death from cancer was found in one study to be 45% less in the group with the highest blood levels of vitamin C. Dr Levy, concerning arthritis, informs us, 'There is no credible argument that oxidative stress is the major culprit in the development of osteoarthritis, polyarthritis and rheumatoid arthritis. Aside from the fact that joints are constructed from vitamin C-dependent collagen and collagen-containing cartilage.'

Vitamin C can protect against poisoning. The link between aluminium and brain dysfunction is becoming more established and many people are suggesting the link with vaccines as being a significant cofactor in autism. Dr Levy inform us that those of you that wish to vaccinate can protect your children, to some degree with vitamin C. In one respect it aids the vaccine's effectiveness, but it can also reduce the chance of some of the more serious problems associated with the vaccine. It supports the immune system and it also can remove aluminium from the body. So if you suspect aluminium is playing a role you might consider using vitamin C. Dr Levy is a good source of information for those wishing further information about this.[240]

What I feel is missing from the debate is the immune system itself. What has to be appreciated is that whether you vaccinate or not it is still the body's own immune system that has to deal with whatever pathogen it happens to become exposed to. The principle of adaptive immunity is based on the principle that once exposed to a pathogen, the body adapts and creates antibodies so that when the body is faced with any renewed attack that the system will create a more powerful response. When you get a wild acquired infection, it stimulates the innate immune system, and you have permanent life-long immunity, this never happens with a vaccine, however. What is missing from the equation is how the body can be assisted in dealing with infection with simple solutions such as high-dose vitamin C, a treatment that is non-toxic and can be used alongside other therapeutic agents, with very minimal cost.

We have already mentioned how Dr Robert Klenner defeated Polio in his town during the 1947 polio epidemic. He published his achievement with 60 patients in Reidsville, North Carolina. He didn't get a Nobel Prize for his discovery, it was at the time they were introducing a vaccination for polio. The tragedy was here was a complete cure that cost dimes and had no side effects. The polio vaccine, however, was contaminated with a monkey virus called simian virus-40 (SV40). Over the last couple of decades this virus has been showing up in human tumours, leading many scientists to believe that this virus may be contributing to these cancers. It has been found in brain and bone tumours, mesotheliomas and lymphomas, and with kidney disease.[241]

Dr Levy describes "an especially incredible case" involving Klenner's treatment of a five-year-old girl who was so stricken with polio that she had been paralyzed in both her lower legs for over four days! Four physicians had diagnosed polio. Klenner treated her with intravenous vitamin C. After four days she started moving her legs again and she was discharged from hospital. By the eleventh day she was able to walk slowly. By the 19th day of treatment there was "a complete return of sensory and motor function." Dr Levy comments, "Vitamin C not only completely cured this case of polio, it completely reversed what would undoubtedly have been a devastating, crippling result for the remainder of this girl's life."[242]

I write this at a time when it has been revealed that fantastic sums are being committed to funding fast-tracked vaccines that may be of dubious benefit and with very little long-term testing.

According to Barbara Loe Fisher, WHO released its COVID-19 R&D Roadmap on March 9ᵗʰ, that BioWorld suggests had been endorsed by "400 experts" and included funding from the European Commission (37.5 million euros), the German government (10 million euros) and an additional 46 million euros from the UK government, with 20 million euros going directly to the Coalition for Epidemic Preparedness (CEPI) for vaccine development. CEPI has committed $100 million to speed up licensure of COVID-19 vaccines but said it was trying to raise $2 billion more to speed vaccines to market.[243]

According to Barbara Fisher, some of the new vaccines now involve mRNA and DNA products made in the lab using synthetic processes which can be produced in large quantities for less money than traditional vaccines. Apparently, the Messenger mRNA vaccines inject human cells with mRNA, usually within lipid nanoparticles, to stimulate cells in the body to become manufacturers of viral proteins. How good is that? I can hardly wait. She points out that neither DNA or mRNA vaccines have been tested in large-scale clinical trials. She informs us that *Chemical and Engineering News* has highlighted the breakneck speed at which COVID-19 vaccines "are moving new technologies from the computer into the clinic at an unprecedented rate." She further reports that what would normally separate pre-licensure phases for proving safety and effectiveness—preclinical animal models, clinical testing, and manufacturing— are now "happening all at once." She also quotes a former vaccine developer who says "It will be the first time that they will be tested in so many people." Well, no doubt, everyone will be getting excited about the idea of being guinea pigs for bid pharma's new vaccine experiments.

According to WHO, the vaccine industry has achieved spectacular growth rates (10-15 % per year compared with 5-7 % for pharmaceuticals). The influenza market has tripled in value from $2.9 billion in 2000 to $3.8 billion by 2018. The global market reached $24.6 billion in 2016 and is expected to grow to $100 billion by 2025. The top earner in the vaccine market in 2017 was GlaxoSmithKline with vaccine revenues of $6.9 billion, closely followed by Merck with $6.5 billion, Sanofi $6.12 and Pfizer with $6.0 billion. WHO informs us, 'Newer and more expensive vaccines are coming into the market faster than ever before.' As previously mentioned there are approximately a further 300 vaccines currently under development. [244]

It could be seen as predictable following the implementation of the National Childhood Vaccine Injury Act of 1986 which protects vaccine manufacturers from lawsuits, that it would create a huge incentive for growth in the vaccine industry—purely to increase business profits—as opposed to necessarily benefit our health prospects. The fact that this protection was given to such pathologically dangerous corporate interests is unlikely to lead to a beneficial health outcome for a great number of people. The US Vaccine Court has awarded over $4.3 billion to date.[245]

The problem the vaccination industry is facing is the general public are losing confidence in vaccines. They are discovering that they are not as effective as has been portrayed, they produce too many side effects and they don't contribute to the general health of the population as much as has been suggested. Anybody that questions the touted benefits of vaccination are labelled "antivaxers." I am not an anti-vaxer by any means. I am anti-pseudoscience, and I believe parents should be told the truth and be allowed to make their own choice whether or not they wish to vaccinate their children.

Many people are alarmed at the dramatic rise of cognitive problems in children, and particularly in autism. In the last five years, autism has increased by 70 %. Dr Lucija Tomljenovic works in neuroscience in the Department of Medicine in the University of British Columbia (UBC). She mentions that when she was in medical school (35 years ago), the incidence of autism was one in 10,000 children, whereas today it is one in 15. She believes that this figure is conservative and that if things don't change that it will soon be 1 in 10. She says that these figures are not due to better diagnostic criteria or some genetic epidemic, 'These arguments are just silly...If you've seen an autistic child from across several gates down an airport, you know it's an autistic child. I mean you do not need to be a rocket scientist to diagnose these children.'

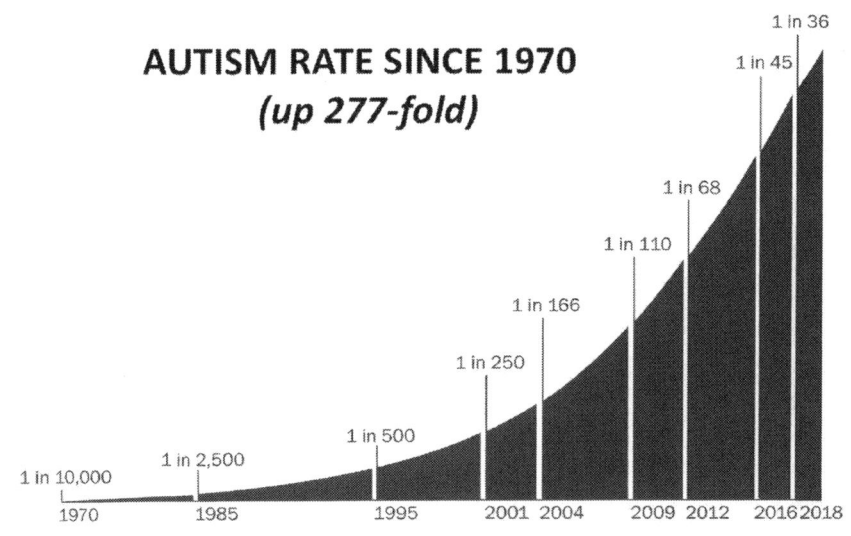

Primary Ingredients of Life

In an interview with Dr Joseph Mercola when asked for her views on the use of aluminum as an adjuvant, she responded, 'Again, the aluminum on its own is a neurotoxin. But the fact is it's not simply aluminum, it's the fact of this exaggerated immune response.' Another aspect that her team investigated was the cross-reactivity between the antibodies that are raised against vaccine antigens: 'Some of them cross-react with our own tissues...We have demonstrated this effect in human papillomavirus (HPV).' In mice studies, they found that there was an inhibition of binding of the anti-HPV antibodies to HPV. 'Why? Because they are preferentially binding the mouse brain protein extract.' Dr Mercola's response was, 'Wow. Does that imply an increased risk for brain autoimmune disorders like multiple sclerosis (MS)?' Dr Tomljenovic replied, 'Exactly. It increases the rate of any immune-mediated nervous system disorders which incidentally appear to be most commonly reported worldwide, following Gardasil. We have done this analysis. We published it in the *Annals of Medicine* where we took vaccines safety databases from various countries, and then we rated the adverse effects based on organ system. We found the most commonly reported are nervous system disorders of immune origin.' Apparently, the Japan Institute of Pharmacovigilance picked up on their paper and asked for the raw data. The match with their data was perfect. This led to them to stop recommending the HPV vaccine in Japan. She mentions that she knows many mothers whose girls have died following HPV.

Dr Mercola in another article revealed how the information regarding the safety of aluminum in vaccines has proved to be based on a substantial flaw. In a 2011 paper comparing aluminium exposure from vaccines in infants to an Agency for Toxic Substances and Disease Registry (ATSDR) safety limit of oral aluminium—which concluded the amount used in vaccines is safe—was found to have made a statistical error according to an erratum published by Physicians for Informed Consent (PIC). The CDC and other health organizations have been using this flawed study as the basis for saying that aluminum adjuvants in childhood vaccines are safe.[246]

According to the PIC 'The paper compared the aluminum exposure from vaccines in infants to a safety limit of oral aluminum determined by the ATSDR. However, this study incorrectly based its calculations on 0.78% of oral aluminum being absorbed into the bloodstream rather than the value of 0.1% used by the ATSDR in its computations. As a result, the FDA paper assumed that nearly 8 (0.78%/0.1%) times more aluminum can safely enter the bloodstream, and this led the authors to incorrectly conclude that aluminum exposure from vaccines was well below the safety limit.'[247]

Dr Mercola also referred to Canadian research questioning the reliability and validity of research into the safety of aluminum in childhood vaccines. Here is what the researchers had to say:

> Aluminum is an experimentally demonstrated neurotoxin and the most commonly used vaccine adjuvant. Despite almost 90 years of widespread use of aluminum adjuvants, medical science's understanding about their mechanisms of action is still remarkably poor. There is also a concerning scarcity of data on toxicology and pharmacokinetics of these compounds. In spite of this, the notion that aluminum in vaccines is safe appears to be widely accepted. Experimental research, however, clearly shows that aluminum adjuvants have a potential to induce serious immunological disorders in humans. In particular, aluminum in adjuvant form carries a risk for autoimmunity, long-term brain inflammation and associated neurological complications and may thus have profound and widespread adverse health consequences. In our opinion, the possibility that vaccine benefits may have been overrated and the risk of potential

adverse effects underestimated, has not been rigorously evaluated in the medical and scientific community.[248]

Dr Mercola also points out that previous efforts to assess the aluminum burden created by vaccines were based on "whole-body clearance rates estimated from a study involving a single human subject." They also used an aluminum citrate solution that is not used in vaccines, which they believe could further affect the excretion rate.

I suspect debate about vaccines is going to heat-up following the covid-19 experience. In the UK, the government has introduced sweeping changes to the Public Health (Control of Disease) Act 1984 that has come into force on the 27th April 2020, regarding vaccinations and covid-19 medical treatment. According to Zed Phoenix, the government now has given itself the power to force medication on its citizens. They have the given themselves the right to take and destroy your personal things, destroy your building, be it place of residence or work, and you no longer have the right to challenge, prosecute or take legal action against their authority, and much more. [249]

The above two sections were in response to the developments of the Covid-19 outbreak. There is more that could be said about this but is beyond the scope of this volume. There is, of course much more that could be said about the use and importance of supplementation of vitamins and minerals in our diet. We could discuss how vitamin D, zinc and magnesium are important in helping fight disease, and contribute to building a strong immune system. This however is not the purpose of this volume, we will however suggest places where you can access this information in the resource section. We wish to look at the bigger picture, how to create optimum health in society as a whole.

How To Survive in the 21st Century

Even with access to fresh fruits and vegetables, there can still be a lack of nutrients for numerous reasons. We are faced with a lot of soil destruction with the industrialization of agriculture, and the crops that are being grown are not grown for the level of nutrients. The majority of food is grown with artificial fertilizers and any number of pesticides, herbicides and fungicides, all of which cause significant challenges with their detoxification and nutrient loss. Even the choice of the plant variety has impacted us, in that many of the new hybrids do not deliver the same nutrient quality as another plant variety but grows more quickly or perhaps is slightly more tolerant to spraying. The simple fact is that the nutrients are not as readily available anymore. If the entire system was organic it would, of course, make a significant difference, as would growing nutrient-dense plants on really fertile soils. Whilst the organic movement is growing, many people still feel forced to exist on the products of industrialized food system. Numerous deficiencies will exist with these foods, notably minerals such as zinc and magnesium, for example; both are lacking in most people's diets, but there is no one size fits all with diets and therefore no one size fits all supplement recommendations are realistically possible.

We have introduced some basic principles that can be applied to all your food choices. I have tried to point out the pitfalls that exist with reliance on a food supply controlled by corporations that are predominantly led by the motive to make money and not to produce health or care about the consequences of their products on our health, some of whom, in fact, can profit from the death of health and the chronic illness that inevitably results from such depleted foods. This situation poses a huge challenge for us all. In my view, it affects the very future of humanity, and it is to this aspect we turn in the next chapter.

Chapter Nine

Shaping Our Future

One common factor, one common organization, is directly responsible for all the challenges that we have discussed so far in this volume that directly affects our health, the health of our children, and even the health of future generations—that is the entity that we know of as the corporation. All the examples of pollution that I have cited—whether it refers to pollution of our water, our soils, the air, or our food—behind it all lies unbridled corporate business interests that put their profits before any other concern. It is to address this issue that we now turn—an issue that I feel is of the utmost importance for us to clearly understand to enable us to create any real fundamental change to the health of our society.

The Rise of the Corporation

The corporation as an entity is a human creation that has existed since the medieval period when monarchs would issue charters to enable expeditions and ventures to promote trade with distant lands. Professor Joel Bakan, informs us that following the spectacular collapse of the 18th century South Sea Company—which was a classic scam and speculative bubble enterprise that involved numerous people from the government and included the king himself—

corporations were banned for more than 50 years. Bakan informs us, 'As for the corporation itself, in 1720, Parliament passed the Bubble Act, which made it a criminal offence to create a company "presuming to be a corporate body," and to issue "transferable stocks without legal authority." [250]

Adam Smith, writing in 1776, in his book *The Wealth of Nations,* warned about ignoring the regulation of commercial entities:

> The proposal of any new law or regulation of commerce which comes from this order [those who live by profit alone] ought always to be listened to with great precaution, and ought never to be adopted till after having been long and carefully examined, not only with the most scrupulous, but with the most suspicious attention. It comes from an order of men, whose interest is never exactly the same with that of the public, who have generally an interest to deceive and even to oppress the public, and who accordingly have, upon many occasions, both deceived and oppressed it.[251]

Back at the time of writing, Adam Smith could have had no idea that one day, corporations would grow to be as big, in terms of turnover, as many countries. Back in 2015, I wrote in *Unhealthy Betrayal,* how of the top 200 financial entities, 161 were corporations. Only seven countries outranked the richest corporations and the revenue of the top 490 corporations in 1999 exceeded $11.5 trillion—approximately 35% of the entire world GDP.[252] The growth and power of corporations seem unstoppable. Researchers at SPERI, the Sheffield Political Economy Research Institute, reported that Walmart sales were around US$500 billion which they compared to the scale of GDP of a rich company like Norway and that a handful of companies including Bayer-Monsanto, PepsiCo, and Nestlé command the global food system. In 2018 the market values of both Amazon and Apple crossed the trillion-dollar line.[253] David Streitfield, of the *New York Times* suggested that this development has created some new super-rich and that Amazon's founder and CEO, Jeff Bezos, is worth nearly as much as Bill Gates and Warren Buffet put together.[254]

However, it is not simply the size nor the wealth of the entity we call a corporation that is of main concern here—it is how they operate and how they use this power and wealth. According to Joel Bakan, writing in his volume, *The Corporation—The Pathological Pursuit of Profit and Power*, the way corporations are administered is fundamentally flawed:

> The corporation's legally defined mandate is to pursue, relentlessly and without exception, its own self-interest, regardless of the often harmful consequences it might cause to others. As a result, I argue, the corporation is a pathological institution, a dangerous possessor of the great power it wields over people and societies.

There are a great many people who feel that corporations are unaccountable institutions that manipulate and control governments and regulatory authorities globally to their advantage with little regard to the consequences to the populations under their influence. There are many who feel that giving them the status of limited liability is a grave error. Here is Bakan again: 'Limited liability had its detractors on both sides of the Atlantic, critics opposed it mainly on moral grounds. Because it allowed investors to escape unscathed from their companies' failures, the critics believed it would undermine personal moral responsibility.'[255]

Another critic of corporations is Professor Kent Greenfield, a corporate lawyer who in his volume, *The Failure of Corporate Law*, where he suggested, 'The existing law governing large corporations in the United States is fundamentally flawed. One aspect of this kind of defect is shareholder supremacy, the rule that managers of a corporation must pursue shareholder benefit above all else…There is an implicit notion that corporations do not have to obey the law as the rest of us—the widespread notion that corporate law is private law, presumptively free of government regulation.' He relates much of the problem with current regulation regarding corporations in the USA with the changes instituted following New Jersey's adoption of a statute in 1889 that released corporations from much of the regulation that existed at that time. He said that there was a rush for many businesses to incorporate in New Jersey, which precipitated actions by other states to deregulate, instituting a "race to the bottom", doing away with more and more regulatory limitations. Delaware is one of the states that pursued this approach and currently 6 in every 10 of the nation's largest corporations choose to incorporate there. Greenfield suggests that 'Delaware offers corporations a way to bypass democratic pressures and to export the costs of its legal structures to other states.' He suggests that far from being a testament to any kind of efficiency, 'It is rather a product of legal rules that are wrongheaded, inefficient, and undemocratic.'[256] It also led to a rush of amalgamations, leading 1800 corporations to be consolidated into just 157 between 1898 and 1904, beginning the rise and dominance of the huge corporations.

Another critic of corporate law is David Korten, who suggested that 'In 1886, in a stunning victory for the proponents of corporate sovereignty, the Chief Justice of the US declared in *Santa Clara County v Southern Pacific Railroad* that a private corporation is a natural person under the US Constitution—although...the Constitution makes no mention of corporations. 'This ruling enabled corporations 'to claim the full rights enjoyed by individual citizens while being exempted from many of the responsibilities and liabilities of citizenship.'

'This ruling enabled corporations 'to claim the full rights enjoyed by individual citizens while being exempted from many of the responsibilities and liabilities of citizenship.'

This evasion of responsibilities is what enables these corporations to generate profits that mere mortals would not be able to create responsibly. It is one of my main criticisms of corporate negligence, the way they feel it is fine to produce a product and dump all the waste by-product created by it onto some other party, just as they did with polluting the Great Lakes, for example, or the oceans with mercury, PCBs and dioxin.

Korten informs us what market theory has to say about this activity: 'Market theory also specifies that for a market to allocate efficiently, the full costs of each product must be borne by the producer and be included in the selling price. Economists call it cost internalization. Externalizing some part of a product's cost to others not a party to the transaction is a form of subsidy that encourages excessive production and use of the product at the expense of others.' He goes further and suggests that 'An unregulated market invariably encourages the externalization of costs because the resulting public costs become private gains.' He quotes the economist Neva Goodwin, who puts it bluntly, "Power is largely what externalities are about. What's the point of having power if you can't use it to externalize your costs—to make them fall on someone else?" He makes a number of suggestions for reform of corporate law but suggests we first need to free our thinking: 'To regain control of our future and bring human societies into balance with Earth, we must reclaim the power we have yielded to these artificial entities. One important step will be to free ourselves from the ideological illusions and policies that free corporations from human accountability.'[257]

'To regain control of our future and bring human societies
into balance with Earth, we must reclaim the power we have yielded
to these artificial entities. One important step will be to free ourselves
from the ideological illusions and policies that free corporations from
human accountability.'

Another corporate lawyer, Harry Glasbeek writing in his book, *Wealth By Stealth—Corporate Crime, Corporate Law, and the Perversion of Democracy,* suggests, 'limited liability leading to limited financial risk and personal immunity for responsibility—has emptied the corporation of moral and ethical constraints that might otherwise inhibit profiteering at any cost.' Glasbeek argues that 'the individuals behind the corporate veil—the executives, directors, and major shareholders—should be identified and characterized as the persons responsible for the corporation's conduct, whether or not they were the hands-on operators.' He acknowledges that the veil of secrecy that so far seems to protect perpetrators of harm must end: 'It must be made clear…that, behind the veil, there are identifiable flesh and blood human beings who are explicitly too willing to profit…without being prepared to pay for it…We must blow away these runaway investors' privacy: it is a privacy that hides ugliness and deceit rather than the intimacy that the legally protected respect for privacy is designed to promote.' As regards to defenders of corporations arguing that they are more economically efficient, he suggests, 'the corporate vehicle is not about economic efficiency but is, rather, nothing but a mechanism for avoiding responsibility.'

Glasbeek quotes Lewis Lapham, the editor of *Harper's* magazine in 1996 when he suggested that 'there are now two governments in the United States' and one of them is 'of course the rule of rich men, rendered virtually invisible by the artifice and the miracle of corporate law.' Glasbeek's review of the world of corporatocracy extends to all areas of business, yet his observations are echoed by many:

> In Anglo-American jurisdictions, capitalists have been blessed by a form of corporate law that promotes irresponsibility, criminality, and the perversion of democracy to advance their goal, the maximization of their wealth and political power. The corporation makes it all seem normal: selfishness, avarice, disregard for others, impersonal, commodified relations, the subjugation of the majority to the whims and caprices of the few. The very normality of it all makes the mediation of the impacts of unequally divided wealth, so characteristic of capitalist economies, all the more difficult to achieve. All of this is to be tolerated because it generates wealth. Greed is elevated to a moral value, supported by massive education campaigns and commercial advertising techniques perfected to wrought changes in expectations and wants. To be a consumer is what citizens are taught. [258]

The Nobel Prize-winning economist Milton Friedman, writing in 1970 in the *New York Times Magazine,* expressed his views on the ideas of "social responsibilities of business". He decried the idea of business with any social conscience: 'businessmen believe that they are defending free enterprise when they declaim that business is not concerned "merely" with profit but also with promoting desirable "social" ends; that business has a "social conscience" and takes seriously its responsibilities for providing employment, eliminating discrimination, avoiding pollution....In fact they are--preaching pure and unadulterated socialism.' For him, there was only duty of business, **"there is one and only one social responsibility of business—to use its resources and engage in activities designed to increase its profits."**[259]

Kent Greenfield quotes other economists who suggest that corporations should seek to maximize profits even if it means breaking the law: 'In their view, the penalties for breaking the law are merely costs of doing business. As long as the expected penalties from illegality are less than expected profits, the corporation should act illegally. The obligation to obey the law is subservient to the obligation to make money.'[260]

Is this behind the pharmaceutical industry's behaviour when they blatantly promote their drugs to children, and drugs that they know are dangerous to us all, even when they know they may cause death? It's not, however, simply one sector of industry affected, the 'pathological' nature of corporate behaviour that Professor Bakan refers to can be found throughout corporatocracy.

Corporations as Pathological Beings?

Bakan suggests 'The "best interests of the corporation" principle is now a feature in the corporate law of most countries…compelling corporate decision makers always to act in the best interests of the corporation, and hence its owners.' He believes 'The law forbids any other motivation for their actions, whether to assist workers, improve the environment, or help consumers save money.'

Corporations have increased the power of their influence as they have increased in size and become global international corporations. Their ability to externalize much of their cost onto society, obtain tax breaks and preferential treatment from governments and, added to this, their continuing amalgamations and consolidation, means their growth has been spectacular. Many see the increasing power of corporations as representing the biggest threat to our democracy that exists and the biggest obstacle we face in trying to create a sustainable future for humanity.

Shaping Our Future

Leo E. Strine, Jr., the Chief Justice of the Delaware Supreme Court, and adjunct faculty member at the University of Pennsylvania and Harvard Law Schools, informs us how recent legal developments, such as the Supreme Court ruling in 2010 *Citizens United vs FEC* (558 U.S. 310) have allowed corporations to further increase their influence on democracy:

> Before Citizens United, bipartisan legislation constrained the influence of huge corporations on our nation's politics. That legislation restricted corporations to spending funds that they raised from voluntary contributions from stockholders and employees. But Citizens United upset that sensible balance, based not just on a newly discovered understanding not only of our Constitution, but an erroneous understanding of corporate law.
>
> Since then, American corporations have helped generate a huge increase in political spending, tilting the playing field much more heavily in favor of the wealthiest interests, and against those of the middle class.

He is also concerned that companies themselves face heightened risks associated with 'the Wild West environment' that now surrounds political spending, and the exposure of corporations 'to the threat of coercion by the rise of secretive organisations associated with powerful interests.' He feels that 'Fundamental reform of this unsavoury reality is overdue.' [261] The Center For Business Accountability suggested that election spending in the USA is 'expected to set new records and the "shadow" of anonymous or so-called political "dark money" [is] growing.' They also mention the recent Business Roundtable announcement redefining the purpose of corporations, that it suggested 'sparked controversy' and 'also left questions unanswered'. They comment that in its statement, the Business Roundtable said that 'signers were committed "to transparency and effective engagement with shareholders," while it did not say what that means. Seventy-three Trendsetter companies, meanwhile, are setting model corporate governance best practices for operating in the most sharply divided political climate in recent memory. These companies choosing sunlight and accountability in their political spending are among the largest and most influential publicly held corporations in the nation.' [262]

The Business Roundtable meeting referred to was on August 19, 2019, involving the participation of 181 CEOs who signed a declaration that they would commit their companies to benefit all stakeholders—customers, employees, suppliers, communities and shareholders. Jamie Dimon, chairman and CEO of JP Morgan Chase and Co, who was chairman of the Business Roundtable, declared, "The American dream is alive, but fraying." He further suggests "Major employers are investing in their workers and communities because they know it is the only way to be successful over the long term. These modernized principles reflect the business community's unwavering commitment to continue to push for an economy that serves all Americans." One of the items they agreed to commit to was:

- Supporting the communities in which we work. We respect the people in our communities and protect the environment by embracing sustainable practices across our businesses.[263]

Many people will be highly sceptical that this declaration will have any impact on our runaway pharmaceutical industry, even though Johnson & Johnson, Pfizer, and Bayer USA were signatories to the document.

As regards to the political influence of the electoral process in the USA, Kenneth Doyle, writing in Bloomberg, informs us that Priorities USA, which collected almost $200 million to help Hillary Clinton in 2016, says it wants to spend that sum or more to help the next democratic candidate. We are informed, however, that this time, Priorities is being funded mostly by undisclosed donations. Apparently, more than three-quarters of the $23.4 million it raised in the first half of that year was collected by a non-profit arm (organized under Section 501(c)(4) of the tax code). The non-profit arm isn't, however, required to report donors to the public. We are informed that the group didn't have a non-profit arm in 2016. Critics of this system call undisclosed donations "dark money", and it is regarded as 'the most damaging cash in a campaign finance system where spending by groups not formally linked to candidates has skyrocketed.' Doyle comments:

> Despite the proliferation of dark money, congressional Democrats, along with the party's presidential contenders, are appealing to voters with messages focused on ending corruption by overhauling election and campaign finance laws and reversing the Supreme Court's 2010 decision in Citizens United v. FEC. That ruling struck down limits on corporate money influencing federal elections and led the way to sharply increased campaign spending.[264]

As regards to the legal status of corporations and whether the Business Roundtable declaration is likely to have any impact, the Program on Corporations, Law and Democracy believe we have to change the law that permits corporations to act irresponsibly and destructively:

> Corporations are not mentioned in the U.S. Constitution. They are legal creations of governments, intended to provide useful goods and services. No voter, citizen, social movement or elected official has ever granted corporations constitutional rights – intended exclusively for human beings. Corporate entities have gained constitutional rights solely from rulings by activist Supreme Court Justices.
>
> Many believe corporate hijacking of the constitution begins and ends with money in elections (i.e. First Amendment 'free speech' rights permitting corporations to spend money to influence elections). But

the threat to people, communities, the environment and democracy itself is much greater and includes additional parts of the First Amendment, as well as other amendments of our constitution.

'Corporations are not mentioned in the U.S. Constitution. They are legal creations of governments, intended to provide useful goods and services. No voter, citizen, social movement or elected official has ever granted corporations constitutional rights – intended exclusively for human beings. Corporate entities have gained constitutional rights solely from rulings by activist Supreme Court Justices.'

Greg Coleridge comments:

Reversing *Citizens United* isn't enough. Simply ending corporate political free speech rights isn't enough. We must abolish all forms of corporate personhood if we expect as self-governing people to assert our authority to protect ourselves, families, communities and what remains of a livable world…not to mention creating a political system for the very first time where *We the People* include <u>All the People</u>.[265]

One of the great issues we face is deciding what kind of world we want to create. It is apparent that our current system is failing. When we are faced with the realization that the pharmaceutical industry, for example, is contributing to the collapse of society, and is the leading cause of death in the USA, we need to reassess our goals and priorities. In the film *The Corporation*, the behaviour of numerous corporations, not just the pharmaceutical corporations, were compared to the behaviour of a psychopath. According to the World Health Organisation's Personality Diagnostic Checklist (based on the Manual of Mental Disorders

DSM IV), there are a number of symptoms that are used to diagnose a psychopath:

- Callous unconcern for the feelings of others.

- Incapacity to maintain enduring relationships.

- Reckless disregard for the safety of others.

- Deceitfulness: repeated lying and conning others for profit.

- Incapacity to experience guilt.

- Failure to conform to social norms with respect to lawful behaviours.

The film documented numerous corporations that exhibited these precise characteristics and came to the conclusion that corporations, under the existing regulatory or lack of regulatory apparatus, was essentially behaving psychopathically in much of its behaviour. [266]

Systemic Corrupting Pathology

Reflecting on Bakan's earlier point that limited liability 'would undermine personal moral responsibility', this point deserves some further exploration. It has already been established that medicine is now the leading cause of death in the USA (this is assuming the deaths due to the opioid epidemic are in included in this category). What is clear is that most doctors are not aware of this situation and are not willingly conspiring to create this collapse of health. For the greater part, they are controlled and manipulated by corporate interests. Corporate interests have infiltrated medicine to such a degree that the medical agenda, the treatment regime, the ideological apparatus, and the training of doctors etc., fully supports pharmaceutical interests and protocols. The pharmaceutical ideology is so embedded that to stand up against this vast industrial stranglehold risks being accused of incompetence and becoming a focus of sustained attack and even being accused of malpractice. There are numerous examples of funds being withdrawn, or only being available for 'approved research' (some examples of which we have already referred to), implicitly corralling people who do not toe the line. Toeing the line means keeping rigidly to the paradigm that utilizes approved drug treatment, surgery, radiation therapy, or chemotherapy as the primary methods of treatment for all illness, and supporting mainstream views such as the cholesterol myth and the huge promotion of statins to treat the myth. In cases where doctors dared challenge the status quo, they were often exposed to media attacks and further personal abuse and ridicule. What we do know, is the industry has been able to employ those they label as 'key opinion leaders' (remember, according to Virapen more than 75% of leading scientists in medicine are paid by the pharmaceutical industry) and key charities and other organisations to support their cause—which is the promotion of their drugs to treat 'disease'.

Melody Petersen, the *New York Times* journalist, in her excellent volume, *Our Daily Meds,* explored the ways the pharmaceutical industry was able to market its products with 'medical education', sponsorship of meetings and seminars and educational conferences, in her experience with examples of medical training she researched in Iowa. She informs us that as a doctor, you could have attended the Iowa Academy of Family Physicians at its summer educational event at The Inn on Lake Okoboji and enjoyed the benefits of the seventeen drug companies who supported the event with their largesse, which aside from the conference included golf tournaments with prizes and gift certificates. Or you could avail yourself of the March educational conference in Silverthorne Colorado, where physicians were told to come and ski and bring the whole family at the five-day event supported by nine pharmaceutical companies. If you were an opinion leader, aside from being paid to give talks at these events, you also were well paid for doing internet seminars, and some opinion leaders actively sought out sponsorship. Dr Satish Rao, a professor of gastroenterology, worked as a consultant and speaker for Novartis and sat on the company's advisory board. He further received "educational grants" from AstraZeneca, Janssen, Novartis, Solvay Pharmaceuticals, and Tap Pharmaceuticals. He also sat on the advisory boards of GlaxoSmithKline, Sanofi-Synthelabo, and Solvay. The extent of control that the pharmaceutical industry had was brought home to Petersen when she called the National Society of Rheumatologists in 2000 and asked to speak to an arthritis expert for an article she was writing. She specifically asked for a physician who was not being paid by the companies she was writing about, at that time the makers of Vioxx and Celebrex: she was informed that there was no-one—all the consultants were consultants or speakers for the companies of these drugs. [267]

Petersen also mentions that in 2004, the University of Iowa boasted that it had 136 scientists managing clinical trials for the industry and that it was involved in so many drug trials that it had negotiated standard written contracts. The drug companies, however, were asking for waivers from the university's requirement that the results be published soon after the trial was completed. Petersen makes the observation that 'Without this rule, there was a risk the public would never learn about a study that found that medicine had dangerous side effects or did not work as expected.' She also mentions that the university tried to get the companies to agree to pay the medical bills of any volunteer in any of the studies who might be injured in the various studies and experiments. She comments, 'If a company refused, the university made sure that it did not promise to pay for the treatment of the volunteers' injuries either.'[268]

We know from the numerous court cases involving most of the pharmaceutical companies that they have all actively sold drugs that they knew to be harmful and in a number of cases caused an unknown and unknowable number of deaths, sometimes of children. There are a considerable number of players in our medical scenario, a web of people not just those directly employed by the pharmaceutical industry. I described the web in *Unhealthy Betrayal* as a form of cancer that was able to permeate its way through society, you could, just as easily, describe it as a parasite that feeds off its host weakening it all the time.

Is it too simplistic simply to say that the pharmaceutical industry is run by people with psychopathic tendencies, or that the industry itself cultivates the expression of such natures in its employees, or even that its policies attract people with psychopathic tendencies, such as its marketing salespeople who knowingly sell ineffective or dangerous drugs? We know now that most pharmaceutical companies are no longer run by medically trained people—they are run and controlled by marketing people. But what about the doctors who simply accept all the gifts and helpfully sign the prescriptions, or the psychiatrists who dole out drugs to children because it pays better than taking the time to evaluate what really is going on in a child's life?

What appears to be evident here is that a state of denial seems to exist, an environment fosters the creation of behaviour that for many of us, may seem reprehensible—but to those in the business who simply become accustomed to being detached and ambivalent about the damage—it just becomes normal, business as usual.

You can draw a parallel between this sector and the economy as a whole. The economist Professor Michael Hudson describes the failings of the economic system in his volume, *Killing the Host—How Financial Parasites and Debt Destroy the Global Economy*. In this volume, which is discussed in my own book *Hijacked,* the workings of the financial system, and the massive debt creation that is exerting huge pressure on the economy, in particular on many if not most countries' ability to fund services adequately and maintain infrastructure—the nature of the corporate domination via private banking interests is seen as both immensely destructive and parasitic.[269]

In an economic system that is increasingly perceived as becoming more predatory, there are people in the industry, even bankers who recognize how the whole system is becoming more pathological. In *Hijacked,* I quoted a former Goldman Sachs partner worth repeating here: 'The good guys got pushed out and the bad guys got pushed up. Those that operated with integrity in the fixed income division began leaving the firm in droves. "Rip your face off" became the Goldman motto.'

'The good guys got pushed out and the bad guys got pushed up. Those that operated with integrity in the fixed income division began leaving the firm in droves. "Rip your face off" became the Goldman motto'. [270]

What has this got to do our story so far? It is not unrealistic to draw a parallel between these industries, all run by corporate interests, all cloaked in layers of secrecy, and all having a direct effect on our health. The 2008 crisis, however, brought home to many how economic collapse does have a direct bearing on our health, and even our ability to simply survive. Aside from the obvious link, that everything we have described so far—that the whole host of factors that affect our health, seemingly not directly connected, yet all orchestrated by corporate interests on every level—is a reflection of a particular state of mind, a similar attitude, a similar aspect of consciousness. The labels that we choose to use to describe this state of consciousness can vary greatly, from simply selfish, and uncaring, to manipulative and destructive, through to sociopathic, psychopathic and even madness. Here is David Korten's view of corporate globalism:

> No sane person seeks a world divided between billions of excluded people living in absolute deprivation and a tiny elite guarding their wealth and luxury behind fortress walls. No one rejoices at the prospect of life in a world of collapsing social and ecological systems. Yet we continue to place human civilization and even the survival of our species at risk mainly to allow a million or so people to accumulate money beyond any conceivable need. We continue to go boldly where no one wants to go.
>
> We are now coming to see that economic globalization has come at a heavy price. In the name of modernity we are creating dysfunctional societies that are breeding pathological behavior—violence, extreme competitiveness, suicide, drug abuse, greed, and environmental degradation—at every hand. Such behavior is an inevitable consequence when a society fails to meet the needs of its members for social bonding, trust affection and a shared sacred meaning. The threefold crisis of deepening poverty, environmental destruction, and social disintegration is a manifestation of this dysfunction.
>
> There is nothing inevitable about the collective madness of pursuing policies that deepen the dysfunction. The idea that we are caught in the grip of irresistible historic forces and inherent human imperfections to which we have no choice but to adapt is pure fabrication. Economic globalization is being advanced by conscious choices by those who see the world through the lens of the corporate interest. There are human alternatives, and those who view the world through the lens of human interest have both the right and the power to choose them.[271]

Shaping Our Future

Does it matter how we choose to label the state of consciousness that is expressed by the actions of people who seem dead set to pillage the planet, pollute the air we breathe, pollute the water we drink, poison the food we eat, poison the land we live on, and destroy the health of millions? I believe that it does. There are many people who do not wish to see themselves as destroyers of the Earth, or participants in the destruction of our health, who yet may be unwitting participants in this very story.

Economic globalization is being advanced by conscious choices by those who see the world through the lens of the corporate interest. There are human alternatives, and those who view the world through the lens of human interest have both the right and the power to choose them.

The predatory behaviour described in the world of finance, and the mercenary behaviour exhibited by many of the players in the pharmaceutical industry are expressions of people who do not appreciate the value of the fact that they are part of a wider community. Such people believe they can pillage, extract, manipulate, destroy, and be intensely selfish to their greater benefit when the reality is that they are practising intense denial of what it is to be truly human. Such gratification as they seek is fleeting: there is no real fulfilment, there is no real happiness to be found in being divorced from the majority of humanity. Whilst some may scorn these views they nevertheless, are acknowledged and reflected in society as a whole when we use terms such as "soul-destroying work", or "depressing work", even "unfulfilling work". At some level, we do know.

How To Survive in the 21ˢᵗ Century

We need to acknowledge as a priority that we change the regulatory apparatus that allows corporations to cause us harm, that also permits them to be able to dump their poisons and waste products, and externalize a significant portion of their costs on us as taxpayers, and that further encourages them to avoid paying their share of taxes by tax avoidance measures, by tax transfer pricing, and creation of bogus offshore companies and such measures. And critically, we need to prevent them undue influence over the political apparatus of all countries such as they currently have, including influence over all the regulatory bodies set up to regulate them. We also, as a society, have to connect with each other and share information and our aspirations to create a better world than we have so far. To do this I believe will take a shift in consciousness.

Global Shift

Change is the natural order of life. Every cell in our body is changed, refreshed, and renewed: none of us is the same person as we were last year. We need to embrace change. To embrace change we need to embrace the possibility of change. For generations, many people held the view that the world was flat, and that if we were to sail too far we would fall off the world. For generations, people believed the Earth was the centre of the universe until Copernicus suggested it was actually the sun.

There are a lot more people who feel there is a real need for change. We need to throw off the corporate yoke. It's not just about one sector of our economy that is failing us, it is a *systemic problem*. That is not to say that all corporations are harmful or inherently bad. Responsible corporations that actually care about their impact on the Earth and their effect on our lives are to be welcomed. In *Unhealthy Betrayal,* I reported on the story of Interface, the international carpet maker, and the company's CEO Ray Anderson. Ray Anderson, says he had an epiphany back in 1994 when his carpet company was a toxic petroleum-based business that created huge amounts of waste. He read a copy of Paul Hawken's book *The Ecology of Commerce—How Business Can Save the Planet* and realised that he was a "plunderer". His company consumed enough energy to light and heat a city, it consumed a billion pounds of petroleum-derived raw materials to create carpet tiles every year and each day just one of his plants sent six tons of carpet trimmings to the local landfill. Following reading Hawken's book (which I also discuss in *Unhealthy Betrayal* in regard to circular economics), he realized that he needed to change his company that had a high-footprint on the Earth to one that had a zero-footprint. According to their website, the company has reached its goal of having a zero-footprint and are working on products that actually absorb carbon dioxide and works with the realities of circular economics.

In *Confessions of a Radical Industrialist—Profits, People, Purpose—Doing Business by Respecting the Earth,* Ray describes his journey from being a destroyer, from 'an old dangerously dysfunctional model to a better one that will operate in balance and harmony with nature.' He says, 'The point of my story is deceptively simple, business and industry—not just American business and industry—must change their ways to survive.' He quotes Hawken when he says ' not only was business and industry the principal instrument of global destruction, it was also the only instrument large enough, wealthy enough, and pervasive and powerful enough to lead humankind out of the mess we were making.' He has a particularly relevant message for academia:

> Change comes slowly in academia, and so the harmful effects of obsolete curricula tend to persist. Here's the decision that you leaders in academia are going to have to make consciously. You can either pass on or perpetuate an old outmoded, and destructive body of knowledge, ensuring that it will remain (and cause more harm) for another generation or two, or three; or you can wake up to the responsibility—and the

satisfaction—of challenging the obsolete status quo in your curricula. To break with that potent opiate, *We've always done it this way.*[272]

No doubt there would be many critics of Anderson's actions: he was not acting with the sole aim of returning profits to shareholders. Ray's actions, however, actually increased the volume of Interstate's business and increased its profits throughout this process. All the measures taken, in the long-term, actually saved the company money, improved worker relations and worker satisfaction, and improved the company's status, not just as a world-class carpet maker, but as a world leader in showing how truly responsible corporate behaviour can benefit society. Ray Anderson is no longer with us, but his legacy will live on. We need more people like him: hopefully, he will inspire more people to bring their consciousness into alignment with the true needs of humanity and inculcate a respect for the amazing planet that we have the privilege of living on.

There are no doubt many among us who feel that without changes in the laws governing corporations the likelihood of the more avaricious companies such as the pharmaceutical industry changing their pathological natures is indeed slim. What kind of a world do we believe we are creating if we encourage people to feel it is okay to invest money into a company that is actively and knowingly causing harm to people, causing death—simply viewing this as the cost of doing business? Glasbeek believes 'We must blow away these runaway investors' privacy: it is a privacy that hides ugliness and deceit.' He makes the important point that we need to deal with what he refers to as 'the central obfuscation: that corporate law promotes the everyday avoidance of personal responsibility' and further:

> Above all, anyone working to devise tactics to help develop an alternative politics must always keep in mind this important point: the obscuring ink sprayed all over us by the octopus-like features of corporate

law produces flesh and blood victors, winners who profit from the unrewarded work and toil of others, who do not care whether their welfare is based on injuries and harms inflicted on others. The wheelers and dealers behind large corporatins should be seen for what they are.

Controlling shareholders of violating corporations should be prosecuted whenever their corporation has violated a regulatory or criminal law rule. [273]

Kent Greenfield believes that corporations need to sign up to a new set of legally binding principles that act as guidance, such as:

1. The Ultimate Purpose of Corporations Should Be to Serve the Interests of Society as a Whole.
2. Corporations are Distinctively Able to Contribute to the Societal Good by Creating Financial Prosperity.[274]

Further principles could be added to prevent further destructive pollution, and they could be required to agree not to cause harm to citizens and negatively affect our health. Joel Bakan discussing corporate charter revocation laws that symbolize the fact that corporations are our creations and that we still have the power to revoke them suggests: 'The time has come to use that power, not only by activating charter revocation laws, but also, more generally, by subjecting corporations to robust democratic controls. The corporation is not an independent "person" with its own rights, needs and desires that regulators must respect. It is a state-created tool for advancing social and economic policy. As such it has only one institutional purpose: to serve the public interest.'[275]

The time has come to use that power, not only by activating charter revocation laws, but also, more generally, by subjecting corporations to robust democratic controls. The corporation is not an independent "person" with its own rights, needs and desires that regulators must respect. It is a state-created tool for advancing social and economic policy. As such it has only one institutional purpose: to serve the public interest.

Post Pandemic Considerations

For those who were hoping that the world would return to some previously experienced 'normality' following the containment of covid-19, I believe will find this not to be the case. The economic considerations will be as profound as anything our society has faced. The health implications are also as profound, and much depends on the lessons we learn.

Evidence that the virus was manmade is persuasive. It is no real secret that one of China's chief virologists, Zhengli-Li Shi, had already created, a chimeric version of a bat virus that was able to cross-species. She was aided by American funding from the NIH to undertake research to do just this, this was after this kind of work was no longer officially sanctioned by the Obama administration, for what was referred to as 'gain-of-function' research. Much of her research was based in the Wuhan laboratory that was close to the fish market, the supposed source of the outbreak. In a 2015 paper, published in *Nature* that she participated in, it states "Using the reverse genetics system, we generated and characterized a chimeric virus expressing the spike of bat coronavirus SHC014 in a mouse-adapted SARS-CoV backbone. The results indicate that group 2b viruses encoding the SHC014 spike in wild-type backbone can efficiently use multiple orthologs of the SARS receptor human angiotensin-converting enzyme II (ACE2), replicate efficiently in primary human airway cells and achieve *in vitro* titers equivalent to epidemic strains of SARS-CoV. Additionally, *in vivo* experiments demonstrate replication of the chimeric virus in mouse lung with notable pathogenesis.'[276]

Shaping Our Future

The 'spike' that is being referred to, is the S-protein that is the important tool for entering human cells, effectively it is like the key to a lock that enables entrance for a virus to invade human cells (via the ACE2 receptor) and propagate and destroy them. The article mentions 'notable pathogenesis' in the mouse lung, which is precisely what was experienced with Covid-19. A further article found that the Wuhan coronavirus is closely related to two viruses (CoVZC45 and CoVZX21) from sample bats from Zhoushan. It was found to have 89.1% nucleotide similarity with the CoVZC45 virus and "shows 100% amino acid similarity to bat CoVZC45 in the nsp7 and E proteins." Dr Judy A Mikovits PhD, Molecular Biologist, and former Director of Lab of antiviral mechanisms NCI. She believes that "the 100% amino acid similarity would mean that it can't possibly be a mutation." This belief was corroborated by Dr Sean Lin, former lab director of the viral disease branch of Walter Reed Army Institute of Research., who suggested, "Maybe the virus was reverse-engineered."[277]

Some people might want to question in the light of this disaster whether it is a good idea to pay for research like this. For whose benefit is this carried out? Another article in Nature, 12th November 2015, questions the sense not just of this type of research in general, but questions the sanity of creating the very chimeric virus that we are referring to above. Simon Wain-Hobson, a virologist at the Pasteur Institute in Paris, points out that the researchers have created a novel virus that "grows remarkably well" in human cells. He also points out, "If the virus escaped, nobody could predict, the trajectory." Another critic of this work was Richard Ebright, a molecular biologist and biodefense expert at Rutgers University in Piscataway. New Jersey who suggests 'The only impact of this work is the creation, in a lab, of a new non-natural risk." Both researchers are long-standing critics of gain-of-function research.[278]

The same researchers question the wisdom of an agency that is supposedly building a stockpile of vaccine treatments against anthrax and avian flu, that also funding the creation of deadlier and more infectious varieties of avian flu, and other animal-borne diseases, which could pose the threat of an outbreak if not handled properly. Professor Ebright suggests "It's hard to imagine that someone thought creating new pandemic pathogens would be a good strategy for defending against pandemic pathogens...It reflects the clear lack of anyone in charge [of US biodefense strategy]." Regarding the moratorium and the temporary suspension of funding for this work, Simon Wain-Hobson suggested, "Rather than use the avian flu moratorium to seek advice, listen and foster debate, many influential scientists engaged in an academic exercise of self justification." Ebright suggested "[The moratorium] was strictly for public relations...No one with a moral compass would propose or perform this work."[279]

The real tragedy of this Covid-19 outbreak was the lack of response to the successful treatment by doctors both in China and the USA of Covid patients with high-dose intravenous vitamin C. Dr Richard Cheng reported the work of Dr Enqian Mao, chief of emergency medicine department at Ruijin Hospital, Shanghai. Mao had been using high-dose intravenous vitamin C (IVC) to treat patients with acute pancreatitis, sepsis, surgical wound healing and other medical conditions for over 10 years. When covid-19 broke out Mao and other medical experts used IVC to successful treat moderate to severe covid-19 cases. As of March 17, 2020, they had successfully treated 358 patients and all patients who received IVC improved and there was no mortality.[280]

There were a number of doctors in the USA successfully treating covid-19 patients with IVC. The Frontline Covid-19 Critical Care Working Group was one group who were using a shared protocol, that included IVC and corticosteroids. According to one of the group, Dr Pierre Kory, the Medical

Director of the Trauma and Life Support Centre, of the Critical Care Service at the University of Wisconsin, "If you can administer intravenous corticosteroids and ascorbic acid starting in the emergency room and every six hours thereafter while in the hospital, the mortality rate of this disease and the need for mechanical ventilators will likely be *greatly* reduced." He further explains that *it is the severe inflammation sparked by the Coronavirus, not the virus itself, that kills patients.* The hyper-inflammation triggered by covid-19, also known as the "cytokine storm" requires the use of the combination of vitamin C and corticosteroids to prevent deterioration into a very severe form of Acute Respiratory Distress Syndrome (ARDS), a condition which causes the lungs to fail. Another physician, Dr Joseph Varon has treated 40 seriously ill covid-19 patients with this protocol in Houston's United Memorial Medical Center. Of these patients, 30 have already gone home, including a 90-year-old woman with a history of colon cancer and sepsis. None of his patients has died.[281] Their website posts "Our MATH+ protocol saves lives. So why isn't the world using it?" Why indeed? I have posted the protocol on my website. I have also posted an article posting how references to the successful treatment of covid-19 using IVC have been blocked by Facebook, Utube and other media sites.

I also reported on the work of Dr Andrew G Weber, a pulmonologist and critical care specialist affiliated with two Northwell Health facilities based on Long Island, New York using IVC treatment, giving 1500mg of vitamin C 3 or 4 times a day. He explains how he has found that vitamin C levels in coronavirus patients drop dramatically when they suffer sepsis and that an inflammatory response occurs when their bodies overreact to the infection. He says. 'It makes all the sense in the world to try and maintain this level of vitamin C.'[282]

How To Survive in the 21st Century

The ability of the pharmaceutical industry to continue to keep people ignorant of the true value of vitamin C is waning even with the huge campaign that they are currently waging. One doctor, based in Detroit fell foul of this campaign when his practice was raided by the FBI, charged with 'health-care fraud'. Dr Mok made the mistake of explaining to FOX 2 how his vitamin C infusions, which also included zinc, glutathione and B complex, helped his patients. Mok said, "I'm mostly seeing people that are mild to moderate illness, and they turn around pretty quick usually after one or two doses they are remarkably better."[283] No doubt they would be better. Their vitamin C levels would likely be non-existent at this stage, adding a further antioxidant like glutathione would contribute to immune function, and adding B vitamins, well, that would be like adding icing on a cake, as it aids in thousands of enzyme operations in the body.

Can Big Pharma keep everybody ignorant forever? As regards to vitamin C, if the sales of vitamin C are anything to go by, they are losing the war. No doubt the media attack will continue. When the results from the difference in the death count become public, will they be able to keep this information hidden? Will people thank their respective national health services for ignoring the value of this life-saving nature of vitamin C at a time that it was most needed? Only time will judge whether they will. There are petitions started to enable the use of intravenous vitamin C in both the USA and the UK hospitals for those who wish to vote for change here.[284] Meanwhile, let's look at another way corporate interests undermine our health.

Unhealthy Agriculture

One of the single most important factors that directly affect our health is our agricultural system. It is not just to do with the quality of food that is being created: our system of agriculture has far-reaching implications for life on earth as we know it. Whilst our agricultural system is associated with, to some extent, individual farmers, what we regard as industrialized agriculture is increasingly associated with farming to mainly support corporate interests. We have briefly reviewed the advent of genetically modified food in chapter five, which is orchestrated by companies such as Monsanto, now part of Bayer. The major part of our food production is based on the intensive application of chemical inputs such as nitrate fertilizers, herbicides, pesticides, and fungicides.

Corporate interests like to portray this form of agriculture as fit-for-purpose 21st-century technology, and not just sustainable but essential to feed and nourish a growing population. The trouble with this view is that is wrong on every count. Industrial agriculture is based on a number of myths that are useful to address:

1. Industrial agriculture is essential to meet the growing demands of an increasing population.
2. Industrial agriculture is more efficient than any other form of agriculture and best placed to meet the requirements of society.
3. Industrial agriculture is able to provide cheap good healthy food, affordable by everyone, whereas other forms of agriculture are not.

Firstly, predictions of global population growth are being challenged by a number of sources. Canadian Darell Bricker, from the market research agency Ipsos, in his recent volume *Empty Planet—The Shock of Global Population Decline,* suggests that our global population is set to plateau and then shrink. He maintains that predictions of population growth by the United Nations are wrong and based on "erroneous assumptions." Part of the change in outlook is based on increasing urbanization and the education of women. When women move to urban areas, children are no longer seen as additional useful labour for the family to work in fields producing food: in this new environment children are found to be an additional financial burden, particularly when finances are scarce.[285] In a vast study on population, fertility, and health by the Gates Foundation, a remarkable decline in fertility has been revealed. This global study found that whereas in 1950 women were having on average 4.7 children in their lifetime, the fertility rate had more or less halved to 2.4 children per woman by 2017. The rate in most European countries has averaged at 1.7. When the rate drops below 2.1, populations shrink predictably. China, the country with one of the biggest populations, had a fertility rate of 1.5 in 2017, even though it has departed from its famous one-child policy.[286]

A number of researchers believe that part of the decreasing fertility is due to the decline of reproductive health, a subject which we have briefly reported on in chapter four. The report published in *The Lancet* in April mentions the 2013 report by WHO and the UN Environment Programme that revealed how the production and exposure to environmental chemicals that could disrupt the endocrine system have increased enormously since World War II. They cite three large Chinese sperm banks that have reported 'steep declines in semen quality from their donors, who predominantly live in cities that are highly polluted.' They report that in Denmark for the last 40 years the fertility rate has been 1.7, and even with assisted reproductive technology (more than 9% of Danish children are born with this help), they suggest that 'more than 20% of Danish men born in the 1960s will never become fathers.'[287]

The next myth that is used to support the continued practice is that more sustainable farming practices such as organic agriculture would be unable to adequately supply enough food to meet our needs.

Shaping Our Future

Peter Rosset challenged the conventional wisdom that small farms are backward and unproductive compared to the large mechanized farms such as exist in America. His study found that smaller farms were "multi-functional" were more productive and efficient, and contributed more to economic development than large farms. Aside from this, he found that small farmers were better stewards of natural resources, and biodiversity, and were able to safeguard the future sustainability of agricultural production. What was important, however, was to abandon simply using yield per acre as a guide for the productivity of a farm, and use total output as a measure. Where a large farm might produce one crop very efficiently, smaller farms produce more products. For example, many farmers intercrop, planting other crops between the rows of their main crop, which controls weeds and can add to the soil structure etc. They also can rear animals along with crops that both contribute to soil fertility and the overall output.[288]

A study by Catherine Badgley and associates undertook a direct comparison between organic agriculture and industrial agriculture. They examined 293 examples of food production and concluded: 'These results indicate that organic agriculture has the potential to contribute quite substantially to the global food supply while reducing the detrimental environmental impacts of conventional agriculture.' Not just did they discover that it was capable of meeting our needs but more than that:

> Our results suggest that organic methods of food production can contribute substantially to feeding the current and future human population on the current agricultural land base, while maintaining soil fertility. In fact, the models suggest the possibility that the agricultural land base could eventually be reduced if organic production methods were employed.

How To Survive in the 21ˢᵗ Century

Currently, industrialized agriculture is supported by significant political support via research and subsidy, whereas organic agriculture has had little investment; in effect, we as taxpayers have been actively supporting the very agricultural system that destroys the soil and our health. Badgley makes the point:

> Also, there is scope for increased production on organic farms, since most agricultural research of the past 50 years has focused on conventional methods. Arguably, comparable efforts focused on organic practices would lead to further improvements in yields as well as in soil fertility and pest management. Production per unit area is greater on small farms than on large farms in both developed and developing countries; thus, an increase in the number of small farms would also enhance food production.[289]

One of the important measures of sustainability is the ability to support biodiversity, both in animals and in plants. A study by Gerold Rahmann in a 2011 meta-analysis reviewed 766 examples of farming systems out of an initial 19,000 and found a higher degree of biodiversity in organic farming. Here are his comments:

> Biodiversity is one of the most important resources on earth, and human activities endanger the total number of species. Large numbers are already extinct or close to being erased. At the Rio-conference 1992, the United Nations agreed to reduce biodiversity losses to zero in 2010. The goals have not been reached. Farming (intensification and land-use change) are the main reasons for biodiversity losses, but agriculture can also protect and enhance biodiversity.

The biologist, author and ecologist Dr Vandana Shiva has been reporting on the work of Navdanya which has promoted diverse ecological agriculture for more than two decades, producing more food and better nutrition. She is critical of the so-called "green revolution."

> The green revolution and genetic engineering have been offered as "intensive" farming, creating a false impression that they produce more food per acre. However, industrial agriculture is chemically intensive and capital intensive. The former produces more toxics, the latter more debt.
>
> To produce more food and nutrition, we need to design production systems which are biodiversity intensive and ecologically intensive. Biodiversity intensive systems produce more food, nutrition and health per acre than industrial chemical monocultures. And by saving on costs of external inputs, they create more wealth per acre for farmers. When measured in terms of contribution to nutrition, health and rural incomes, industrial systems have very low productivity.

Like Peter Roset, she is critical of comparative yield figures that the proponents of industrial agriculture like to trot out to portray small farmers as inefficient: 'Green revolution systems have high "yield", but low output. And it is output that feeds the soil and the people, not the yield of globally traded commodities, which are used for biofuel or animal feed.' She also explains how industrial agriculture actually is counterproductive and increases the pressure on land use:

> India's experience tells us that instead of more land being released for conservation, by destroying diversity and multiple uses of land, the industrial system actually increases pressure on the land since each acre of a monoculture provides a single output, and the displaced outputs have to be grown on additional acres. And globally, the chemical intensive land extensive system has had to spread to the Amazon rainforest. This is not land saving or biodiversity conserving, it is land destroying and biodiversity destroying agriculture.

How To Survive in the 21ˢᵗ Century

Dr Shiva reports on multi-cropping and polyculture systems that have been developed that are leading the way in agricultural production without the use of destructive chemical sprays that are not just more sustainable, the food produced is healthier, tastier, and far more nutritious. She gives numerous examples of this type of food system:

> The polycultures of ecological agricultural systems have evolved because more output can be harvested from a given area planted with diverse crops than from an equivalent area consisting of separate patches of monocultures. For example, in plantings of sorghum and pigeon pea mixtures, one hectare will produce the same yields as 0.94 hectares of sorghum monoculture and 0.68 hectares of pigeon pea monoculture. Thus one hectare of polyculture produces what 1.62 hectares of monoculture can produce. This is called the land equivalent ratio (LER).
>
> Planting multiple crops in a mixture will have low yields of individual crops but will have a higher total output of food. In the terraced fields of the Himalayas, women farmers produce, even in a bad year, six times more total output than industrially farmed rice monocultures.

She cites the example of a mixed organic farm in the Himalaya that produces 9,000 kg of maize, radish, mustard greens and peas. A chemically farmed maize monoculture yields 5,000kg. This is 1,000kg more maize than the biodiverse system but 4,000kg less food in terms of nutrition per acre.

She informs us, 'In terms of nutrition per acre, the biodiverse farming system is much more productive than the chemical monocultures, it provides 305 (g) of calcium and 29.3 (g) of iron compared to the monoculture.' She cites what is referred to as the *baranaja* (twelve crop) system, which produces 2680 kg of food per acre compared to 2186 of a maize monoculture, and gives us an accurate idea of the nutritional difference:

In terms of protein the production is 4214 vs 242 kg, carbohydrate 1622.94 vs 1447.14, fat 131.8 kg vs 78.7 kg, and energy 9359470 kcal vs 7476120 kcal. In terms of vitamins, banana produces 1360.9 mg vs 1967 mg beta carotene in case of maize monoculture, folic acid 2206.3 mg to 437 mg. Minerals are – calcium 5052 g vs 218 g, iron 143.9 g vs 50.3 g, phosphorus 9505 g vs 7607 g, magnesium 3604 g vs 3038 g, potassium 11186 g vs 6252 g.

She suggests that Navdanya's work on biodiversity-based organic farming shows India could feed twice its population through biodiversity intensification. She cites the UN report submitted to the General Assembly on 20th December 2010 (report submitted to the Special Rapporteur on the Right to Food, Olivier de Schutter) that confirms that ecological agriculture produces more food (p.8), "resource conserving, low-external-input techniques have a proven potential to significantly improve yields", and "ecological interventions on 12.6 million farms increased crop yields of 79 percent".[290]

There are numerous examples of farmers' innovative approaches to crop-growing that negates the use of spraying chemicals that destroy the soil. Fred Pearce informs us that thousands of farmers across east Africa raise yields by planting weeds with their crops. The insect pests are attracted to napier grass and get caught up in their sticky honey traps: this enables farmers to defeat the stem borer. Their maize crop, however, was also under attack from a parasitic plant, the striga, or witch-weed, which wrecks more than $10 billion worth of crops every year. Their solution to this problem was to plant another weed called Desmodium in between the maize, and the parasitic striga will no longer grow there. It apparently does not like the Desmodium plant. These two strategies resulted in increased yields of 60-70%. Poly-cropping is being used to raise productivity all over the world: 'The success of sustainable agriculture is dispelling the myth that modern techno-farming is the most productive method', says Miguel Altieri of the University of California, Berkeley. 'In Mexico, it takes 1.73 hectares of land planted with maize to produce as much food as one hectare planted with a mixture of maize, squash and beans.' Pearce quotes another study into sustainable agriculture by Jules Pretty of the University of Essex, involving more than 200 projects in 52 countries and more than 4 million farmers, covering an area the size of Italy where crop yields increased by an average of 73%. In all cases, it involved simple farming developments that did not involve the use of chemical sprays of any kind.[291]

The great agronomist Sir Albert Howard, biologist and farmer, former director of the Institute of Plant Industry Indore, and agricultural adviser to states in central India and Rajputana, spent years researching how to improve crop yields and health and developed a system of agriculture that did not rely on chemical sprays and artificial fertilizers. He developed a system of composting that he called the Indore method that he used successfully throughout the world. It was a method that utilized creating a mixture of plant humus and animal manure and with some starter soil that would combine and compost down into usable humus in approximately three months that by itself would protect plants from pests and diseases and increase yields significantly. He would create approximately 8,000 tons a year of this compost at his Indore farm and grew crops that were healthy and robust and the soil would be enriched year after year. Instead of draining and impoverishing soil using sprays and artificial fertilizer his soil actually became more productive over time, not less, as is the case with current agricultural practice.

Howard worked on a number of estates improving the productivity of tea, cotton, maize, rice, sugar cane and vegetable production using his knowledge and creating a healthier soil condition with the production of humus by the Indore process. In one of the previous paragraphs, we discussed the parasitic witch-weed problem of striga infested maize fields—Howard believed this was just an infestation that was only found to exist in poor soil conditions such as he found in Rhodesia: 'This parasite promises to prove a valuable sensor for indicating whether or not the maize soils of Rhodesia are fertile. If witch-weed appears, the land needs humus; if it is absent, the soil contains sufficient organic matter. Good farming will, therefore, provide an automatic method of control.' Howard found pests and disease were a problem created by poor farming technique. He noted that as the advancement of the chemicalization of agriculture progressed, new diseases and pests were increasingly being presented as soil was becoming further impoverished and destroyed, risking more serious problems with health not just of the plants and the soil, but of the animals and populations that relied on this form of agriculture for sustenance.

The third myth that is industrial agriculture is able to provide cheap, good, healthy food, affordable by everyone, whereas other forms of agriculture are not. This statement raises so many points that deserve a response: it is simplistic and betrays the way the industry is massively subsidized by public money; it ignores the way its massive chemical reliance destroys soil health, plant health, and animal health and its consequential disastrous effect of humanity's health: and further, it ignores its immensely harmful ecological impact not just affecting greenhouse gas emissions but water supplies, pollution of the sea, and much more. Whilst this discussion, in itself, could deserve a book in its own right (which is not the intention of this volume), we can review some of the problems that are becoming more apparent to some agronomists and scientists.

In *Unhealthy Betrayal,* I wrote about the work of one of America's great agronomists, Don Huber, emeritus professor at Purdue University and senior scientist on USDA's National Plant Disease Recovery System. He has been a plant physiologist and pathologist for over 50 years, and specialized in soil-borne diseases, microbial ecology, and host-parasitic relationships. For the past 20 years, he has conducted extensive research into the effects of glyphosate on crops. In the process, he and other scientists discovered some very alarming facts about glyphosate the major component of Roundup and, the most widely used herbicide worldwide. In January 2011 he was so concerned by what he was finding that he wrote to the secretary of Agriculture, Tom Vilsack warning of his findings, particularly the discovery of a new, and then unidentified pathogenic organism. At precisely this time Vilsack, a known enthusiast for genetically modified crops and genetic engineering in general, was preparing to approve two new Roundup-Ready alfalfa applications. There was a concerted lobbying effort by the industry to push this through.

Huber was disturbed about the effects of glyphosate, particularly in the soil and the creation of some dangerous new pathogens. His letter to Vilsack was made public, and some of his comments are worth repeating here:

> For the past 40 years, I have been a scientist in the professional and military agencies that evaluate and prepare for natural and man-made biological threats, including germ warfare and disease outbreaks. Based on this experience, I believe the threat we are facing from this pathogen is unique and of a high risk status. In layman's terms, it should be treated as an emergency.
>
> I have studied plant pathogens for more than 50 years. We are now seeing an unprecedented trend of increasing plant and animal diseases and disorders. This pathogen may be instrumental to understanding and solving this problem. It deserves immediate attention with significant resources to avoid a general collapse of our critical agricultural infrastructure.

Shaping Our Future

He explains to Vilsack that glyphosate, the main ingredient in Roundup, is a chelator, in that it binds with minerals, leading to plants being deprived of nutrients, which in turn leads to their demise, and also affects the main crop and animals grazing the land:

> You have to realize all that mode of action is immobilizing a critical essential nutrient. Those nutrients aren't just required by the weed, but they're required by microorganisms. They're required by us for our own physiologic functions. So if it's immobilized, it may be present if we do a regular test. But it's not necessarily physiologically available in the same efficiency that would have been if it wasn't chelated with that glyphosate or other chemical chelator.

He emphasizes how this herbicide is systemic in the plant and accumulates in most of its growth points:

> It's going to be in your root tips, your shoot tips, your legume nodules, and in the food that we eat. Because it's in those reproductive structures, that's where it accumulates. The later it is supplied, now that they're using glyphosate—as ripening agents to kill a plant to kind of speed up its harvest process—the only place that it can go is right into the seed.

Huber expresses his concern for how this herbicide is creating serious ecological problems by destroying the very organisms that make up soil:

> Glyphosate is extremely toxic to all of those organisms. What we see with our continued use and abuse of this powerful pesticide, this powerful weed killer, is it is also totally eliminating many of those organisms from the soil. We no longer have the same balance that we used to have.

Consequently, we see an increase of over 40 new diseases or 40 diseases that we used to have managed under fairly effective control, but all of a sudden are another serious problem for us.

One of the issues that provoked Huber to write to the secretary of agriculture was the development of dangerous forms of fungi that caused sudden death syndrome in soybeans and instituted significant changes in the gut flora of animals grazing and being fed food systemically treated with glyphosate.

The other thing we see is that the normal biological control organisms, even in the animal, are very sensitive to the residual glyphosate levels. I was just reviewing a paper–as I flew out here yesterday–on chronic botulism or toxic botulism type problem. This is where you have the Clostridium botulinum in the intestinal tract. It's a common soil organism everywhere.

But all of a sudden we're seeing cases now, especially in dairy and other situations, where the animals are dying and becoming impaired from the botulism toxin from the Clostridium in the intestinal tract, and rumen in the stomach. That normally didn't occur before, because you have all of those organisms that provided the natural biological control.

In this paper, what they show is that residues of glyphosate that are permitted in our feed and food products are high enough to kill those normal biological control organisms--your Lactobacillus, your Alcaligenes. The numbers of those organisms are very effective in preventing the toxin production by Clostridium that those organisms are eliminated by glyphosate levels that can be in our food and feed supply. Then the animals suffer the same effects as with giving them treatment of this very intense biological warfare chemical that is produced naturally in the intestine, without that balance again.... I saw again that there's enough residual glyphosate potential in our feed and food to all of a sudden make an extremely benign organism fatal or lethal in that process.[292]

Dr Joseph Mercola interviewed Professor Huber and asked him about the organism that was causing serious concern in the agricultural community:

> We're not sure what it is. It was first identified by veterinarians who were confronted with very high reproductive failure in animals…It's not a fungus. It's not bacteria. It's not a mycoplasma or a virus—about the same size of a small virus. You have to magnify it from 38 to 40,000 times.

He expresses his concern about the high levels of abortion rates (70%) in the dairy herds and the high glyphosate levels:

> You put that on top of 10 to 15% of infertility to start with, and you're not going to have a dairy very long. In fact, a lot of our veterinarians are now becoming very concerned at the failure for being able to have to have replacement animals.
>
> But what we do know is that it causes reproductive failure, infertility, as well as miscarriage for cattle, horses, pigs, sheep, and poultry. We can anticipate with that broad spectrum of animal species, which is extremely unusual, that it will also be with humans.
>
> We see an increasing frequency of miscarriage and a dramatic increase in infertility in human populations in just the last eight to 10 years.
>
> If you look at where this entity is—again, with the veterinarians when they have identified it and the American Cattlemen's Association testified to it before Congress in 2002–there were two conditions that were threatening the industry. One was this reproductive failure—as many as 40 to 50% of the pregnant animals losing their offspring. The other one was premature ageing.[293]

Worldwide, around 650,000 tons of glyphosate products were used in 2011 and sales were worth around US$6.5 billion in 2010, more than the value of all other herbicides combined. Global agricultural use of glyphosate mushroomed following the adoption of GE-HT crops in 1996. The total volume applied by farmers rose 14.6-fold, from 51 million kg (113 million pounds) in 1995 to 747 million kg (1.65 billion pounds/ 747,000 metric tons) in 2014. And its use keeps increasing, in large part because of the production of GM crops.[294]

Monsanto has sold glyphosate as a perfectly harmless herbicide, but the truth does not bear this out. Professor Don Huber has no doubt as to the importance of understanding how dangerous glyphosate, the main component of Roundup, is: 'The future historians aren't going to judge us by how many tons or pounds of pesticides we apply or don't apply, but how willing we are to sacrifice future generations, as well as jeopardize the very basis of our own existence, all based upon failed promises and flawed science. The only benefit is that it affects the bottom line of a few companies. There's no nutritional value.'[295]

'The future historians aren't going to judge us by how many tons or pounds of pesticides we apply or don't apply, but how willing we are to sacrifice future generations, as well as jeopardize the very basis of our own existence, all based upon failed promises and flawed science. The only benefit is that it affects the bottom line of a few companies. There's no nutritional value.'

Professor Don Huber is not alone in his concern on our over-reliance of pesticides and herbicides, particularly glyphosate. Dr Zach Bush, a triple-certified board physician with expertise in internal medicine, endocrinology and metabolism, and hospice/palliative care, has a particular interest in glyphosate. For a number of years he has been researching the link between health and the gut biome, and in more recent times the link between the gut biome and the soil microbiome. One area of concern is the rise of mental problems in the young, such as autism. In an interview with Daniel Schmachtenberger, he explains his concern: 'We had a very stable rate of autism in the population until about 1975 and then things started to rise a little bit. Then in the 1990s, things just really took off furtively. We had 1 in 5000 children with autism in 1975. Today, we have 1 in 40. The vast majority of that increase we doubled between 2012 and 2015. We are just seeing this extraordinarily vertical rise in a really devastating neurologic condition in the very young. On the other side of the population, we had a very steady rate of Parkinson's and Alzheimer's that was really traced in the geriatric population until the 1990s. Then we see this steady climb of Parkinson's in males and Alzheimer's in females. That phenomenon has tracked very closely with our autism phenomenon'.

Dr Bush has been concerned about the overuse of antibiotics for some time now. 'In the USA an amazing 7.7 million antibiotics are prescribed every year. On top of that as of 2014, the US use in agriculture approximated to 30 million pounds in the production of chickens, pigs and cows, and right up to the time of death so their feces and urine is contaminated with it. This means that approximately four times as much antibiotic is going into the food chain as from doctors.' But this is less significant than what we are doing to the plants according to Dr Bush: 'Again, that all pales in comparison to what we're doing to our plants and the soils around them. The number one antibiotic on the planet right now is a chemical called glyphosate. Glyphosate is the active ingredient in Roundup...we're using 4 ½ billion pounds of that antibiotic worldwide. It's interesting because it's never been patented as a weed-killer. That's what they tell us it is, but, in fact, it's an antibiotic. It was patented as an antibiotic, antifungal, antiparasite that can kill single-celled life that it touches. It also kills the plants and it does both the bacteria and the plants through the same mechanism. It blocks an important enzyme pathway called the shikimate pathway. This enzyme pathway produces the ringed aromatic amino acids. The three that it blocks are phenylalanine, tyrosine and tryptophan, all three of which are critical for brain function'. Dr Bush's concern here is that these are essential amino acids, which means the body cannot manufacture them; they are among the nine amino acids that have to be imported into the body. But they are now less available, and he believes it is not just affecting neurodevelopment: 'so we denuded the environment of bacteria by spraying 4 billion pounds of antibiotic on our soil, so we killed the soil, creating lack of nutrients now in the soil. Then we sprayed a chemical, the same chemical that would block the essential building blocks for a healthy human body and brain.' The effect of this also has far-reaching implications on the gut, as his laboratory has revealed that glyphosate has been shown to disrupt the gut membrane itself, which creates a very inflammatory situation. Dr Bush informs us: 'We now know that everything from your neurodegenerative disorders to asthma to allergies, all the way down to cancer and Alzheimer's to mention the rest of the end of life, all of this is just a spectrum of chronic inflammation manifesting in different organ systems'.[296]

On another occasion, Dr Bush expressed concern as to where the environmental destruction and the chemicalization of our agricultural system was leading us, with the rate of cancer in women catching up and now almost equal to the rate of men: 'The survival of the species is hanging in the balance right now, and we are teetering on the edge of real collapse of own biology's capacity to live here on this blue planet of ours.' When asked about the cancer statistics he suggested, 'The numbers keep shifting, one in two men certainly and one in three women, but in the last few weeks we have heard that the statistics are now approximately even, a stunning statistic, we are one degree of separation from cancer at this point.'

'The survival of the species is hanging in the balance right now, and we are teetering on the edge of real collapse of own biology's capacity to live here on this blue planet of ours.'

Dr Bush offers another reason he is concerned for our future as a race: 'A stunning statistic has recently been revealed is as a whole a population of men over the last generation of the last 22 years we have seen a halving of the sperm counts of the entire population. To lose fifty percent of our sperm capacity in just one generation is a stunning look at why many of us are looking at 60 to 70 years maximum left for our species. We can't reproduce anymore, you fast forward 30 or 40 years.' As regards to the alarming rise in a number of diseases in our population, Dr Bush adds an interesting observation: 'But bizarrely the good news is it is actually cancer, heart disease, autoimmune diseases, neurologic diseases, mood disorders, all of them went berserk at the same time in history. All of them have this big uptake in the early 1990s and then really acceleration in 2000/2005 and now we are on this vertical climb in the late teens of our millennium here. And so that trajectory of all the systems going down at once suggests something really reassuring actually, we must have one root-cause to what we did, we must have put something literally in the water to cause such a diversity of diseases and syndromes in such a short period of time in such a heterogeneous population.' He further explains his thinking, 'This singularity of disease phenomena means we should be able to turn our attention quickly to say what happened between 1998 and 2002 to change everything. So the punchline here is up for debate still, but to my knowledge, no other science group has done as much work as we have done to correlate the times in history that these events have happened and the chemicals that have entered our water and food systems during that time. The single largest contributor to the chemical destruction of our food chain is the chemical called glyphosate which is the active ingredient in the famous weed-killer Roundup.' He mentions that since the patent expired on glyphosate, and the vast majority of it now being manufactured in China 'sold on the international market for pennies on the dollar', he suggests: 'so we have this molecule…now just being made en masse by chemical companies all over the world and poured into our waterways. This has spelt a disaster for topsoil, first of all. It kills the microbiome which is bacteria, fungi and this diverse ecosystem of hundreds of thousands of species of bacteria, parasites, single-celled organisms and millions, five million species of fungi followed by probably tens of millions if not billions of species of viruses all being affected by this chemical now. So this huge biome, which is really the way life happened. I don't care whether you are an earthworm, a dog or a human, you rely on the microbiome for the nutrient delivery in your body. And what our lab has been working on is to understand the communication network between the bacteria, the fungi and the human cells. And it turns out that that microbiome regulates your own genome, it determines which human you create from the genes your mum and dad handed you.'

Dr Bush questions the sense of letting a company like Monsanto, that developed Agent Orange used to destroy much of the jungles of Vietnam during the Vietnam War, supply its chemicals for our food: 'so we have now hired a chemical warfare company to grow our food chain and should we expect anything but death to come out of that experience?' Following the development of GMOs, the use of Roundup increased dramatically, particularly in the US. 'Roundup Ready can handle direct spraying. So that weed-killer became a crop treatment in 1996. Suddenly we are eating this stuff days after spraying this chemical. And, of course, we are accelerating and it is now in drinking water and in breastmilk and it's everywhere and we have to realise we simply built a concept of warfare against the microbiome and the result of that is ultimately going to be human death.'

Aside from working with clients to restore their health, Dr Bush is also working with the farming community to restore soil health and become part of the regenerative movement in agriculture. When asked about what we as consumers could do to protect ourselves from the worst effects of the dysfunctional agricultural system he had this to add, firstly, that he was 'Super optimistic in the end… So what do we do now? From a food standpoint it's quite simple we can reconnect consumers with farmers.'[297]

There will some people who might say that the goal of creating quality food, such as organically-grown food on real, fertile land is an unrealistic goal that it will cost too much: that people will not be able to afford it. This point needs to be addressed. The question really is, why is it that human beings living on this bountiful Earth, with already much more food produced than can be eaten, are unable to access the basic sustenance to provide basic health?

The answer to this question can take a book in its own right and is discussed in my previous book *Hijacked*. We can, however, briefly review some of the ideas that were addressed in this volume. In this previous volume, we traced how our economy evolved from its feudal roots into its current form that is more like a casino-style economy than a useful functioning economy. The economy can be regarded as a vehicle that is used to enable transactions to enable trade between people, organisations and countries, and facilitate the exchange of goods and services. Our economy is based on a system whereby private corporate interests create money out of nothing and charges us interest for giving them this privilege that then issues this money as debt. Governments have given up their sovereign right to create money and have effectively given this right to private corporate interests, and they allow this to occur and even allow themselves to be burdened with debt—which is now so vast it is considered completely unrepayable. On top of this, by giving up this sovereign right, governments are further burdened with vast payments of interest to these private corporate banks to support this system. Following deregulation finance and banking have moved off-shore to tax havens and developed new ways to gamble using products such as collateralized debt obligations (CDOs), repos, and a whole host of new securitization products.

Whilst this has led to a much more complex system, the reality is that it is completely unsustainable, and it basically transfers wealth from the real economy to a very small minority, generally referred to as the 1%, but in reality, is more commonly the 0.01%. Aided by a taxation system that actively supports a more predatory economy and more of a gambling mentality, we now have a system that is highly unstable and not conducive to supporting the real needs of society. It is a setup that supports predatory corporate development, penalizing most other forms of business. It is not a healthy form of capitalism. People who criticize this system, however, are often labelled 'marxists', 'lefties', or given other abusive labels. But the reality is it is simply a very inefficient, destructive, lopsided, and fundamentally flawed system. Capitalism does not have to be destructive: it can be a vehicle for usefully serving the greater creative potential of humanity.

It doesn't, however, have to be based on fake money and phoney wealth, as it currently is. The collapse of 2008 was a perfect expression of its destructive nature. That was just another taster of its destructive power. Being that it is totally unsustainable—it will not get 'better' or return to 'normal'—there is no 'normal' with such an unsustainable system. It is also no accident that we are dealing with an unsustainable healthcare system, founded on an unsustainable agricultural system, supported by an unsustainable economic system—this is no mere accident or play on words—this is the reality we have created. This is the reality that has been created by almost totally unregulated corporate domination of our lives, obsessively seeking simply to maximise returns and increase growth, is inherently unsustainable and destructive.

The fact that many people cannot afford to eat food that will supply real health even when they are happy to supply their labour to society is more of an expression of how unequal our food and money distribution system is, which is reflected in the dysfunctional nature of our political apparatus that allows this dysfunction to continue to allow the super-wealthy 0.1% to gain even more wealth. The *Financial Times,* in their article "Widening Disparity—Wealthiest 1% strengthens grip over corporate America", informs us that the richest 1% of Americans now account for more than half the value of equities owned by US households, according to Goldman Sachs. Apparently, since 1990, the wealthiest have bought a net $1.2 trillion in shares whilst the rest of the population has sold more than $1 trillion: by the end of September 2019, the top 1% controlled a record $21.4 trillion representing 56% of US equities.[298] This kind of disparity can only be addressed by reforming our economies.

Judging how we count the real cost of a highly chemically-based agricultural system and deal with its professions of being able to supply 'cheap food', we have to look beyond simply the cost we might have to pay at a supermarket. We don't just pay for it once. We have already paid for it many times over in other ways, such as the direct subsidies. The costs are many, many fold more than the simple shop price. The environmental costs are not immediately obvious: however, they are more apparent when you look for them.

How To Survive in the 21ˢᵗ Century

Insect Apocalypse

In November 2019, *The Guardian* reported on a recent study by Dave Goulson, professor of biology, at the University of Sussex, that highlighted the massive decline of the insect population. In their article titled: 'Insect apocalypse poses risk to all life on Earth, conservationists warn,' it suggested that 'half of all insects may have been lost since 1970 as a result of the destruction of nature and heavy use of pesticides.'[299]

In a release by the University of Sussex, Dave Goulson informs us, 'Insects make up the bulk of known species on earth and are integral to the functioning of terrestrial and freshwater ecosystems, performing vital roles such as pollination, seed dispersal and nutrient cycling. They are also food for numerous larger animals, including birds, bats, fish, amphibians and lizards. If we don't stop the decline of our insects there will be profound consequences for all life on earth.' The report brings together scientific research studies from around the world, with findings indicating that we may have lost 50% or more of our insects since 1970, while 41% of the Earth's remaining five million insect species are now 'threatened with extinction'. As for the evidence for the cause of the decline he says, "What we do know however is that the main causes of decline include habitat loss and fragmentation, and the overuse of pesticides. Wild insects are routinely exposed to complex cocktails of toxins which can cause either death or disorientation and weakened immune and digestive systems."[300]

In his actual report, he informs us that approximately three-quarters of the crop types grown by humans require pollination by insects. Of the pollinators, 23 bee and flower-visiting wasp species have become extinct in the UK since 1850. He says: 'We are witnessing the largest extinction event on Earth since the late Permian [a geological epoch 250 million years ago].'

Shaping Our Future

'We are witnessing the largest extinction event on Earth
since the late Permian [a geological epoch 250 million years ago].'

He informs us that the number of flying insects has fallen by three-quarters in 27 years. "It's terrifying," said Goulson commenting on the research. "Insects are at the heart of everything. They pollinate most of the crops we grow – they pollinate more than 80% of wildflowers. They help recycle nutrients. They are predators of pests. If we lose insects, life on earth will collapse."

According to Suzanne Fisher-Murray from the university, 'The research provided important evidence to the European Food Standards Agency, which was commissioned by the European Parliament to review the impacts of the chemicals. The review directly led to a 2013 European Union moratorium preventing the use of the three pesticides – clothianidin, imidacloprid and thiamethoxam – on flowering crops such as oilseed rape and sunflowers that appeal to bees and other pollinating insects.'

The study mentions that France is one of Europe's biggest consumers of pesticides (per unit of agricultural area). It reveals that 'In 2013, after controversy over levels of pesticide concentration in drinking water, the French government set a target of a 50% decrease in pesticide use, promoting the principles of agroecology and advocating integrated pest management for a reduction of pesticide reliance.' What is useful to know is what the result of this implementation by the French farmers actually was. 'We demonstrated that low pesticide use rarely decreases productivity and profitability in arable farms. We analysed the potential conflicts between pesticide use and productivity or profitability with data from 946 non-organic arable commercial farms showing contrasting levels of pesticide use and covering a wide range of production situations in France.' The report adds that they 'failed to detect any conflict between low pesticide use and both high productivity and profitability in 77% of the farms.' This is encouraging, as this would be the main reason that many farmers would be reluctant to reduce their use of pesticides.[301] This review follows on from a similar international review published in April 2019, by Francisco Sánchez-Bayoa and Kris Wyckhuys, where they acknowledged that over 40% of insect species are threatened with extinction. Their review highlights 'the dreadful state of insect biodiversity in the world, as almost half of the species are rapidly declining and a third are being threatened with extinction.'

Their review looked at the causes for this decline and concluded that 'The main drivers of species declines appear to be in order of importance: i) habitat loss and conversion to intensive agriculture and urbanisation; ii) pollution, mainly that by synthetic pesticides and fertilisers; iii) biological factors, including pathogens and introduced species; and iv) climate change.'

To put this into perspective they point out, 'The repercussions this will have for the planet's ecosystems are catastrophic, to say the least, as insects are at the structural and functional base of many of the world's ecosystems since their rise at the end of the Devonian period, almost 400 million years ago.' [302]

Navdanya International, an organisation that is devoted to reclaiming Earth democracy and food sovereignty, suggests, 'Life on this planet, our own future, is under severe threat of the sixth mass extinction and climate catastrophe.' They have started a campaign 'Poison-free Food and Farming 2030' to prevent what they perceive as a serious challenge to life on Earth: 'It is clear that the sixth mass extinction has now begun, driven by the limitless greed of the 1% and their total disregard of the ecological limits set by the Earth, and the inherent limits for social justice and human rights.' Not just that, they see the extinction of much more than insects. 'The poison-based industrial and monoculture paradigm of growing food is responsible for the destruction of biodiversity, extinction of species and is driving climate change. 50% of the greenhouse gas emissions come from an industrial food system which is also uprooting the small peasants who provide 80% of the food.'[303] These are some of the costs not evident in the idea of cheap food, that industrial agriculture would like us to ignore. But can we? As regards to whether consuming the products of the industrialized high-chemical input system produce health, we have to ask what is your measure for health?

What Is Real Health?

How do we create a healthy world? Is it possible to create a healthy world? I believe that it is. But first, we need to be clear what we mean. What is health? Is health simply the absence of any obvious disease process?

I knew a man who told me that he never had a day's illness in his life. Some would say he was healthy, but they would be wrong; he died three weeks later from cancer. According to the United Health Foundation, half of adult Americans (50.1%) perceive their health as very good or excellent. Life expectancy in the USA is ranked 27th out of 33 countries within its peer group of OECD countries. In 2008, 107 million Americans—almost 1 out of every 2 adults age 18 or older—had at least 1 of 6 reported chronic illnesses that included: cardiovascular disease, arthritis, diabetes, asthma, cancer, and chronic obstructive pulmonary disease. Since 2012 obesity has increased by 11% to 30.9% in adults and low birthweight babies have increased more than 50% in the last three years to 8.3% of live births.[304]

According to the Centers for Disease Control and Prevention (CDC), in 2015-2016, 45.8 % of the US population used prescription drugs in the previous 30 days. Prescription drug use can vary with age: the CDC informs us that 18 % of children under the age of 12 years used prescription drugs, whereas it rose to 85 % for adults aged 60 and over. Today 1 in 2 Americans will be diagnosed with cancer before they die. In a separate report, the CDC informs us that dementia and Parkinson's continue to rise and that now 1 in 38 boys are diagnosed with autism compared to a mere 1 in 5,000 in the 1970s. We are also informed that developmental disabilities in general are on the rise in the USA among children, and are significant at 17.8 % of the general population.[305]

The above information does not paint a picture of glowing health in America. It simply suggests that some people may be considered "healthy". What could aid us is to have a comparison of a population that might be considered truly healthy. The Hunza, for example, a population who live in the hills of Northern India, who were renowned for their health and their complete lack of most of the diseases that affected Western civilisation. Sir Albert Howard visited these people to review their agricultural system and found their system to be in perfect harmony with his own views, in that they recycled all their food and waste products back into the soil, and observed the Law of Return, which basically meant they returned fertility to the earth and did not deplete it. I remember reading about these people and found an amusing anecdote about them and their abilities. A Western reporter arrived to do an article on these people, and was delayed in his task by an elderly man, in his 80's. Apparently, the man he hoped to interview had gone to the next village, 5 miles away. The man apparently ran all the way back from the other village but came across his wife who further delayed him due to feelings of passion for her, that so overpowered him he had to make love with her before going to the interview. The Hunzas don't have such a regard for time as Westerners do. However, he did make it to the interview. Pretty good energy for a man reputedly 86 years old don't you think?

It is difficult to analyse precisely how healthy a population of any given country is. Most statistics do not take into account all the factors of health. They don't, for example, consider the levels of infertility or disability due to drug problems, or the loss of IQ or mental health issues etc. Studies of groups like the Hunza, however, can be a useful comparative guide. Linking our health to the state of soil fertility is not something that is easy to do, which the proponents of industrial agriculture have used to their advantage so far, but it is becoming obvious to many more researchers that our health is indelibly linked to soil fertility. So how fertile are our soils?

Soil Degradation

More people are coming to realize that the fertility of human beings is linked to the very soil that nourishes our bodies—that nourishment begins with the soil that produces the food we all consume. One of the biological principles of life teaches us that if we nurture and feed the soil that enables the billions of microorganisms to feed the plants they, with adequate supplies of water and sunlight, will thrive and convert the energy of the sun and supplies of carbon dioxide via photosynthesis into food that will sustain life and create an abundance of health.

Globally, we have lost 33 % of arable topsoil to erosion or degradation in the past 40 years. In the EU, nearly a billion tons of soils are lost *each year*. Soil degradation globally is considered to cost our economies $10 trillion per annum. A UK collaborative study estimated soil degradation in England and Wales cost the economy £1.2 billion per year, mainly due to loss of organic content of soils (47%), compaction (39%), and erosion (12%). Lancrop, a company that performs 15,000 soil tests a year in the UK, reports that over 70% of UK arable soils analysed have less than 4% organic matter, and they inform us that loss of organic matter leads to soil compaction.[306] In 2011, the non-profit organisation the

Environmental Working Group, released a report that was critical of the USDA's estimates for soil erosion in the USA. Referring to the estimates given out by the USDA's Natural Resources Conservation Service they suggested, 'There is compelling evidence, however, that soil erosion and runoff from cropland are far worse than these estimates suggest. Indeed, it appears that the nation is losing ground in the decades-old fight to gain control over this most fundamental and damaging environmental problem in agriculture. In some places in Iowa, recent storms have triggered soil losses that were twelve times greater than the federal government's average for the state, stripping up to 64 tons of soil per acre from the land.' The report finds the government subsidy payment scheme sorely lacking; they noted 'Between 1997 and 2009, the government paid Iowa farmers $2.6 billion to put conservation practices in place. It paid six times as much—$16.8 billion—in income, production and insurance subsidies that encouraged maximum-intensity planting, not conservation. Across the Corn Belt the gap was even greater—$7.0 billion for conservation and $51.2 billion for income, production and insurance subsidies.'[307]

A report in *Scientific American* explained that creating topsoil is no simple matter, and that generating three centimetres of topsoil globally takes 1,000 years: if current rates of degradation continue, all the world's topsoil could be gone within 60 years, according to senior UN officials. The report warns that 'unless new approaches are adopted, the global amount of arable and productive land per person in 2050 will only be a quarter of the level in 1960,' according to the FAO.[308]

It's not just the loss of soil that we need to consider, it's all the consequences of poor agricultural practice that needs to be understood. Dr Christine Jones, an internationally renowned and highly respected groundcover and soils ecologist, explains some of the more obvious consequences:

Over the last 150 years, many of the world's prime agricultural soils have lost between 30% and 75% of their carbon, adding billions of tonnes of CO_2 to the atmosphere. Losses of soil carbon significantly reduce the productive potential of the land and the profitability of farming. Soil degradation has intensified in recent decades, with around 30% of the world's cropland abandoned in the last 40 years due to soil decline. With the global population predicted to peak close to 10 billion by 2050, the need for soil restoration has never been more pressing.

Soil dysfunction also impacts on human and animal health. It is sobering to reflect that over the last seventy years, the level of every nutrient in almost every kind of food has fallen between 10 and 100%. An individual today would need to consume twice as much meat, three times as much fruit and four to five times as many vegetables to obtain the same amount of minerals and trace elements as available in those same foods in 1940.[309]

A report by the UK Environment Agency informs us that soil holds 3 times as much carbon as the atmosphere, it also reduces the risk of flooding by absorbing water; it is a wildlife habitat and delivers 95% of global food supplies. UK soils contain approximately 10 billion tons of carbon that the agency equates with roughly 80 years of annual greenhouse gas emissions. They inform us, 'Intensive agriculture has caused arable soils to lose 40 to 60% of their organic carbon, and the impacts of climate change pose further risks.' They comment that 'Soil carbon loss is an act of economic and environmental self-harm.' [310]

In a section on soil biology, the agency points out that in just one gram of soil there can be as many as a billion bacteria, which would work out at approximately 5 tons of soil organisms per hectare. They are composed of 11 million species of soil organisms of which less than 2 % have been named and classified. They also reveal that the soil invertebrate community has only been surveyed nationally twice (in 1998 and 2007). The subject of what actually is soil is worth further discussion, not just because it is the basis of life, but because there have been some amazing discoveries about the very basis of life as we know it. This we will review in the next section.

Sir Albert Howard, in another volume, *The Soil and Health--A Study of Organic Agriculture,* which was published just before his death in 1947, reported on the 1938 USDA yearbook study on soil erosion in America. This revealed that more than 250 million acres or 61 % of the total area under crops in the USA had suffered either complete or partial destruction. Effectively 'three-fifths of the original agricultural capital of this great country has been forfeited in less than a century.' [311] We, of course, know of the degradation that occurred in the 1930's Dust Bowl days, when vast areas of America were completely denuded of topsoil leaving virtual desert in its wake. The US Secretary of Agriculture in 1937 was Henry A. Wallace; he was prompted to make the following comments as a foreword in the above-mentioned USDA yearbook:

> THE EARTH is the mother of us all—plants, animals, and men. The phosphorus and calcium of the earth build our skeletons and nervous systems. Everything else our bodies need except air and sun comes from the earth.
>
> Nature treats the earth kindly. Man treats her harshly. He overplows the cropland, overgrazes the pastureland, and overcuts the timberland. He destroys millions of acres completely. He pours fertility year after year into the cities, which in turn pour what they do not use down the sewers into the rivers and the ocean. The flood problem insofar as it is man-made is chiefly the result of overplowing, overgrazing, and overcutting of timber.
>
> This terribly destructive process is excusable in a young civilization. It is not excusable in the United States in the year 1938...

Shaping Our Future

> The social lesson of soil waste is that no man has the right to destroy soil even if he does own it in fee simple. The soil requires a duty of man which we have been slow to recognize.[312]

No doubt if Wallace could see the state of American agriculture, with its infamous feedlot system, where animal manure, which has historically been regarded as a precious asset and fundamental resource to be returned to the earth to aid its fertility, is now regarded as pollution, he might turn in his grave. The same might be said of the massive lakes of pig excrement in the huge industrial plants which rear animals indoors in metal crates on concrete floors—they have become no more than industrial waste, now more regarded as pollution to deal with. Sir Howard's view about this rash irresponsibility was straight forward and echoed Wallace's comments: 'No one generation has a right to exhaust the soil from which humanity must draw its sustenance. The resources of the earth should be used as God's gifts to the whole human race and used with due consideration for the needs of the present and future generations.'

'No one generation has a right to exhaust the soil from which humanity must draw its sustenance. The resources of the earth should be used as God's gifts to the whole human race and used with due consideration for the needs of the present and future generations.'

He believed that the duty to the soil, and hence the Earth was fundamental to health and should supersede short-term profit-taking:

> Perhaps mankind will have learnt the great lesson—how to subordinate the profit motive to the sacred duty of handing over unimpaired to the next generation the heritage of fertile soil.

How To Survive in the 21ˢᵗ Century

He believed that a significant change in attitude would be required to achieve this goal:

> One of the great tasks before the world has been outlined…It is to found our civilization on a fresh basis—on the full utilization of the earth's green carpet. This will provide the food we need: it will prevent much present-day disease at the source and at the same time confer robust health and contentment on the population; it will do much to put an end automatically to the remnants of this age of banditry now coming to a disastrous close. Does mankind possess the understanding to grasp the possibilities which this simple truth unfolds? If it does and if it has the audacity and the courage to tread the new road, then civilization will take a step forward and the solar age will replace this era of rapacity which is already entering into its twilight. [313]

In the UK a few years later the issue of how we run agriculture was raised in the House of Lords, in the autumn of 1943 during the war, by Lords Teviot, Bledisloe, Glentanar, Portsmouth, and Warwick, who were critical of the way the UK Ministry of Agriculture was blindly pursuing the promotion of artificial fertilizers. I add some of their comments purely to illustrate that total acceptance of this system of agriculture was not universal even with people such as these lords, who were, after all, members of the English aristocracy, and therefore landowners themselves and representatives of the ruling class. Lord Teviot gave his reasons for introducing a motion requesting that the ministers for Agriculture, Health and Food should establish studies to look into the long-term consequences for health with the introduction of artificial fertilizers, and the resultant use of pesticides, herbicides, and fungicides that inevitably followed:

> Only a few days ago I was talking to a friend who works among hospitals, and she was very perturbed at the enormous increase in the number of young people who have cancer. I remember that in my young

312

days it was only old people who were thought to have cancer, but to-day such troubles seem to be on the increase. Then take the animals of our country. I do not think any of us who are connected in any way with agriculture can be other than perturbed at the number of diseases there are among our farm stocks. Take foot-and-mouth disease, Johne's disease, mastitis, abortion, swine fever and many others that one could mention. Lastly, I come to the crops. We are well aware that the diseases among our crops are legion. Yet it seems to me that we accept all these afflictions as part of our existence; and while immense sums are expended in trying to cure them, I am afraid there is no doubt whatever that disease is increasing.

Every day we hear a great deal about planning. The real object behind this Motion is to see that we put planning for the health of our people, the animals, the plants and the crops of our country, first.

One of his concerns was the lack of resources that were being allotted to what he considered to be an important issue, being particularly ignored by the British Medical Association that of disease prevention. 'While hundreds of millions are expended in trying to cure, only one-fifth of one per cent of the natural expenditure and waste through ill-health is expended on research to find out, not how to cure but how to prevent.' He further mentions, 'We hear a great deal about a balanced diet. With this naturally I am in entire agreement, but unless the components come from a healthy soil rich in humus, life-giving and disease-resisting properties must be deficient.'

The Earl of Portsmouth added his observations: 'vigorous abounding health, normal health, and not merely the average freedom from disease, can come only from proper treatment of the soil in the beginning...If, therefore, there is complaint from time to time, when care is taken to prepare good food, that the cost of it is high, I would like to reply that the high cost of ill-health equals the low cost of food, and the low cost of food, as my noble friend has just said, equals exploitation of the soil.' He further makes the comparison with spraying harmful chemicals on human tissue with the way we treat soil: 'But we are doing exactly that to the soil. With lethal sprays we are destroying the soil's power of resistance and we are at the same time giving continuous doses of chemical food and chemical stimulants so that the infinite complex of bacterial and mycelial life in the soil is being upset, and we are upsetting the vitamins content, that is the capacity of the soil to produce food, by destroying the humus within the soil itself.' He makes a final point with regard to the use of life's waste products to enrich soil and health, and also refers to the chemist who is attributed to promoting the ideology behind the reliance on artificial fertilizer and man-made chemicals in agriculture: 'That the use of the wastes of life in accordance with natural laws is at the root of national health, seems to us to issue from a contemplation of the whole subject. Even when wastes are returned to the land merely to get rid of them, they assert their power of conferring fertility …. It would seem that the marriage of agriculture to a foreign partner, chemistry, arranged by Baron Liebig in 1840, was a mistake.' I further add a comment by the Earl of Warwick regarding what he believes is required to truly support the strength of Britain: 'The first bulwark of our national safety here is our land. The first certain guarantee of the continuation of the great quality which has made the British nation what it is depends on our land, and I am sure that, if only we can keep the soil fertile, disease can and will disappear in plant, in beast and in man.' [314]

These views by members of the House of Lords were from men who were all familiar with Sir Albert Howard's work and his book *An Agricultural Testament,* published in 1940, which they referred to in their speeches, and can be regarded as the views of educated politicians. What may further be of interest is that Baron Justus von Liebig, referred to above, and considered the father of industrial agriculture, in his last major work published in 1863, *The Natural Laws of Husbandry,* gave a very different perspective on the use of chemical fertilizers than he has previously been attributed with. According to David Montgomery, professor of geomorphology and supporter of soil regeneration, Liebig recommended returning organic matter to the fields to provide crops with a full complement of nutrients. Montgomery comments: 'It turns out that the patron saint of chemical fertilizers thought that soil organic matter *was* the key to sustaining civilization… He advocated for a large-scale return to organic matter to farms because "a soil deficient in organic matter must necessarily be less productive than a soil abounding in it."'[315]

Lord Teviot withdrew his motion, following the commitment by the Duke of Norfolk, the Joint Parliamentary Secretary of the Ministry of Agriculture and Fisheries to act on their recommendations. In reality, no serious action was undertaken, the Ministry of Agriculture pursued a relentless policy, as did the US Department of Agriculture, to promote the use of artificial fertilizers and the resultant use of pesticides, herbicides, and fungicides that were required to support this use.

Many view the reliance on chemicals as a conflict between chemists on one hand who had this reductionist view of nature, and biologists who looked at the deeper relationship of soil, the relationship between the soil biota and the plants and the complex nutrient relationships involved. Others believed that it was all about the power of corporate interests and their control over farming.

Montgomery, in his book *Growing A Revolution—Bringing Our Soil Back to Life,* gives a geologist's view after examining agricultural practices around the globe. He is a total convert to reforming agriculture into a system that he calls 'conservation agriculture', where creating soil fertility is prime. He makes the comment that I feel is useful here that 'the people making the most of the money from farming are not the farmers. It's those who sell stuff to farmers who are doing really well under the current system—the companies who sell the inputs on which conventional farming rests.' I also like his comment: 'restoring healthy soil to the world's agricultural lands is one of the best investments we can make in humanity's future. And so as we grapple with the daunting problems of how to feed the world, cool the planet, and stem the losses in the natural world, let's not lose sight of a simple truth. Sometimes answers we seek are closer than we might think—right beneath our feet.'[316] That conveniently takes us to the next section where we invite you to visit one of the most incredible aspects of our world.

The Magic of Soil Biota

Sir Albert Howard was convinced that health could only be created by firstly creating a healthy soil that promoted a healthy biota of soil organisms, including bacteria and fungi. This world was little understood back in his day, and, even today, too few people know or understand the significance of the soil biota. Howard was a pioneer and a biologist with a real understanding of the importance of soil health and its relationship to the health of plants and all animals. Of the huge diversity of organisms that make up our soil, he found the fungi, in particular, the mycorrhizae, responded readily to compost production and interacted with most of the plants he studied, physically attaching themselves to plant roots. They formed a symbiotic relationship and actively fed the host plant in return for nutrients from the plant. In much like the way our gut flora have become essential to our digestion and health so, it seems, has the soil biota also become essential to optimizing plant health, contributing to our health; in fact, we now know some of the bacteria involved are, incredibly *the same bacteria*. Howard found that the animals thrived feeding on plants grown on humus-rich soil. He was so confident of his animals' health that on numerous occasions, when faced with a neighbouring farm's animals suffering from outbreaks of foot-and-mouth disease, he would let his animals rub noses with infected animals, yet not one of his animals ever succumbed to the disease.

In *An Agricultural Testament,* Sir Albert Howard discussed his findings after decades of research into farming and his Indore method of composting. He never found the need to revert to the use of synthetic chemicals; his policy was to always to increase the fertility of the soil and let nature take care of the rest. The only problem he faced was a matter of the timing of his book's release—there was a war on. When World War II was over there was a shortage of food: in the UK, for example, rationing was worse after the war than during the conflict. And much the same as after the First World War, the factories that had amassed large supplies of ammonia used for bomb-making had surplus ammonia that was no longer needed, and it was decided to promote their use as a nitrogen supplement on farmland. This prompted a virtual stampede into the use of synthetic chemicals, particularly the artificial fertilizers, which produced instantaneous yields with little labour—labour being a cost that few farmers could afford at this critical time, particularly in Western countries. His ideas were therefore easily marginalized, and many people have never to this day come across his work—thus it led the way for corporate interests to be able to prevail over the development of agriculture with the use of their biocides and artificial fertilizers.

There are many people who are beginning to realize that Sir Albert Howard was a man before his time and that his ideas and knowledge are not simply ideas that time passed by, but a more fundamental understanding of agriculture that has now—come of age. Take, for example, his views on the mycorrhizae. He suggested, back in 1931, that this symbiotic relationship was a critically important process and was found to increase under the application of his Indore compost. Contemporary research by leading biologists have found that 80% of plants have this relationship with the mycorrhizae, and the fungi are found to efficiently deliver soil nutrients to their host plants, including proteins and minerals, particularly phosphorus and nitrogen, and the plants reward the mycorrhizae with energizing sugars. Modern researchers have also found that the fungal threads can connect with more than one plant and that nutrients can be transferred between plants, shaping whole plant communities. Biologists now understand that this symbiotic relationship is ancient, that these fungi have existed for more than 400 million years, and have had a crucial role in the development of plants. They have been shown to protect plants against heavy metals and have been found to play a significant role in the rejuvenation of land after catastrophic fires. The interconnection between plants and mycorrhizae has led to the understanding that a large oak tree, for example, maybe feeding not just its fungal partners but also other plants in its neighbourhood, particularly during dry spells and droughts, with essential water for survival. Biologists have, surprisingly, discovered some plant families that don't even use photosynthesis to create the nourishment they need; they simply rely on the fungus network.[317] One of the reasons there is so little understanding of the fungal network in the soil that we refer to as the mycorrhizae is that it is mostly invisible to the naked eye. Howard, however, was well aware of the role of the mycorrhizae, as he supported his research with extensive use of the microscope.

Howard consistently argued that trees play a crucial role in supporting the health of the soil and the fertility of crops. Their deep roots bring up minerals from far below the earth's surface, and when they shed their leaves, this foliage provides mineral-rich humus that does not just maintain the level of nutrients available but provides more fertility and organic matter. They also protect the land from soil erosion, as the rich biomass created absorbs water, and protects soil against hard rain falling directly onto it. As well, they provide shade that protects animals from intense heat and storms and reduces soil temperature, which can be important in warmer climates. As I write this we have been hearing about the fires in Australia. Howard would have observed that part of the cause of the intense temperatures has been aggravation by the massive loss of trees and the intense use of tillage that leaves soil exposed, which can easily raise the temperature of the soil by 20 degrees, translating into warmer air temperatures and making a significant difference to the weather on large landmasses. What he also discovered was if you cut down enough trees, flooding and soil erosion are sure to follow.

Michael Philips, in his volume *Mycorrhizal Planet,* describes the intricate relationship between plants, fungi, bacteria, and all the organisms that make up what we loosely call soil. He points out one of the most important things to understand about the mycorrhizae is its ability to sequester carbon which is hugely useful for reducing CO_2 levels: 'Root fungi provide *the solution* for our current climate change impasse. Free of charge. No carbon credits involved… Mycorrhizae sequester carbon. Big time. Here lies a future and a hope'. One of the ways that the arbuscular mycorrhizae sequester carbon is by the way it forms the gooey glycoprotein glomalin that it creates to seal off intercellular spaces in the soil. According to Phillips this important secretion completely eluded detection until the 1990s: 'What stunned soil ecologists ever since is that glomalin contains as much as 40 percent carbon in its molecular structure— representing nearly a third of carbon storage in soils worldwide. Humic substances, by comparison, hold only about 8 percent of soil carbon reserves.' What researchers have found is that the CO_2 levels in the atmosphere will actually stimulate fungi to produce more glomalin. This is incredible: it seems that these fungi could be considered to be a balancing mechanism for CO2 levels for the earth if only we would have the sense not to destroy them and allow them to do their work—all for free! Aside from this immense benefit, they also give fertile soil its rich crumbly texture that makes the soil so absorbent, instead of being impervious and compacted as the degraded soils of industrialized agriculture tend to be. Such compacted soils tend to create massive runoffs with high rainfall which results in flooding and erosion of the precious topsoil. The relationship of the mycorrhizae to trees has now been traced back to some 160 million years and has been shown to be much bigger than expected. Scientists have discovered networks in undisturbed areas that cover more than 2300 acres (965 hectares), more than 4 square miles. This would make it the largest organism in the known world!

Scientists are learning this relationship is much more complex than was previously believed. It seems that the fungus also provides moisture in times of drought. So aside from creating a soil structure that holds more water, during extended dry weather and even drought they send down roots to bring up moisture from the depths, some reaching 12 feet (4 metres) deep. They also can bring up minerals from the depths, not just from the subsoil, but even deeper levels that they obtain by attacking rock with acids, just to supply minerals required by their host plants. What has also been discovered is that, in the larger established networks interconnecting many plants, the mycorrhizae act as a distribution network delivering nutrients from one plant to another. Researchers list phosphorus and nitrogen as the principle nutrients that are delivered by the mycorrhizae, followed by calcium in depleted soils. They also supply iron, copper, zinc, potassium, and magnesium, along with sulphate from the organic matter. Analysis of the root connections shows that the mycorrhizae establish storage structures called vesicles in the roots of the host plant which contain large amounts of lipids and often nuclei. The fungi also interreact with bacteria: they trade hard-won carbon for phosphate from the phosphate-solubilizing bacteria. Secretions by the fungi can stimulate the bacteria to produce organic acids which can attack rock, freeing potassium, calcium, and magnesium ions.[318]

It seems what we have going on below ground involving the vast network of fungi, bacteria, worms, nematodes, viruses, and the range of biota that inhabit the soil is immensely more complex than previously thought. The symbiotic relationships are more entangled, and the nutrient exchanges more extensive and diverse. Aside from the fungi, bacteria also play an important role in plant health. The bacteria able to colonize plant root systems and promote plant growth are referred to as plant growth-promoting rhizobacteria. Aside from their well-known ability to fix nitrogen for plants, they are now known to provide a wide range of growth-enhancing materials to plants, including essential minerals such as phosphorus, potassium, and calcium, as well as other useful nutrients. They also protect plants from pathogens mineralize organic compounds and aid in the production of phytohormones. Scientists from McGill University in Montreal, Quebec, suggest: 'Plants growing in field soil cannot be viewed as single organisms. They are a source of solar-derived reduced carbon and, as such, are colonized, for good or ill, by a wide range of microbes and other organisms—these plants are communities of organisms, and we do not understand the nature of the communities to any great extent.' [319]

No discussion of soil biota, particularly the creation of real fertile soil could be undertaken without the mention of the contribution of the earthworm. Its contribution to soil fertility is immense. Its constant burrowing through the soil aerates the soil, making it more pliable and water-absorbing, all of which aid plants to grow healthily. But by far their greatest addition is via their excretions, what is commonly referred to as vermicast a highly nutritive organic fertilizer rich in humus, beneficial soil microbes and a host of useful compounds. Its benefit in enriching the soil is such that there are entire industries now devoted to exploiting its usefulness turning waste products into vermicompost, what some researchers call 'organic gold'.

> A revolution is unfolding in vermiculture studies for vermicomposting of diverse organic wastes by waste eater earthworms into a nutritive "organic fertilizer" and using them for production of chemical free safe food in both quantity & quality without recourse to agrochemicals. Heavy use of agrochemicals since the "green revolution" of the 1960s boosted food productivity at the cost of environment & society. It killed the beneficial soil organisms & destroyed their natural fertility, impaired the power of 'biological resistance' in crops making them more susceptible to pests & diseases. Chemically grown foods have adversely affected human health. The scientific community all over the world is desperately looking for an economically viable, socially safe & environmentally sustainable alternative to the agrochemicals.[320]

The mighty worm is now seen as a valuable contributor to plant health, not just by the fantastic quality of readily available nutrients it supplies to plants as it breaks down organic material—it has high levels of nitrogen—according to Sujit Adhikary 'the resulting earthworm castings (worm manure) are rich in microbial activity and plant growth regulators and fortified with pest repellence attributes as well. In short, earthworms through a type of biological alchemy are capable of transforming garbage into "gold".' There is much more that could be said about this fine creature, it even gets rid of weeds, for example. Many farmers are unaware of how this little helper will take seeds expressed by weeds and burrow them deeper into the earth where they will not be able to germinate, in order to save as a winter food store. However, we can now turn to one of the more promising advances in agriculture with regard to soil creation, that of no-till farming.

No-Till Farming and Regeneration Agriculture

For generations, one implement that we inextricably associate with agriculture is the plough (plow in America). However, there are many who now even question how wise it is to continue its indiscriminate use. David Montgomery, the geologist and agrarian writer whom we have previously referred to suggests, 'it is perfectly clear that of all our world-changing inventions, the plow was, and remains, one of the most destructive'. As we mentioned previously Montgomery has travelled the world studying agricultural techniques and found that wherever the plow was used, soil fertility has been compromised. Inevitably, more fertilizer would be required and plants would succumb to pests and diseases that previously were not a problem. When it came to regenerating the soils no-till systems were much faster, yields improved, cost of inputs dropped significantly as did labour inputs.[321]

The good news is we are perfectly capable of restoring health to our soils, our agricultural system, and to our animals and ourselves. Whilst the dire predictions of the collapse of agriculture may be realistic if we don't change our ways—we are perfectly capable of changing how we grow food. There are farmers in our midst who are already creating real fertility, and not just creating real fertility, they are actually earning better incomes creating that fertility than those trapped on the treadmill of using artificial fertilizers and the chemical pesticides, herbicides, and fungicides that are destroying their soils, and contributing to CO_2 admissions as they are all based on intensive reliance on fossil fuels.

There are a number of systems of agriculture that are regenerating soil, Regenerative Agriculture is one of the most successful. Regenerative Agriculture is mostly based on no-till farming. Farmers using this system have found that they can produce much better fertility a lot faster with little or no chemical inputs without using the plough. They have found that conventional ploughing destroys the very mycorrhizae that exist in fertile soils, actually nourishing plant life. By not ploughing and with extensive use of cover crops they have found they can increase soil fertility year on year and also produce nutrient-dense, quality food. Gabe Brown, a farmer based in North Dakota, started farming with little previous experience, on a farm with poor soils with less than 2% organic matter and a rain infiltration rate of ½ inch per hour. He quickly built up the organic matter to 6% and when he had his infiltration rate re-tested it had increased to 16 inches per hour. As his knowledge improved he found he was able to increase the organic matter in his soils to over 10% adding 1% a year in newly-acquired land. He has added several inches of topsoil to his land, increased its water holding capacity, increased its soil carbon levels and fertility to such a degree that he can produce far superior food in more abundance than conventional growers using the synthetics. Although he regularly produces yields of 20 % in excess of the conventional growers, he prefers to look at profit per acre, as this is his benchmark. He mentions how one year the farmer with the record for growing corn actually lost money on his crop due to all the input costs: he, however, is considered to have one of the most profitable farming operations in his county. One of the added bonuses of using the no-till system is you have more time to yourself; in Gabe's case, he has used some of that time to write about his experience of transforming a farm with exhausted soils after being farmed conventionally for decades to a farming system that increases fertility year on year and is very profitable to boot. His book is called *Dirt to Soil—One Family's Journey into Regenerative Agriculture.* [322]

Gabe Brown is one of an increasing number of farmers discovering that changing farming practice from reliance on artificial fertilizers and pesticides to no-till farming methods and using more diverse cover crops enriches the soil, produces excellent yields, and pays better than the treadmill and dependence of the industrial system. In *Unhealthy Betrayal*, I reported on another farmer, Joe Salatin, from Polyface farm, Swope, Virginia, who took over a farm destroyed by industrial farming. He restored the soils and considers himself a grass farmer, as he grows mainly grass and rears animals, like Gabe Brown he has a profitable enterprise using a similar approach. He raises 40,000 pounds of beef, 30,000 pounds of pork, 10,000 broiler chickens, 1200 turkeys, 1000 rabbits and 35,000 eggs on 100 acres of grassland and some 450 acres of woodland. His grass is a diverse mix of grasses and fobs that gives his animals much more than just a 2 or 3-type grass mix it contains clovers and herbs that the animals use to keep healthy, and it produces highly sought-after meats, as well as creating very fertile soils.

It's not just good news that alternative agricultural practices such as Regenerative Agriculture and Conservation Agriculture, can be profitable and create better food, without harmful pesticides there is so much more at stake. How we choose to farm and what we choose to eat has huge implications for humanity's future. Dr Christine Jones, the internationally renowned soil ecologist we introduced earlier, expresses the situation we face:

> Technological developments since the Industrial Revolution have produced machinery capable of extracting vast quantities of fossil fuels from beneath the Earth's surface - as well as machinery capable of laying bare large tracts of grasslands and forests. Taken together, these factors have resulted in the release of increasing quantities of CO_2 to the atmosphere while simultaneously destroying the largest natural sink over which we have control...The potential for reversing the net movement of CO_2 to the atmosphere through improved plant and soil management is immense. Indeed, managing vegetative cover in ways that enhance the capacity of soil to sequester and store large volumes of atmospheric carbon

in a stable form offers a practical and almost immediate solution to some of the most challenging issues currently facing humankind.

The movement of carbon from the atmosphere to soil—via green plants—represents the most powerful tool we have at our disposal for the restoration of soil function and reduction in atmospheric levels of CO_2 [323]

Most of the carbon drawn down by plants connected to the mycorrhizae and their bacterial friends is sent down via the roots to feed this underground biome, estimated at 80 to 90 % of the plant's production. This is converted into liquid carbon and sugars. Some question why it is that the plant kingdom is willing to divert so much of their resources into the soil biome the answer is simple—these organisms, through this symbiosis, produce nutrient-dense high-vitality crops. If we were all to wake up to this great gift that nature offers us on a plate for free, we could radically change this world and create real health in our communities.

The ability of the plants to draw down carbon and to donate it to the soil biota is a critically important process, not just for the creation of fertility in the soil and in the plants themselves but also the ability to reduce atmospheric CO_2 levels. Seth Itzkan calculated that the potential for SOC sequestration on grasslands is 88 to 210 Gt [Giga tons]. He suggests that 'This is the atmospheric CO_2 equivalency of 41 to 99 ppm, enough to dramatically mitigate global warming.' This is just on the grasslands. If you also include all cropland and the possibility of the regeneration and the creation of really fertile soil this leads to the ability of sequestration of CO_2 that no one has been able to accurately calculate.

Dr Vandana Shiva is a biologist and ecologist who believes that we are facing a simple choice: we can continue on our path to further collapse of health or choose to farm in ways that truly support the soil and our health. She believes that there are but two paths open to the future of farming:

The first path is made by walking with nature, co-creating and co-producing with diverse species, the living earth and her complex web of life, with sensitivity, intelligence and care. This is the path of life which has sustained humanity in its diversity over millennia.

The second path is the industrial path based on fossil fuels and poisons. This path is the path of death. It goes against the principles of nature and life. It violates the principle of diversity and imposes monocultures and uniformity. It violates the principle of giving back and extracts from nature and farmers, disrupting ecological sustainability and social justice. It is the path to extinction and climate catastrophe, of destruction of small farms and displacement of farmers and the spread of hunger, malnutrition and chronic diseases.

She further adds:

Two Paths to the Future Fake Knowledge, Fake Food, Fake Economies vs Real Knowledge, Real Food, Real Economies. [324]

Corporate Domination of Life

We have looked at a number of ways corporate domination of our life has led not just to the health destruction of our society, but the destruction of our environment and in the process the corruption of science and the political structures that govern us. I believe that it is inevitable that we reform agriculture, ignorance of the destructive nature of the industrialization of agricultural practice cannot prevail forever. However, agriculture is but one aspect of how corporate interests dominate our lives, but to ignore the power we have invested in corporations with limited liability and no real regulation would be a grave error.

How To Survive in the 21st Century

If you create an institution that has no real legal responsibility, whose only real directive is to make money at all costs, by any means possible—and you then let it set up and control the rules of the game—are we supposed to be surprised at the outcome? They create their own money, lend it to their favoured corporations on a preferential basis, set up the tax rules to limit their liability, set up the legal system to promote their own development, and set up international trade rules that allow them to peddle their wares dealing death and destruction as a corporate right (such as selling tobacco, pesticides, drugs or other harmful products). With their ability to create profits unhindered by any real norms they have been able to grow at unprecedented rates, becoming ever more powerful and wealthy, exert immense control over political systems via their lobbyists and political donations. The bigger corporations learned quite quickly that size mattered: the bigger they became, the more power they had, the more they could create monopolies, and have less competition to deal with.

It's like a runaway train. You can see that if nothing is done there is a grave likelihood of disaster. Corporations left unregulated and unconstrained in this economic environment will take over every aspect of life that they deem profitable. Eventually, there will be nothing outside of corporate control— nothing at all. Corporations can simply continue to takeover, buy-out or amalgamate with other companies as they have been doing successfully for decades, using borrowed money as debt, and we as taxpayers effectively actively fund this behaviour by giving them an immense tax-break by allowing them to set all this new debt against their expenses. The unregulated tax-break of the interest charges even spawned organisations such as KKR (Kohlberg, Kravis & Roberts) to use the debt break to take over companies, load them with debt, and eventually resell them reaping immense profits.[325] Amalgamations reduce competition and create immense power; they can hold countries to ransom, as they demand tax breaks and favourable legislation and threaten to leave if their demands are not met leaving massive unemployment and economic disaster in their wake. The problem we face is that as the economy stalls and deteriorates competition between the various corporate entities will intensify: they will become even more pathological and predatory, which will affect us all.

Post-Pandemic Economy

It is difficult to predict what will be considered the worst aspect of the covid-19 pandemic. Obviously, the direct health consequences of the virus can be eventually ascertained. What however is difficult to evaluate is the economic consequences. There are now 30 million Americans without work (as of May 5th, 2020). Many of these people do not have health insurance and we do not know what impact this will have on their ability to adequately feed themselves and their families, and the consequences to their overall health.

As regards to the greater economy, we know that corporate debt has been growing to gigantic levels but was mostly being ignored except for repeated warnings by the Federal Reserve (Fed) in its financial stability reports. The worry is that this massive debt bubble will eventually implode, exacerbating what is already a huge economic shock into further economic meltdown. In my previous volume *Hijacked,* I suggested that the way our economy has evolved from its feudal roots into its neo-feudal casino-styled, minimally regulated version of an economy, where private corporations are freely allowed to create money out of nothing via debt creation has created an unstable economy. I suggested that the 2008 crisis, whilst a very significant economic crash, was in my view, just a taster of what was likely to come. What is difficult to predict is when it will become a new crisis, and how bad will it get. This is still the case. Hopefully, this crisis will wake up a few more people to the inherently destructive nature of our so-called 'modern economy'. No doubt, all the blame for the coming economic damage will be laid at the feet of the pandemic, and the decisions made to isolate people and curtail normal economic activity. Discussion of this is beyond the scope of this volume, however, some mention of the economic circumstances behind the destructive debt process might be useful.

Wolf Richter explains how the corporate debt mountain has become more of an issue, 'Corporate leverage was gigantic. But no-one cared. And then comes February 20th when it began to unravel, and suddenly people cared. By early March junk bond issuance was freezing up and it became clear that these overleveraged companies couldn't refinance their debt, couldn't borrow money to fund their losses and would run out of cash soon, and would default.' He explains how the Fed plowed $2.3 trillion into Wall Street in seven weeks, and further by "jawboning" about buying corporate bonds and junk bond ETFs created a massive buying spree of junk bonds and junk bond ETFs, and a rally in stocks and bonds. Much of this buying spree was in the hope that buyers would be able to sell to the Fed at a profit, but the Fed wasn't buying. It provoked an increase of commercial and industrial (C&I) loans of such an amount as has not be seen before. It eight weeks they jumped from over $600 billion to $3 trillion in C&I loans. Here is Richter's take on the situation:

> So now we have this crazy situation where the next crisis has arrived, the next downturn is here, and it's a bad one, and likely the worst one we will see in our lifetimes, and the record amount of corporate debt that everyone had warned about, and the Fed had fretted about publically did what it was expected to do, and it started blowing up and the credit markets did what they were expected to do and they started freezing it. And then the Fed came out with about $3.2 trillion QE in a few weeks and cut its interest rates to zero and added a lot of jawboning about buying corporate bonds. And this has cost and enabled corporate America to load up on even more debt than ever before.[326]

As he further mentions, 'That record pile of debt has become a lot more explosive and much bigger in just a couple of months than it already was before, and that's where we are at now. Nothing has been solved.' Richter, in my view, is a very astute economist, and he tends to say it as it is. This debt problem is not due to the pandemic, it's due to poor business management, and reliance on using debt for takeovers, and obtaining tax relief, etc. What it means for you and me is that the economic fallout will be hugely exacerbated by this debt, and will create corporate collapses leading to further chaos.

Many people will tend to see this economic chaos as separate from all the other issues that we have so far discussed in this volume. I would argue that this is not separate, this directly affects your health and is, in fact, all part of the same corporate pathology. In my view, it's not just inseparable, it's fundamental to the whole problem we have. Banking is based on creating money out of nothing and creating debt. By allowing banks to do this, governments are giving up the sovereign right to create money. This creates the situation where they have to 'borrow' money from the banks at interest, which creates debts and the subsequent need to pay interest which grows, and grows, and grows. This continues until you have a debt mountain so vast that most of human endeavour is geared towards servicing this debt—a form of debt slavery. For those who would like a more in-depth discussion of this, *Hijacked* is recommended.[327]

The financial fallout for most of us will be dramatic, not, however, if you are a billionaire. Between 1990 and 2020, US billionaire wealth soared by 1,130% (in 2020 dollars). Three US billionaires—Jeff Bezos, Bill Gates, and Warren Buffett continue to own as much wealth as the bottom half of all US households combined. Between January 1 and April 10, 30 of the nation's wealthiest 170 billionaires have seen their wealth increase by tens of millions of dollars. Eight of them have seen their net worth surge by over $1 billion. Jeff

Bezos (Amazon) has seen his fortune increase by an estimated $25 billion according to an Institute for Policy Studies report, they point out that, 'This is larger the Gross Domestic Product of Honduras, $23.9 billion in 2018.' This is due to being in a system that has the scales tipped towards the super-wealthy who can hide their wealth in tax havens and see that the taxes they pay as measured by a percentage of their wealth decrease by 79 percent between 1980 and 2018.[328] It is also due to the massive Fed bailout, where since March 11, the Fed has printed $2.41 trillion. According to Wolf Richter, the purpose of this massive amount was to inflate asset prices across the spectrum, it was a 'gift to Wall Street and asset holders—the wealthier the asset holder, the bigger the gift.' He adds the further comment:

> If the Fed had spread that $2.34 trillion equally over the 130 million households in the US, each household would have received $18,535. For many households, this would have been welcome help to get through the crisis. But no. This was helicopter money for Wall Street.[329]

For many people getting a payment of $18,535 would be a life-saver. It just goes to show who is really running the show. For most of us, it will be a struggle to get back on our feet.

Suffice it to say here that how governments choose to offer economic support to overcome the economic consequences of this pandemic will have profound implications for our future. Whether they decide to 'borrow' the money and create more debt for future taxpayers or use their sovereign right to create money will have implications for generations to come. The question is, are we going to be suppliant citizens and let businesses and banks be bailed out again, just like the last time and allow ourselves to become deeper in debt—and submit to further debt slavery—this remains to be seen.

Shaping Our Future

The choices we make today will affect us and future generations.

Our choice is simple. We have to decide whether to let unregulated, mostly pathological corporations control our lives and humanity's destiny, or create a true democracy run for the interests of humanity, not simply for corporate interests or the 0.1 percent, the super-wealthy.

Our choice is simple. We have to decide whether to let mostly, unregulated pathological corporations control our lives and humanity's destiny, or create a true democracy run for the interests of humanity, not simply for corporate interests.

Sustainable Future

We already know that Big Agra will never be able to regenerate agriculture. Small farmers, growing mixed crops, some with animals of various sorts can produce more food of better quality than the large industrialized farms, and not just do this, but are also better able to support the health of the soil. This is already happening, increasingly globally. This needs to be recognized. Everyone needs to understand this so that when corporate apologists try to bamboozle us with their propaganda, their fake studies, their fake projections, their fearful predictions of catastrophe if we abandon their artificial chemical model—we can all appreciate that by supporting our smaller farmers, encouraging them to increase their soil fertility and produce healthier crops without artificial chemicals, we will produce healthier plants in abundance, and healthier animals and people.

We know that this may not happen overnight. There can be a transitionary period of adjustment, where farmers may need to be financially supported, generally, this can mean changing the emphasis of subsidies that already exist. In *Hijacked,* I reported on a tax system less-based on harmful taxes such as the value-added tax (VAT) that exists in Europe to one based on an Earth Resource Fee, loosely-based on Henry George's idea of a land tax. Instituted correctly, this would not penalize farmers who significantly increase the fertility of their land that would be providing us with a supportive health structure, it would also be providing fertile land for our children and future generations—this needs to be recognized. Under our current economic system, farmers are mostly impoverished except for a few of the large growers most of them have been facing diminishing returns for years. Farmers who care for the land are arguably one of our most important and valuable assets: they need our support and encouragement to create truly healthy soil which will provide healthy plants and support animal health and our health.

Supporters of the industrial model will argue that prices, particularly for meat will rise substantially. What has to be remembered is that this system is heavily subsidized, both directly and indirectly—and the consequential health impacts are not costed into their 'cheap' meat. If the artificial subsidies were to be removed and organic agriculture was given a level playing field, perhaps people would be content to eat meat a little less often, knowing that what they were now eating was free of harmful chemicals and significantly healthier for their families.

Unleashing Humanity's True Creative Potential

One of the challenges we face will be being able to create a real dialogue. The corporations that most directly affect our futures are the most-wealthy. They use their wealth to dominate the media, they spend vast sums on advertising, public relations etc. They substantially control information.

The very fact that you are reading this book, however, and have made it through much of the less admirable aspects of corporate enterprise that I have so far reviewed, is testament to your resilience and gives me hope that we can do this. Whilst I have made a study of this less admirable side of human activity, I am an abiding optimist. I believe that humanity is born for better things than simply being fodder for corporate exploitation. Everyone is affected by the health crisis that is consuming our societies in one way or another.

We need to channel our energies into creating useful change.

How we respond to our current predicament will no doubt be based on our own particular circumstances. We all, however, have the power to create change. Changing how we think and what we put on our plates can have profound implications. Whether to choose organic or not, for some people, is not a simple option. Whilst, for a food choice, I would always suggest choosing organic over non-organic food as it means a reduction in the chemical exposure for ourselves and our families and it no longer supports industrialized agriculture—it's not, however, the end goal. Just because crops are organic does not necessarily mean they are all going to be nutrient-dense, grown in rich fertile soils. Some organic growers have impoverished soils and there is no huge incentive for them to create more fertility, which takes time and resources, and much of the understanding of how to do this is not as widely known as it should be. We need to better connect with our food supply in whatever way we can, supporting local markets, farmer's markets, local suppliers, etc.

I believe the expression 'if you are not part of the solution you are part of the problem,' has relevance to the situation we face. Our ability to be part of the solution may be reflected by our personal circumstances, our sphere of influence and other factors. Inaction, however, risks further deterioration of social conditions and environmental conditions—which many people feel is already at a critically desperate stage. I am hoping that this volume will provoke positive discussion and constructive action on a number of levels.

No doubt some will see that reform will require significant changes to the way we regard our respective democracies. There are already moves to change the way big money can buy elections and control politicians. The organisation *Wolf-PAC* is a grass-roots political action committee that has introduced a free and fair elections resolution to call for an Article V convention, to propose an amendment to the American Constitution to restore balance and integrity to elections in the USA. They suggest that 'A convention would give us an opportunity to have a national conversation, somewhere other than Congress, about how to make our elections work better for the average American.' As a real grass-roots organization, it is getting significant support and it believes that it will be able to break the stranglehold of big money over the political system. This is to be welcomed and is one way that change can be created. [330] Another organization, based in the USA, *Indivisible,* is also having a significant impact, in trying to reshape the way elections are run. Candidates for election are given scorecards to show the degree that their policies reflect the true requirements of their membership. Building a real grass-roots movement recognises that real change will not come from any one leader, but through a movement of real inclusive people power. [331]

Shaping Our Future

George Monbiot in his book *Out of the Wreckage—A New Politics for an Age of Crisis*, suggests that a combination of these groups and the lessons learnt by Becky Bond and Zack Exley, who helped run a grass-roots campaign for the election of Bernie Saunders would be a supremely effective format for achieving change. Bond and Exley wrote about their experiences in a volume of their own, *Rules for Revolutionaries: How Big Organizing Can Change Everything*. They identified twenty-two rules of Big Organizing that can be used to drive social change movements of any kind. And they tell the inside story of one of the most amazing grassroots political campaigns ever run. [332]

There are many ways, as individuals, we can generate change that will lead to a better world, whether it is simply by changing how we think, or by changing what we put on our plates, by changing laws, or by changing farming methods. We can all participate in one way or another. Reining in the power of corporations and making them *and their investors* responsible for the carnage they create will take a concerted effort, which would include changing laws, but, more than anything needs the realization from us that things have to change, and can change. All is possible. Human beings have the creative potential to create a better world. Creating dialogue is a beginning and the purpose of this book. Thank you for reading this book.

RESOURCES

My Websites:

https://fundamental-health.com/   https://fundamental-wealth.com/

Nutritional resources

Journal of Orthomolecular Nutrition: http://orthomolecular.org/index.shtml

Vitamin C Foundation: http://vitamincfoundation.org/

Agriculture

Regeneration International: Mission: To promote, facilitate and accelerate the global transition to regenerative food, farming and land management for the purpose of restoring climate stability, ending world hunger and rebuilding deteriorated social, ecological and economic systems.
https://regenerationinternational.org/our-network/

Christine Jones PhD, Soil Ecologist: www.amazingcarbon.com

Vaccine information

Barbara Loe Fisher: Vaccine Information Center https://www.nvic.org/

Financial

Wall Street On Parade is a financial news site created and maintained by Russ and Pam Martens. https://wallstreetonparade.com/

Wolf Street The Stories Behind Business Finance & Money. Published by Wolf Richter. https://wolfstreet.com/

Michael Hudson, Economist and writer: https://michael-hudson.com/

Resources

On Banking

Public Banking Institute: Banking in the Public Interest:
https://www.publicbankinginstitute.org/

American Monetary Institute, Info on money reform.
https://www.monetary.org/

Positive Money—Making money and banking work for people:
https://positivemoney.org/

REFERENCES

[1] Andrew Burgoyne, *Unhealthy Betrayal—How the Manipulation of Science and Politics by Corporate Interests Destroys Health and Threatens the Future of Humanity.* Fundamental Press, 2015.

[2] Andrew A D Burgoyne, *Hijacked—How the Banking Industry, Finance, and Corporate Interests Have Hijacked our Economy and Corrupted Democracy.* Fundamental Press, 2018.

[3] Ibid. Since 1980, the overall US economy has grown 145 percent, whereas the median (average) income has only grown by 9 percent. The average income of the top 10 percent, however has grown by 178 percent, and corporate profits (after taxation) have grown by a phenomenal 239 percent. See also: David C Korten, *When Corporations Rule the World,* Berrett-Koehler Publishers Inc., 2015.

[4] Andrew Burgoyne, 2015.

[5] Evaggelos Vallianatos, with McKay Jenkins. *Poison Spring—The Secret History of Pollution and the EPA,* Bloomsbury Press, New York, 2014, p178.

[6] Ibid.

[7] Andrew Burgoyne, 2015. See also "Unsound Science, Politics and Obesity–The Threat to Our Health." A series of papers on this topic, available at: https://fundamentalhealth.org/unsound-science-politics-and-obesity-the-threat-to-our-health/

[8] Gary Taubes, *The Diet Delusion,* Ebury Publishing, 2007, p20.

[9] John Yudkin, *Pure White and Deadly—How Sugar is Killing Us and What We Can Do About It,* 1972.

[10] American Heart Association, "Trans Fats", https://www.heart.org/en/healthy-living/healthy-eating/eat-smart/fats/trans-fat See also the work of Mary Enig who campaigned against trans fats at the

References

Weston Price Foundation:https://www.westonaprice.org/health-topics/soy-alert/the-brilliance-and-courage-of-dr-mary-enig/

[11] For more information about fats try: John Finnegan, *The Facts About Fats,* First Celestial Arts Printing, 1993. Also Udo Erasmus, *Fats that Heal, Fats that Kill.* Alive Books, 1986. Mary G. Enig, Ph.D, *Know Your Fats; The Complete Primer for Understanding the Nutrition of Fats, Oils, and Cholesterol,* Bethseda Press, 2000.

[12] Robert Mendick, "Cooking with vegetable oils releases toxic cancer-causing chemicals, say experts." *The Telegraph,* Thursday 04 July 2019.

[13] Martin Grootveld, Benita C. Percival, Kerry L. Grootveld, "Chronic non-communicable disease risks presented by lipid oxidation products in fried foods."Leicester School of Pharmacy, De Montfort University, The Gateway, Leicester, UK. Apr 04, 2018.
http://hbsn.amegroups.com/article/view/19226/20413 doi: 10.21037/hbsn.2018.04.01

[14] Robert Mendick, "Cooking with vegetable oils releases toxic cancer-causing chemicals, say experts." *The Telegraph,* Thursday 04 July 2019.

[15] E. Patterson, et al., "Health Implications of High Dietary Omega-6 Polyunsaturated Fatty Acids", *J Nutr Metab.* 2012; 2012: 539426. Published online 2012 Apr 5. doi: 10.1155/2012/539426 PMCID: PMC3335257 PMID: 22570770 https://www.ncbi.nlm.nih.gov/pmc/articles/PMC3335257/

[16] A. P. Simopoulos, "The omega-6/omega-3 fatty acid ratio, genetic variation, and cardiovascular disease. *Asia Pac J Clin Nutr.* 2008;17 Suppl 1:131-4. https://www.ncbi.nlm.nih.gov/pubmed/18296320

[17] Brian Scott Peskin, *The Hidden Story of Cancer.* Pinnacle Press, 2006.

[18] Michael Moss, *Salt Sugar Fat—How the Food Giants Hooked Us,* W H Allen, 2013.

[19] Ibid.

[20]Marie Ng, PhD et. al., "Global, regional, and national prevalence of overweight and obesity in children and adults during 1980–2013: a systematic

analysis for the Global Burden of Disease Study 2013". *The Lancet*, Volume 384, Issue 9945, p766-781, August 30, 2014. https://www.thelancet.com/journals/lancet/article/PIIS0140-6736(14)60460-8/fulltext 2014DOI:https://doi.org/10.1016/S0140-6736(14)60460-8

[21] Global Report on Diabetes, World Health Organisation, 2016. See also Fact Sheet:

https://www.who.int/news-room/fact-sheets/detail/diabetes

[22] Dr Robert Lustig, *Fat Chance—The bitter truth about sugar,* Fourth Estate, London, 2013, p125.

[23] Andrew Burgoyne, *Unhealthy Betrayal—How the Manipulation of Science and Politics by Corporate Interests Destroys Health and Threatens the Future of Humanity.* Fundamental Press, 2015. Also see www.FundamentalHealth.org, Unsound Science, Politics and Obesity—the Threat to our Health.

[24] Jean A. Welsh, Andrea Sharma, Solveig A. Cunningham, and Miriam B. Vos "Consumption of Added Sugars and Indicators of Cardiovascular Disease Risk Among US Adolescents." *Circulation.* 2011;123:249–257

https://doi.org/10.1161/CIRCULATIONAHA.110.972166

[25] Kimber L. Stanhope, et al., "Consumption of Fructose and High Fructose Corn Syrup Increase Postprandial Triglycerides, LDL-Cholesterol, and Apolipoprotein-B in Young Men and Women." *Journal of Clinical Endocrinology & Metabolism,* Volume 96, Issue 10, 1 October 2011, pE1596–E1605, https://doi.org/10.1210/jc.2011-1251

[26] Harvard School of Public Health, The Nutrition Source—Sugary Drinks.

https://www.hsph.harvard.edu/nutritionsource/healthy-drinks/sugary-drinks/

[27] Aseem Malhotra, "Sugar is now enemy number one in the western diet." *The Guardian*, Sat 11th Jan, 2014.

[28] Helen Hunt, "Sugar is the new tobacco - Liverpool professor in row with former health secretary"

Liverpool Echo, 9 Jan 2014.

References

[29] Aseem Malhotra, "Sugar is now enemy number one in the western diet." *The Guardian*, Sat 11th Jan, 2014.

[30] Cristin E. Kearns, DDS, MBA, Laura A. Schmidt, PhD, MSW, MPH, and Stanton A. Glantz, PhD. "Sugar Industry and Coronary Heart Disease Research. A Historical Analysis of Internal Industry Documents". *JAMA Intern Med.* 2016 Nov 1; 176(11): 1680–1685. doi: 10.1001/jamainternmed.2016.5394.

[31] Dr Robert Lustig, *Fat Chance—The bitter truth about sugar,* Fourth Estate, London, 2013, p94.

[32] Gerald Reaven M.D., *Syndrome X—The Silent Killer—The New Heart Disease Risk.* Fireside, 2000, p22.

[33] John Yudkin, *Pure White and Deadly—How Sugar is Killing Us and What We Can Do About it,* 1972.

[34] Lustig 2013.

[35] Gary Taubes, *The Diet Delusion,* Vermilion, 2008, p191.

[36] Uffe Ravnskov et al., "LDL-C does not cause cardiovascular disease: a comprehensive review of the current literature." *Journal Expert Review of Clinical Pharmacology.* Volume 11, 2018 - Issue 10. https://doi.org/10.1080/17512433.2018.1519391. https://www.tandfonline.com/doi/full/10.1080/17512433.2018.1519391

[37] Andrew Burgoyne, 2015. See also further info at www.FundamentalHealth.org, videos and articles.

[38] Uffe Ravnskov et al., 2018.

[39] Uffe Ravnskov, M.D., PhD, "Big Pharma Mafia Continue Their Misleading", 22/09/2018. http://www.ravnskov.nu/2018/09/22/september-2018-big-pharma-mafia-continue-misleading/

[40] Duane Graveline, MD., *The Dark Side of Statins,* Spacedoc Media LLC, 2017, p77.

⁴¹ B. Joseph, and Hannah Yoseph, MD, *How Statin Drugs Really Lower Cholesterol—And Kill You One Cell at a Time.* 2012, p182.

⁴² Lee Know, ND, *Mitochondria and the Future of Medicine—The Key to Understanding Disease, Chronic Illness, Aging, and Life Itself.* Chelsea Green Publishing, 2018.

⁴³ Ibid.

⁴⁴ https://www.drperlmutter.com/brain-needs-cholesterol/ See also: West R. et al. "Better memory functioning associated with higher total and low-density lipoprotein cholesterol levels in very elderly subjects without the apolipoprotein e4 allele". *Am J Geriatr Psychiatry.* Sept;16(9):781-5, 2008. https://www.ncbi.nlm.nih.gov/pubmed/18757771 doi: 10.1097/JGP.0b013e3181812790.

⁴⁵ Uffe Ravnskov, M.D., PhD, *Fat and Cholesterol are Good for You*, GB Publishing, Sweden. 2009, p1.

⁴⁶ Ravnskov et al., 2018.

⁴⁷ Samuel S. Epstein, M.D. *The Politics of Cancer Revisited,* East Ridge Press, 1998, p2.

⁴⁸ A Burgoyne, 2015

⁴⁹ Andrew A D Burgoyne, *Hijacked—How the Banking Industry, Finance, and Corporate Interests Have Hijacked our Economy and Corrupted Democracy.* Fundamental Press, 2018.

⁵⁰ Cancer Research UK. "Worldwide cancer statistics" https://www.cancerresearchuk.org/health-professional/cancer-statistics/worldwide-cancer#heading-Zero Cancer Research UK. "1 in 2 people in the UK will get cancer." 4 February 2015. https://www.cancerresearchuk.org/about-us/cancer-news/press-release/2015-02-04-1-in-2-people-in-the-uk-will-get-cancer

⁵¹ Samuel S Epstein M.D. *The Politics of Cancer Revisited,* East Ridge Press, 1998, p298.

References

52 "Cancer causing Chemicals in Food," Subcommittee on Oversight and Investigations of the House Committee on Interstate and Foreign Commerce, Ninety-Fifth Congress, Second Session. December 1978, p iii. https://babel.hathitrust.org/cgi/pt?id=mdp.39015078682914&view=1up&seq=3

53 Marie-Monique Robin, *Our Daily Poison—From Pesticides to Packaging, How Chemicals Have Contaminated the Food Chain and are Making Us Sick.* The New Press, 2014.

54 A Burgoyne, 2015, p118.

55 Environmental Working Group, "Body Burden: The Pollution in Newborns. A benchmark investigation of industrial chemicals, pollutants and pesticides in umbilical cord blood." July 14, 2005 https://www.ewg.org/research/body-burden-pollution-newborns

56 Ibid.

57Executive Summary, "Fourth National Report on Human Exposure to Environmental Chemicals 2009", Department of Health and Human Services, Centers for Disease Control and Prevention.

58 EPA Fines Teflon Maker DuPont for Chemical Cover-up, Environmental Working Group, Dec 14 2005. https://www.ewg.org/news/news-releases/2005/12/14/epa-fines-teflon-maker-dupont-chemical-cover

59 World Wide Fund for Nature (WWF) Detox Campaign "Chemical Check Up—An analysis of chemicals in the blood of Members of the European Parliament. April 2004.

60 Marie-Monique Robin, *Our Daily Poison—From Pesticides to Packaging, How Chemicals Have Contaminated the Food Chain and are Making Us Sick.* The New Press, 2014, p 369.

61 Rachel Carson, *Silent Spring,* Haughton Mifflin Company, 1962.

62 A Burgoyne, 2015, p140-50.

63 Theo Colborn, *Our Stolen Future,* Dutton, 1996, p187.

64 Brieger, Katharine K., "PCB-Contaminated Food in the Canadian Arctic: Interactions between Environmental Policy, Cultural Values, and the Healthcare System" (2011).Pomona Senior Theses. Paper 95. http://scholarship.claremont.edu/Pomona_theses/95

65 Evaggelos Vallianatos, with McKay Jenkins. *Poison Spring—The Secret History of Pollution and the EPA,* Bloomsbury Press, New York, 2014, p62.

66 Marie-Monique Robin, 2014, p227.

67André Leu,, *Poisoning Our Children—The Parent's Guide to the Myths of Safe Pesticides,* Acres USA, 2018, p20.

68 Robin Messange et al., "Major Pesticides Are More Toxic to Human Cells than Their Declared Active Principles." *Bio Med Research International* (December 2013). https://www.hindawi.com/journals/bmri/2014/179691/

69 Theo Colborn. "A Case for Revisiting the Safety of Pesticides. A Closer Look at Neurodevelopment." *Environmental Health Perspectives* 114, no.1 (January 2006): 10-17. https://www.ncbi.nlm.nih.gov/pmc/articles/PMC1332649/

70 Wingspread Statement on the Precautionary Principle--Racine, WI, January 20, 1998. http://www.rachel.org/?q=en/node/3357

71 2010 Annual Report. President's Cancer Panel. *Reducing Environmental Cancer Risk.* U.S. Department of Health and Human Services, National Institutes of Health, National Cancer Institute.

72 A Burgoyne 2015,p 215. For more on this story try: Leila McNeill. May 8, 2017 "The Woman Who Stood Between America and a Generation of 'Thalidomide Babies' How the United States escaped a national tragedy in the 1960s." Smithsonian.com May 8, 2017.

73 Dan Fagin, & Marianne Lavelle. *Toxic Deception-How the Chemical Industry Manipulates Science, Bends the Law and Endangers Your Health.* Center for Public Integrity, Common Courage Press, 1999, p35.

[74] Jeffrey Smith, for example, *Genetic Roulette—The Documented Health Risks of Genetically Engineered Foods,* Yes Books, 2007.

[75] "Statement of Policy: Foods Derived From New Plant Varieties," *FDA Federal Register* May 29, 1992, Volume 57, no 104, Sec. VI.

[76] Kurt Eichenwald, Gina Kolata & Melody Petersen. "Biotechnology Food: From the Lab to a Debacle," *New York Times*, January 25, 2001.

[77] Henryk Behr, *A Momentary Lapse of Reason—Living With L-Tryptophan Induced EMS and the Hidden Dangers of Genetic Modification of our Foods,* Xlibris Corporation, 2011.

[78] Tomoko Inose & Kousaku Murata. "Enhanced accumulation of toxic compound in yeast cells having high glycolytic activity: a case study on the safety of genetically engineered yeast." *International Journal of Food Science and Technology* (1995) 30, 141-146 1 April 1995.

[79] Steven M. Drucker, *Altered Genes Twisted Truth—How the Venture to Genetically Engineer Our Food Has Subverted Science, Corrupted Government, and Systematically Deceived the Public.* Clear River Press, 2015, p 230.

[80] Amy Dean, D.O. and Jennifer Armstrong, M.D. Genetically Modified Foods, *American Academy of Environmental Medicine* , May 8, 2009.) Available at: http://aaemonline.org/gmopost.html

[81] Elements of Precaution: Recommendations for the Regulation of Food Biotechnology in Canada, An Expert Panel Report on the Future of Food Biotechnology, *The Royal Society of Canada*, January 2001.

[82]Caroline Cox, Glyphosate (Roundup), Herbicide Factsheet, *Journal of Pesticide Reform*, Fall 1998, Vol 18, No 3. http://www.eastbaypesticidealert.org/Glyphosate%20Factsheet%201.htm

[83] T. Bøhn et al, "Compositional differences in soybeans on the market: Glyphosate accumulates in Roundup Ready GM soybeans." *Food Chemistry*, Volume 153, 15 June 2014, pp207-215.

[84] Vandana Shiva, in the foreword to André Leu's book, *Poisoning Our Children—The Patent's Guide to the Myths of Safe Pesticides.* Acres USA, 2018.

[85] F William Engdahl, *Seeds of Destruction, The Hidden Agenda of Genetic Manipulation,* Global Research, 2007.

[86] Andrew Rowell "The Sinister Sacking of the World's Leading GM Expert- and the Trail that leads to Tony Blair and the White House. *The Daily Mail,* July 7,2003.

[87] F. William Engdahl, *Seeds of Destruction—The Hidden Agenda of Genetic Manipulation,* Global Reseach, Centre for Research on Globalization. 2007, p 24.

[88] Amy Dean, D.O. and Jennifer Armstrong, M.D. "Genetically Modified Foods". *American Academy of Environmental Medicine.* May 8th 2009. https://www.aaemonline.org/gmo.php

[89] "Recent Trends in GE Adoption", United States Department of Agriculture Economic Research Service. https://www.ers.usda.gov/data-products/adoption-of-genetically-engineered-crops-in-the-us/recent-trends-in-ge-adoption.aspx

[90] Jonathan R. Latham, PhD. "GMO Dangers: Facts You Need to Know". T Colin Campbell Center for Nutritional Studies. https://nutritionstudies.org/gmo-dangers-facts-you-need-to-know/

[91] Yanfang Fu et al, "High-frequency off-target mutagenisis induced by CRISPR.Cas nucleases in human cells." Nature Biotechnology. 31, 9 (2013), pp822-26. doi.org/10.1038/nbt.2623.

[92] Vandana Shiva with Kartikey Shiva, *Oneness vs The 1%--Shattering Illusions, Seeding Freedom.* New Internationalist Publications Ltd. 2019, p104.

[93] Ibid.

[94] Genetically modified crops breed economic dependence, new form of slavery, says Cardinal Turkson, *Catholic Review,* January 19, 2012. https://www.archbalt.org/genetically-modified-crops-breed-economic-dependence-new-form-of-slavery-says-cardinal-turkson/

[95] A Burgoyne, 2015 p386.

References

⁹⁶ Frances Moore Lappé and Joseph Collins, *World Hunger—10 Myths,* Grove Press, 2015, p 4.

⁹⁷ Allison Wilson, PhD and Jonathan Latham, PhD."GMO Golden Rice Offers No Nutritional Benefits Says FDA." *Independent Science News.* June 3, 2018. https://www.independentsciencenews.org/news/gmo-golden-rice-offers-no-nutritional-benefits-says-fda/

⁹⁸ Jeffrey M. Smith, *Genetic Roulette—The Documented Health Risks of Genetically Engineered Foods,* Yes Books, 2007, p33.

⁹⁹ Ibid.

¹⁰⁰ Jonathan Latham, PhD., "Have Monsanto and the Biotech Industry Turned Natural Bt Pesticides into GMO "Super toxins"? " Biotechnology, Commentaries, *Environment* October 9, 2017 https://www.independentsciencenews.org/environment/have-monsanto-and-the-biotech-industry-turned-natural-bt-pesticides-into-gmo-super-toxins/

¹⁰¹ Dr Joseph Mercola, "Eating This Could Turn Your Gut Into a Living Pesticide Factory", 31 May 29, 2012. https://articles.mercola.com/sites/articles/archive/2012/05/29/genetically-modified-crops-insects-emerged.aspx?e_cid=20120529_DNL_art_1

¹⁰² Bhat, M.S., P. Parimala, S. Rama Lakshmi and K. Muthuchelian. "In-Vitro cytotoxic and genotoxicity studies of Cry1Ac toxin isolated from Bt cotton (RCH2 Bt) on human lymphocytes." *Acad. J. Plant Sci.,* 4(3): 64-68. 2011.

¹⁰³ US President's Cancer Panel's Annual Report, 2010, p 45.

¹⁰⁴ Vandana Shiva, in the foreword to André Leu's book, *Poisoning Our Children—The Patent's Guide to the Myths of Safe Pesticides.* Acres USA, 2018.

¹⁰⁵ Mohan Manikkam et al., "Transgenerational Actions of Environmental Compounds on Reproductive Disease and Identification of Epigenetic Biomarkers of Ancestral Exposures." PlosOne, 7, no. 2 (February 2012.

¹⁰⁶ Michael K Skinner, Carlos Guerrero-Bosagna, & M Muksitul Haque, "Environmentally induced epigenetic transgenerational inheritance of sperm

epimutations promote genetic mutations." *Epigenetics*. 2015 Aug; 10(8): 762–771. doi: 10.1080/15592294.2015.1062207 PMCID: PMC4622673 https://www.ncbi.nlm.nih.gov/pmc/articles/PMC4622673/

[107] Philippe Grandjean and Philip Landrigan, "Neurobehavioural effects of developmental toxicity." *Lancet Neurol*, 2014:13: 330-38. https://www.ncbi.nlm.nih.gov/pubmed/24556010

[108] Matej Mikulic, "Global Pharmaceutical Industry - Statistics & Facts," *Statista*, Aug 13, 2019. https://www.statista.com/topics/1764/global-pharmaceutical-industry/

[109] "Global pharma spending will hit $1.5 trillion in 2023, says IQVIA", *Pharmaceutical Commerce*, January 29, 2019. https://pharmaceuticalcommerce.com/business-and-finance/global-pharma-spending-will-hit-1-5-trillion-in-2023-says-iqvia/

[110] Ray D Strand, M.D., *Death By Prescription—The Shocking Truth behind an Overmedicated Nation,* Thomas Nelson Publishers, 2003.

[111] Ibid.

[112] Gary Null, PhD, Martin Feldman, MD, Debora Rasio, M.D., & Carolyn Dean, M.D., ND. *Death By Medicine,* Praktikos Books, 2010.

[113] Ibid. US Senate Finance Committee. Testimony of David J. Graham, MD, MPH, November 18, 2004.

[114] Andrew Burgoyne, *Unhealthy Betrayal—How the Manipulation of Science and Politics by Corporate Interests Destroys Health and Threatens the Future of Humanity.* Fundamental Press, 2015.

[115] Drugbank Statistics 2019. https://www.drugbank.ca/stats

[116] Marcia Angell, M.D. *The Truth About Drug Companies—How They Deceive Us and What to Do About It.* Random House, 2004. See also Dr. Marcia Angell, former editor in chief of the *New England Journal of Medicine* on health corruption. https://www.wanttoknow.info/health/health-corruption

[117] Peter C Gøtzsche, *Deadly Medicines and Organised Crime—How big pharma has corrupted healthcare.* Radcliffe Publishing, 2013.

References

[118] Ibid.

[119] John Abramson, M.D., *OVERDO$ED AMERICA—The Broken Promise of American Medicine. How the Pharmaceutical Companies are Corrupting Science, Misleading Doctors, and Threatening Your Health.* Harper Collins, 2005.

[120] Ray D Strand, M.D., *Death By Prescription—The Shocking Truth behind an Overmedicated Nation,* Thomas Nelson Publishers, 2003.

[121] Ibid.

[122] Ben Goldacre, *Bad Pharma—How medicine is broken, and how we can fix it,* Fourth Estate, 2013.

[123] This was SmithKline Beecham, before they merged with Glaxo Welcome and became GSK.

[124] Ben Goldacre, *Bad Pharma—How medicine is broken, and how we can fix it,* Fourth Estate, 2013.

[125] Peter C Gøtzsche, *Deadly Medicines and Organised Crime—How big pharma has corrupted healthcare.* Radcliffe Publishing, 2013, p19.

[126] Ibid, p130.

[127] Ray D Strand, M.D., *Death By Prescription—The Shocking Truth behind an Overmedicated Nation,* Thomas Nelson Publishers, 2003, p74.

[128] Terry Turner, "Proton Pump Inhibitor (PPI) Side Effects."*Drugwatch.* September 12, 2019.
https://www.drugwatch.com/proton-pump-inhibitors/side-effects/

[129]Terry Turner, "Proton Pump Inhibitor (PPI) Lawsuits," *Drugwatch, September 12, 2019.*
https://www.drugwatch.com/proton-pump-inhibitors/lawsuits/

[130] Leading antacid tablet brands in the United States in 2018, based on sales (in million U.S. dollars), *Statista,* 2019.
https://www.statista.com/statistics/194544/leading-us-antacid-tablet-brands-in-2013-based-on-sales/

[131] Alexander Cockburn." When half a million Americans died and nobody noticed." *The Week,* Apr 27, 2012

https://www.theweek.co.uk/us/46535/when-half-million-americans-died-and-nobody-noticed

[132] David Brodwin, "Money for Nothing. The U.S. spends big bucks on mental illness treatments that may not even work." *U.S. News,* July 22, 2015

[133] Lea Winerman, "By the numbers: Antidepressant use on the rise." *American Psychological Association*, November 2017, Vol 48, No. 10.

[134] Alan Schwarz, "Thousands of Toddlers Are Medicated for A.D.H.D., Report Finds, Raising Worries."
New York Times, May 16, 2014.

[135] Peter C. Gøtzsche, *Deadly Psychiatry and Organised Denial,* People Press, 2015.

[136] Gardiner Harris & Benedict Carey, "Reasearchers Fail to Reveal Full Drug Pay." *New York Times,* June 8, 2008.

[137] Peter C. Gøtzsche, *Deadly Psychiatry and Organised Denial,* People Press, 2015, p36.

[138] John Virapen, *Side Effects Death: Confessions of an Pharma-Insider.* Virtual Book Worm Publishing Inc. 2010.

[139] Peter Breggin, *Toxic Psychiaty—Drugs and Electroconvulsive Therapy: The Truth and the Better Alternatives.* Harper Collins, 1993 pp356, 450-453.

[140] Peter R. Breggin, M D. *Medicating Madness—The Role of Psychiatric Drugs in Cases of Violence, Suicide, and Crime,* St Martin's Griffin, New York, 2008, p 96.

[141] Peter C Gøtzsche, *Deadly Medicines and Organised Crime—How big pharma has corrupted healthcare.* Radcliffe Publishing, 2013, p112.

[142] Ray Moynihan, Jenny Doust, David Henry, "Medicalisation-Preventing overdiagnosis: how to stop harming the healthy." *BMJ*, 2012; 344: e3502.

[143] John Virapen, *Side Effects: Death—Confessions of a Pharma-Insider,* Virtual Worm.com Publishing Inc., 2010, p100.

[144] Joseph Glenmullen, M.D., *Prozac Backlash—Overcoming the Dangers of Prozac, Zoloft, Paxil, and other Antidepressants with Safe, Effective Alternatives,* Simon & Shuster, 2000, p15.

[145] Ann Blake Tracy PhD, *Prozac—Panacea or Pandora,* Cassia Publications 2001.

[146] Robert Whitaker, *Anatomy of an Epidemic—Magic Bullets, Psychiatric Drugs, and the Astonishing Rise of Mental Illness in America.* Broadway Paperbacks, 2010, p246.

[147] Peter R. Breggin, " Rational Principles of Psychopharmacology for Therapists, Healthcare Providers and Clients." *J Contemp Psychother* (2016) 46: 1-13

[148] Sarah Boseley, "They Said it was Safe", *The Guardian,* Saturday October 30, 1999.

[149] David Healy, *Let Them Eat Prozac—The Unhealthy Relationship between the Pharmaceutical Industry and Depression.* New York University Press, 2004, p76.

[150] Jon Rappoport, "Prozac Maker Eli Lilly Subverted Mass Murder Trial." *Principia Scientific International (PSI),* October 4, 2019. https://principia-scientific.org/prozac-maker-eli-lilly-subverted-mass-murder-trial/

[151] Ann Blake Tracy PhD, *Prozac—Panacea or Pandora,* Cassia Publications 2001. p59.

[152] Peter C. Gøtzsche, *Deadly Psychiatry and Organised Denial,* People Press, 2015, p14.

[153] Andrew Burgoyne, *Unhealthy Betrayal-How the Manipulation of Science and Politics By Corporate Interests Destroys Health and Threatens the Future of Humanity,* Fundamental Press, 2015.

[154] Chris McGreal, *American Overdose—The Opioid Tragedy in Three Acts,* Faber & Faber Ltd, 2019.

[155] Judith Feinberg. "Tackle the epidemic, not the opioids." *Nature,* 09 September 2019.

156 Chris McGreal, *American Overdose—The Opioid Tragedy in Three Acts,* Faber & Faber Ltd, 2019, p166.

157Chris McGreal, "Drug makers conspired to worsen the opioid crisis. They have blood on their hands." The Guardian, Thu 29 Aug 2019.

158 Jan Hoffman, "Johnson & Johnson Ordered to Pay $572 Million in Landmark Opioid Trial." *New York Times*, Aug. 26, 2019

159 Hannah Kuchler in New York "Johnson & Johnson hit with $8bn court order over antipsychotic drug." *Financial Times*, October 9, 2019.

160 Edward Helmore in New York. "Lawsuits, payouts, opioids crisis: What happened to Johnson & Johnson?" *The Guardian* Fri 18 Oct. 2019.

161 Harriet Ryan, Lisa Girion and Scott Glover. "OxyContin goes global — "We're only just getting started." *LA Times*. Dec. 18, 2016.

162 Kenan Malik. "America's opioid catastrophe has lessons for us all, about greed and racial division." *The Guardian* Sun 1 Sep 2019

163 Jan Hoffman, "Purdue Pharma Tentatively Settles Thousands of Opioid Cases". New York Times Sept 13, 2019.

164 Chris McGreal, *American Overdose—The Opioid Tragedy in Three Acts,* Faber & Faber Ltd, 2019, p300.

165 Guardian staff and agencies "Purdue Pharma agrees $12bn settlement in opioids case, plaintiffs' lawyers say". *The Guardian* Weds 11 Sept 2019

166 Jan Hoffman, "Would a Purdue Bankruptcy Protect the Sacklers? Good Question." *New York Times*, Sept. 16, 2019.

167 Chris McGreal, *American Overdose—The Opioid Tragedy in Three Acts,* Faber & Faber Ltd, 2019, p166.

168 Tracy Seipel, "Election 2016: Big Pharma's $70 million tops California campaign contributions." *The Mercury News*, July 11, 2016.

169 Barbara Kollmeyer, "$1bn here we come.' — Martin Shkreli told Turing board as Daraprim buy got closer," *Market Watch*, Feb 3 2016.

170Actuarial Outpost, "Pharma and Arbitrary Drug Prices," *Actuarial Outpost*, 20 Sept 2015

References

http://www.actuarialoutpost.com/actuarial_discussion_forum/archive/index.php/t-299668.html

[171] Leslie E. Sekerka, Lauren Benishek, "Thick as Thieves? Big Pharma Wields its Power with the Help of Government Regulation." *Emory Corporate Governance and Accountability Review,* 2019. http://law.emory.edu/ecgar/content/volume-5/issue-2/essays/thieves-pharma-power-help-government-regulation.html

[172] Ray Moynihan, Iona Heath, and David Henry, "Selling Sickness: The pharmaceutical industry and disease mongering." *BMJ.* 2002 Apr 13; 324(7342): 886–891. doi: 10.1136/bmj.324.7342.886. PMCID: PMC1122833 PMID: 11950740

[173] Melody Petersen, *Our Daily Meds,* Picador, 2008, p33.

[174] Susan Kelleher & Duff Wilson, "Suddenly Sick. The hidden big business behind your doctor's diagnosis". *The Seattle Times Co,* June 26-30, 2005.

[175] Ibid.

[176] Andrew Burgoyne, *Unhealthy Betrayal—How the Manipulation of Science and Politics by Corporate Interests Destroys Health and Threatens the Future of Humanity.* Fundamental Press, 2015.

[177] Leslie E. Sekerka and, Lauren Benishek, "Thick as Thieves? Big Pharma Wields its Power with the Help of Government Regulation." *Emory Corporate Governance and Accountability Review,* 2019.

[178] Roxanne Nelson, BSN, RN. "Is direct-to-consumer advertising leading practice?" AJN October 2007 Vol. 107, No. 1025. https://www.nursingcenter.com/pdfjournal?AID=743814&an=00000446-200710000-00018&Journal_ID=54030&Issue_ID=743761

[179] Leslie E. Sekerka, Lauren Benishek, 2019.

[180] Marion Nestle, *Food Politics—How the Food Industry Influences Nutrition and Health.* University of California Press, 2007, p124.

[181] American Heart Association. "Heart-Healthy Foods." https://www.heart.org/en/healthy-living/company-collaboration/heart-check-

certification/heart-check-in-the-grocery-store/heart-check-food-certification-program-nutrition-requirements

[182]John Casey, "The Truth About Fats. Web MD". Feature Reviewed by Louise Chang, MD on February 03, 2003. https://www.webmd.com/women/features/benefits-of-essential-fats-and-oils#1

[183] Ibid.

[184] Marcella Garsetti et.al. "Fat composition of vegetable oil spreads and margarines in the USA in 2013: A national marketplace analysis." *Int J Food Sci Nutr.* 2016 May 18; 67(4): 372–382. doi: 10.3109/09637486.2016.1161012 PMCID: PMC4898149 PMID: 27046021

[185] Robert Mendick, "Cooking with vegetable oils releases toxic cancer-causing chemicals, say experts." *The Telegraph,* Thursday 04 July 2019. See also: Esterbauer H, "Cytotoxicity and genotoxicity of lipid-oxidation products." *Am J Clin Nutr.* 1993 May; 57(5 Suppl): 779S-785S; doi: 10.1093/ajcn/57.5.779S. See also:

Sarah Moumtaz, et al. "Toxic aldehyde generation in and food uptake from culinary oils during frying practices: peroxidative resistance of a monounsaturate-rich algae oil" *Nature, Scientific Reports* vol.9, Article number: 4125 (2019), Published: 11 March 2019 https://www.nature.com/articles/s41598-019-39767-1#Sec7

[186] Joanna Blythman, *Swallow This—Serving Up the Food Industry's Darkest Secrets,* Fourth Estate, 2015.

[187] Eric Schlosser, *Fast Food Nation-What the All-American Meal is Doing to the World,* Allen Lane, Penguin Press, 2001.

[188] *Reports and Data*, October 10, 2019. https://www.globenewswire.com/news-release/2019/10/10/1928250/0/en/Food-Flavors-Market-To-Reach-USD-19-72-Billion-By-2026-Reports-And-Data.html

[189] Eric Schlosser, *Fast Food Nation-What the All-American Meal is Doing to the World,* Allen Lane, Penguin Press, 2001.

[190] Michael Moss, *Salt Sugar Fat—How the Food Giants Hooked Us.* WH Allen, 2014.

[191] Qing Yang, "Gain weight by 'going diet?' Artificial sweeteners and the neurobiology of sugar cravings." *Neuroscience,* June, 2010. See also "Why artificial sweeteners can increase appetite" *Science Daily,* July 12, 2016 https://www.sciencedaily.com/releases/2016/07/160712130107.htm Qiao-Ping Wang et al., "Sucralose Promotes Food Intake through NPY and a Neuronal Fasting Response." *Cell Metabolism,* 2016; 24 (1): 75. DOI: 10.1016/j.cmet.2016.06.010

[192] Thiago Magalhães Cabral et al. "Artificial Sweeteners as a Cause of Obesity: Weight Gain Mechanisms and Current Evidence." *Health,* Vol.10 No.5, May 2018

DOI: 10.4236/health.2018.105054

[193] Bernard Jensen, D.C., PhD., Co-authored with Sylvia Bell *Tissue Cleansing Through Bowel Management,* Bernard Jensen, 1981.

[194] Leon Chaitow, *Probiotics—How 'Friendly Bacteria' can Restore Health and Vitality*, Thorsons, 1990.

[195] Erin Ferranti, PhD, MPH, RN, et al. "20 Things you Didn't Know About the Human gut Microbiome." *J Cardiovasc Nurs.* 2014 Nov-Dec; 29(6): 479–481.

[196] Michael Pollan, "Say Hello to the 100 Trillion Bacteria That Make Up Your Microbiome – Some of My Best Friends are Germs," *New York Times*, May 16, 2013.

[197] Sayer Ji, "7 Ways Probiotics DETOXIFY Your Body", GreenMed Info LLC, Friday March 30, 2018, This work is reproduced and distributed with the permission of GreenMedInfo LLC. Want to learn more from GreenMedInfo? Sign up for the newsletter here //www.greenmedinfo.com/greenmed/newsletter.

[198] Arlene Semeco, MS, RD, "The 19 Best Prebiotic Foods You Should Eat, Healthline," June 8, 2016.

https://www.healthline.com/nutrition/19-best-prebiotic-foods#section14

[199] Russell Blaylock, M.D., *Excitotoxins—The Taste That Kills,* Health Press, 1995.

[200] Janet Starr Hull, *Sweet Poison—How the World's Most Popular Artificial Sweetener Is Killing Us My Story,* New Horizon Press, 1998.

[201] Joanna Blythman, *Swallow This—Serving Up the Food Industry's Darkest Secrets,* Fourth Estate, 2015, p250.

[202] Ibid.

[203] Deepak Kumar Verma, Prem Prakash Srivastav, Ami Rameshbhai Patel, Kimmy G. "Genetically Modified Organisms (GMOs) Produced Enzymes: Multifarious Applications in Food Manufacturing Industries". *Bioprocess Technology in Food and Health: Potential Applications and Emerging Scope*, Publisher: Apple Academic Press, Inc., [AAP]- CRC Press, pp.77-12. September 2018.

https://www.researchgate.net/publication/328381367_Genetically_Modified_Organisms_GMOs_Produced_Enzymes_Multifarious_Applications_in_Food_Manufacturing_Industries

[204] Jenni Russell, "Could these foods be giving us cancer?", *The Guardian,* Thurs 15 Aug, 2002

[205] Md. Abul Haider Shipar, "A General Review on Maillard Reactions in Foods."
Toronto Institute of Pharmaceutical Technology, Sept 2009.

[206] Lauane Nunes, et al. "The Maillard Reaction in Powdered Infant Formula." *Journal of Food and Nutrition Research*. 2019, 7(1), 33-40. January 23, 2019. DOI: 10.12691/jfnr-7-1-5

[207] Ibid.

[208] Tim aus der Beek, Frank-Andreas Weber, Axel Bergmann et al. "Pharmaceuticals in the environment: Global occurrence and potential

cooperative action under the Strategic Approach to International Chemicals Management (SAICM) 2016". German Environment Agency. 2016.

[209] Joe Thornton, *Pandora's Poison—Chlorine, Health, and a New Environmental Strategy,* MIT Press, 2000, p19.

[210] Ibid. p139.

[211] Carl C. Pfeiffer, PhD, M.D., *Nutrition and Mental Illness—An Orthomolecular Approach to Balancing Body Chemistry.* Healing Arts Press, 1987.

[212] William Dufty, *Sugar Blues,* Chilton Book Company, 1975, p94.

[213] Sally Pacholok,RN., BSN., Jeffrey Stuart, DO., *Could It Be B12?-An Epidemic of Misdiagnoses.* Quill Driver Books, 2011.

[214] William Dufty, *Sugar Blues,* Chilton Book Company, 1975, p92.

[215] Abram Hoffer, M.D., PhD., Writing in the Foreword to *Vitamin C: The Real Story*, by Steve Hickey, PhD, and Andrew Saul, PhD, Basic Health Publications, 2008.

[216] Thomas E. Levy, MD, JD. *Curing the Incurable-Vitamin C, Infectious Diseases, and Toxins,* Livon Books, 2002.

[217] PhilipWashko, & Mark Levine, "Inhibition of Ascorbic Acid Transport in Human Neutrophils by Glucose." *Biol Chem* 273 :33 (1992): 23568-23574.

[218] Andrew Saul PhD., and Steve Hickey PhD., *Vitamin C: The Real Story.* Basic Health Publications, Inc. 2008.

[219] Sander Rozemeijer, et al. "Estimating Vitamin C Status in Critically Ill Patients with a Novel Point-of-Care Oxidation-Reduction Potential Measurement." *Nutrients.* 2019 May 8;11(5). pii: E1031. doi: 10.3390/nu11051031.

[220] Aileen Hill, et al., "Vitamin C to Improve Organ Dysfunction in Cardiac Surgery Patients—Review and Pragmatic Approach." *Nutrients,* 2018 Aug; 10(8): 974. doi: 10.3390/nu10080974 PMCID: PMC6115862 PMID: 30060468

[221] *American Journal of Clinical Nutrition*: https://academic.oup.com/ajcn *Journal of Orthomolecular Nutrition:* http://orthomolecular.org/index.shtml

[222] James M. May and Fiona E. Harrison, "Role of Vitamin C in the Function of the Vascular Endothelium." *Antioxid Redox Signal.* 2013 Dec 10; 19(17): 2068–2083. PMCID: PMC3869438 PMID: 23581713 doi: 10.1089/ars.2013.5205

[223] B Frei, L England, and B N Ames. "Ascorbate is an outstanding antioxidant in human blood plasma."

Proc Natl Acad Sci U S A. 1989 Aug; 86(16): 6377–6381. doi: 10.1073/pnas.86.16.6377PMCID: PMC297842 PMID: 2762330

[224] Fiona E. Harrison, James M. May, "Vitamin C function in the brain: vital role of the ascorbate transporter SVCT2." *Free Radic Biol Med.* 2009 Mar 15;46(6):719-30. doi: 10.1016/j.freeradbiomed.2008.12.018. Epub 2009 Jan 6.

[225] Andrew W Saul, PhD, as a reference for the book by Dr Steve Hickey and Dr Hilary Roberts, *Ascorbate: The Science of Vitamin C,* 2004, posted on Amazon.

[226] Thomas E.Levy, MD, JD. *Primal Panacea*, MedFox Publishing, 2011, p17.

[227] Andrew W. Saul and Atsuo Yanagisawa, MD, PhD. "Hospital-based Intravenous Vitamin C Treatment for Coronavirus and Related Illnesses." *Orthomolecular Medicine News Service*, **Feb 2, 2020.**

[228] Andrew W. Saul, Editor, "Coronavirus Patients in China to be Treated with High-Dose Vitamin C." *Orthomolecular Medicine News Service*, Feb 13, 2020

[229] Andrew W Saul, "Tons of Vitamin C to Wuhan. China Using Vitamin C against COVID," *Othomolecular Medicine News Service*, Feb 23, 2020.

[230] Christina Farr & Salvador Rodriguez, "Facebook, Amazon, Google and more met with WHO to figure out how to stop coronavirus misinformation" CNBC Fri, Feb 14, 2020 2:19 pm.

Updated Fri, Feb 14 2020 3:53 PM EST

[231] Robert F Cathcart, III, MD, "Vitamin C, Titrating to Bowel Tolerance, Anascorbemia, and Acute Induced Scurvy." *Medical Hypotheses*, 7:1359-1376, 1981.

References

[232] BIOtechNOW. "New PhRMA Report: Nearly 300 Vaccines Currently in Development." September 11, 2013. https://www.bio.org/blogs/new-phrma-report-nearly-300-vaccines-currently-development

[233] Dr Joseph Mercola, "Vitamin C Works for Sepsis. Will it Work for Coronavirus? Mercola.com, Feb 24, 2020.
https://articles.mercola.com/sites/articles/archive/2020/02/24/iv-vitamin-c.aspx

[234] Phil Archer, "Local hospital using experimental drug treatment in hopes of saving lives of COVID-19patients." Click2Houston.com April 16, 2020. Frontline COVID-19 Critical Care Working Group.
Physician Contact, New York: Keith Berkowitz, M.D., Member, FLCCC Working Group keith@centerforbalancedhealth.com
Physician Contact, California: Howard Kornfeld, M.D., Member, FLCCC Working Group info@pharmacologypolicy.org , 415-383-2949

[235] Dr Pierre Kory's Testimony to the US Senate Committee Hearing, Homeland Security and Government Affairs, May 6th, 2020.

[236] Lorena Mongelli & Bruce Golding, "New York hospitals treating coronavirus patients with vitamin C," *New York Post,* March 24, 2020.

[237] For more information regarding supplementation, see: Andrew W Saul, Editor. "Vitamin C Protects Against Coronavirus." *Orthomolecular Medicine News Service,* Jan 26' 2020.
http://orthomolecular.org/resources/omns/v16n04.shtml

[238] The Protocol can be found here: evms.edu/covidcare

[239] Doris Loh, "COVID-19, ARDS & Cytokine Storms – The Recycling of Ascorbic Acid by Macrophages, Neutrophils and Lymphocytes." *Evolutamente,* 5th April, 2020. https://www.evolutamente.it/covid-19-ards-cytokine-storms-the-recycling-of-ascorbic-acid-by-macrophages-neutrophils-and-lymphocytes/

[240] Thomas E. Levy, MD, JD. *Primal Panacea*, MedFox Publishing, 2011.

[241] Fernanda Martini et al., "Simian virus 40 in humans," *Infect Agent Cancer,* 2007: 2: 13. Jul 9. doi: 10.1186/1750-9378-2-13 PMCID: PMC1941725

242 Andrew Saul, "Hidden in Plain Sight: The Pioneering Work of Frederick Robert Klenner MD. *J Orthomolecular Med,* 2007, Vol 22, No 1, p31-38. Also available at www.doctoryourself.com

243 Barbara Loe Fisher," Meet the New Billionaires Club: COVID-19 Vaccine Developers." *Health Impact News,* April 21, 2020. Also: Nuala Moran, "WHO releases COVID-19 roadmap: funding efforts in progress." *BioWorld,* March 9, 2020.

244 Miloud Kaddar, Global Vaccine Market Features and Trends, World Health Organisation. Also: Eric Sagonowski, "The top 5 vaccine companies by 2017 revenue," *Fierce Pharma,* Aug 1, 2018.

245 Health Resources & Services Administration, Vaccine Injury Compensation Program Data Report, Updated April 1 2020.

246 Dr Joseph Mercola, "Major Error Found in Vaccine Aluminum Safety Calculation." April 7, 2020. https://articles.mercola.com/sites/articles/archive/2020/04/07/vaccine-aluminum-safety-calculation-error.aspx

247 Physicians for Informed Consent Reports on ResearchGate: Landmark FDA Paper on Aluminum Safety in Vaccines Has Crucial Math Error. *Physicians for Informed Consent.* March 6th, 2020.

248 Tomljenovic L, Shaw CA, "Aluminum vaccine adjuvants: are they safe?" *Curr Med Chem,* 2011: 18 (17): 2630-7. DOI:10.2174/092986711795933740

249 Zed Phoenix: Public Health (Control of Disease) Act 1984. https://www.youtube.com/watch?v=HzJpRvSUbl4&feature=youtu.be https://www.legislation.gov.uk/ukpga/

250 Joel Bakan, *The Corporation—The Pathological Pursuit of Profit and Power,* Constable & Robinson Ltd, 2005, p6.

251 Adam Smith, *The Wealth of Nations,* 1776.

252 Andrew Burgoyne, *Unhealthy Betrayal—How the Manipulation of Science and Politics by Corporate Interests Destroys Health and Threatens the Future of Humanity,* p367.

[253] Corporate Power & the Global Economy, SPERI Sheffield Political Economy Research Institute.

3 January, 2019. http://speri.dept.shef.ac.uk/2019/01/03/corporate-power-the-global-economy/

[254] David Streitfield, "Amazon Hits $1,000,000,000,000 in Value, Following Apple." *New York Times,* Sept 4, 2018.

[255] Joel Bakan, *The Corporation—The Pathological Pursuit of Profit and Power,* Constable & Robinson Ltd, 2005, p12.

[256] Kent Greenfield, *The Failure of Corporate Law—Fundamental Flaws and Progressive Possibilities,* University of Chicago Press, 2006, p2.

[257] David C Korten, *When Corporations Rule the World,* Earthscan Publications Ltd., 1995.

[258] Harry Glasbeek, *Wealth By Stealth—Corporate Crime, Corporate Law, and the Perversion of Democracy,* Between The Lines, 2002, p282.

[259] Milton Friedman, "The Social Responsibility of Business Is to Increase Its Profits." *New York Times Magazine*, September 13 1970

[260] Greenfield 2006.

[261] Leo E. Strine, Jr. In the Foreword to "The 2019 CPA-Zicklin Index of Corporate Political Disclosure and Accountability", Center For Political Accountability, Oct 24, 2019.

[262] "The 2019 CPA-Zicklin Index of Corporate Political Disclosure and Accountability", Center For Political Accountability", Oct 24, 2019.

[263] Corporate Governance Business Roundtable Redefines the Purpose of a Corporation to Promote 'An Economy That Serves All Americans' Aug 19, 2019.

https://www.businessroundtable.org/business-roundtable-redefines-the-purpose-of-a-corporation-to-promote-an-economy-that-serves-all-americans

[264] Kenneth P. Doyle, "Shadow of Dark Money Grows as 2020 Groups Shun Donor Disclosure." *Bloomberg Government,* August 2, 2019

265 Program on Corporations, Law & Democracy, "Corporate Hijacking of the U.S. Constitution", Featured Poclad Article Oct 2019 http://www.poclad.org/

266 The Corporation, A film by Mark Achbar, Jennifer Abbot and Joel Bakan. www.thecorporation.com

267 Melody Petersen, *Our Daily Meds,* Sarah Cricton Books, 2008, p75. For more examples see: A Burgoyne, *Unhealthy Betrayal.*

268 Ibid.

269 Michael Hudson, *Killing the Host—How Financial Parasites and Debt Destroy the Global Economy.* ISLET-Verlag 2015.

270 Monika Mitchell, 'Ripping your Face Off: Goldman Sachs vs. The World', *Huffington Post*, March 14, 2012.

271 David C Korten, *When Corporations Rule the World,* Earthscan Publications Ltd., 1995, p261.

272 Ray C. Anderson, with Robbin White, *Confessions of a Radical Industrialist— Profits, People, Purpose—Doing Business by Respecting the Earth,* McClelland & Stewart Ltd, 2009.

273 Harry Glasbeek, *Wealth By Stealth—Corporate Crime, Corporate Law, and the Perversion of Democracy,* Between The Lines, 2002, p271.

274 Kent Greenfield, *The Failure of Corporate Law—Fundamental Flaws and Progressive Possibilities,* University of Chicago Press, 2006, p127.

275 Joel Bakan, *The Corporation—The Pathological Pursuit of Profit and Power,* Constable & Robinson Ltd, 2005, p158.

276 Vineet D Menachery et al. "A SARS-like cluster of circulating bat coronaviruses shows potential for human emergence." *Nat Med,* 2015; 21(12): 1508-1513. PMCID: PMC4797993 NIHMSID: NIHMS766724 PMID: 26552008

277 Joshua Philipp, ""The first documentary movie on CCP virus, Tracking Down the Origin of the Wuhan Coronavirus." *Epoch Times*, Aired on April 7th, 2020. https://www.youtube.com/watch?v=3bXWGxhd7ic Fan Wu, Su Zheo et al. "A

new coronavirus associated with human respiratory disease in China." 7th Jan 2020. Feb 3rd Published. Nature, 579, 265-269 (2020). Dan Hu et al.

"Genomic characterization and infectivity of a novel SARS-like coronavirus in Chinese bats." Sept 12, 2018, *Emerg Microbes Infect.* **2018: 7 : 174 PMCID: PMC613831**

[278] Declan Butler, "Engineered bat virus stirs debate over risky research." *Nature,* 12th November, 2015.

[279] Carl Franzen, "Killer cure: why is the US creating new viruses and stockpiling the vaccines?" *The Verge,* April 17, 2013.

[280]Richard Cheng, MD, PhD, "Successful High-Dose Vitamin C Treatment of Patients with Serious and Critical COVID-19 Infection." *Orthomolecular Medicine News Service,* Mar 18, 2020.

http://www.orthomolecular.org/resources/omns/v16n18.shtml

See also: Richard Cheng, MD, PhD, "Can early and high intravenous dose of vitamin C prevent and treat coronavirus disease 2019 (COVID-19)?" *Medicine in Drug Discovery* Volume 5, March 2020.

[281] https://covid19criticalcare.com/

[282] Lorenga Mongelli & bruce Golding, "New York hospitals treating coronavirus patients with vitamin C." *New York Post,* March 24, 2020.

[283] Arjun Walia, "FBI raids Doctor Using Vitamin C To Help Treat & Prevent Coronavirus While China Is Still Using It." *Collective Evolution,* April 30, 2020.

[284] Sign a petition to get the FDA: Approve High Dose IV Vitamin C for Coronavirus Patients: https://www.change.org/p/explore-high-dose-iv-vitamin-c-for-coronavirus-patients Sign a petition to enable the NHS in the UK the use of Vitamin C for protecting both the staff and for IV use for patients: www.change.org C4UK.

[285] Darrell Bricker & John Ibbitson, *Empty Planet—The Shock of Global Population Decline,* Robinson, 2019.

[286] GBD 2017 Population and Fertility Collaborators, Population and fertility by age and sex for 195 countries and territories, 1950–2017: a systematic analysis

for the Global Burden of Disease Study 2017, *Global Health Metrics|* Volume 392, ISSUE 10159, P1995-2051, November 10, 2018.

2018DOI:https://doi.org/10.1016/S0140-6736(18)32278-5

Also published in *The Lancet;*

https://www.thelancet.com/journals/lancet/article/PIIS0140-6736(18)32278-5/fulltext#%20

See also a BBC Review: James Gallagher Health and science correspondent, BBC News

"Remarkable' decline in fertility rates" 9 November 2018.

https://www.bbc.co.uk/news/health-46118103

[287] Niels E Skakkebaek. Niels Jørgensen. Anna-Maria Andersson. Anders Juul. Katharina M Main, Tina Kold Jensen et al. "Populations, decreasing fertility, and reproductive health." *Correspondence, Lancet*, Volume 393, Issue 10180, P1500-1501, April 13, 2019 DOI:https://doi.org/10.1016/S0140-6736(19)30690-7

[288] Peter Rosset, "The multiple functions and benefits of small farm agriculture in the context of global trade negotiations." Food First Policy Brief no. 4. Sept 1999.

[289] Catherine Badgley et al., "Organic agriculture and the global food supply." *Renewable Agriculture and Food Systems:* 22(2); 86–108, June 2006 doi:10.1017/S1742170507001640

[290] Vandana Shiva, "Health Per Acre: Organic Solutions to Hunger." *BIJA, The Seed,* Volume 58, Summer 2011.

Research Foundation for Science Technology and Ecology (RFSTE)

[291] Fred Pearce, "An ordinary miracle. Bigger harvests, without pesticides or genetically modified crops? Farmers can make it happen by letting weeds do the work. *New Scientist* Vol 169 Issue 2276 - 03 February 2001, p 16.

[292] Professor Don Huber "Worse than DDT: When You Eat This, it Ends Up Lingering in Your Gut: A One on One Interview with Dr Don Huber." (Part 2) January 15, 2012. Available at:

http://articles.mercola.com/sites/articles/archive/2012/01/15/dr-don-huber-interview-part-2.aspx

[293] Ibid.

[294] Friends of the Earth Europe "Introducing Glyphosate, the world's biggest selling herbicide." June 2013.

Charles M Benbrook, "Trends in glyphosate herbicide use in the United States and globally." Environ Sci Eur. 2016; 28(1): 3. doi: 10.1186/s12302-016-0070-0 PMCID: PMC5044953 PMID: 27752438

[295] Professor Don Huber, "Worse than DDT: When You Eat This, it Ends Up Lingering in Your Gut: A One on One Interview with Dr Don Huber," (Part 2) January 15, 2012. Available at:

http://articles.mercola.com/sites/articles/archive/2012/01/15/dr-don-huber-interview-part-2.aspx

[296] Daniel Schmachtenberger , "Gut Health and the Microbiome with Dr. Zach Bush M.D." *Neurohacker Collective,* December 28, 2017. https://neurohacker.com/gut-health-microbiome-dr-zach-bush-m-d

[297] Zack Bush MD. Goop Podcast www.zachbushmd.com https://zachbushmd.com/podcast/goop/ She also his www.Farmersfootprint.us site for further info.

[298] "Widening Disparity—Wealthiest 1% strengthens grip over corporate America" *The Financial Times,* Tues 11 Feb, 2020.

[299] Damian Carrington, "Insect apocalypse' poses risk to all life on Earth, conservationists warn." *The Guardian,* Weds 13 Nov, 2019.

[300] Broadcast: News items "New report reveals true impact of insect apocalypse and calls for urgent action" University of Sussex. http://www.sussex.ac.uk/broadcast/read/50282

[301] Prof Dave Goulson, FRES, "Insect declines and why they matter". Report for the South West Wildlife Trusts. 2019. See also: Suzanne Fisher-Murray, "Shining a light on the impact of pesticides on bees." University of Sussex, 2019.

https://www.sussex.ac.uk/research/explore-our-research/life-sciences/impact-of-pesticides-on-bees-dave-goulson

[302] Francisco Sánchez-Bayoa, Kris A.G. Wyckhuys. "Worldwide decline of the entomofauna: A review of its drivers." *Biological Conservation,* Volume 232, April 2019, Pages 8-27.

https://www.sciencedirect.com/science/article/pii/S0006320718313636

https://doi.org/10.1016/j.biocon.2019.01.020

[303] Navdanya International, "Poison Free, Fossil Fuel Free, Food and Farming 2030." https://navdanyainternational.org/publications/pledge-for-poison-free-food-and-farming/

[304] "Health Status USA: America's Health rankings", Annual report. United Health Foundation. 2020.

https://www.americashealthrankings.org/explore/annual/measure/Health_Status/state/ALL

"International Comparison of Life Expectancy", Office of Disease Prevention and Health Promotion

https://www.healthypeople.gov/2020/about/foundation-health-measures/General-Health-Status#life

[305] "Prescription Drug Use in the United States, 2015–2016," National Center for Health Statistics, Centers for Disease Control and Prevention (CDC). See also Zablotsky B. et al., "Prevalence and Trends of Developmental Disabilities among Children in the United States: 2009–2017," *Pediatrics,* October 2019, 144 (4) e20190811; DOI: https://doi.org/10.1542/peds.2019-0811 A full copy of the report, Prevalence of Autism Spectrum Disorder Among Children Aged 8 Years - Autism and Developmental Disabilities Monitoring Network, 11 Sites, United States, 2014" is available on the CDC website: www.cdc.gov/mmwr/volumes/67/ss/ss6706a1.htm

[306] Jonathon Leake Professor of Plant-Soil Interactions, "Soil degradation by intensive UK agriculture and how to reverse it." University of Sheffield.

References

307 Craig Cox, Andrew Hug, Nils Bruzelius, "Losing Ground", *Environmental Working Group*, April 2011

308 Chris Arsenault, "Only 60 Years of Farming Left If Soil Degradation Continues." *Scientific American,* December 5, 2014.

309 Christine Jones PhD., "Light Farming: Restoring carbon, organic nitrogen and biodiversity to agricultural soils." https://www.amazingcarbon.com/

310 The Environment Agency: "The State of the environment: Soil." June 2019.

311 Sir Albert Howard, *The Soil and Health—A Study of Organic Agriculture,* 1947.

312 Henry A. Wallace, US Secretary of Agriculture, *Soils and Men, Yearbook of Agriculture* 1938, USDA.

313 Sir Albert Howard, *The Soil and Health—A Study of Organic Agriculture,* 1947.

314 House of Lords Hansard, Agriculture And Food Values : 26 October, Vol. 129, 1943.

https://hansard.parliament.uk/Lords/1943-10-26/debates/d894d48a-4fc6-4f6d-9849-ad4ce1ec1b25/LordsChamber

315 David R Montgomery, *Growing A Revolution—Bringing Our Soil Back to Life,* W W Norton & Company, 2017, p246.

316 Montgomery 2017, p 273.

317 Elizabeth Pennisi, "The Secret Life of Fungi", *Science,* 11 June, 2004, Vol 304.

318 Michael Philips *Mycorrhizal Planet-How Symbiotic Fungi Work with Roots to Support Plant Health and Build Soil Fertility,* Chelsea Green Publishing 2017.

319 E.J.Gray & D.L.Smith. "Intracellular and extracellular PGPR: Commonalities and distinctions in the plant–bacterium signaling processes". *Soil Biology and Biochemistry.* Vol. 37, Issue 3, March 2005, Pages 395-412

320 Sujit Adhikary, "Vermicompost, the story of organic gold: A review," *Agricultural Sciences,* January 2012, Vol.3, No.7, 905-917 DOI:10.4236/as.2012.37110

321 David R Montgomery, *Growing A Revolution—Bringing Our Soil Back to Life,* W W Norton & Company, 2017, p20.

322 Gabe Brown, *Dirt to Soil—One Family's Journey into Regenerative Agriculture,* Chelsea Green Publishing, 2018.

323 Christine Jones PhD., "Light Farming: Restoring carbon, organic nitrogen and biodiversity to agricultural soils." Amazing Carbon. https://www.amazingcarbon.com/

324 Vandana Shiva, "Farming with Nature, Cultivating the Future, Two Paths to the Future." *Navdanya International* 2019.

325 As reported in *Unhealthy Betrayal, 2015,* p363.

326 Wolf Richter, "Nothing's Fixed – What's Behind the Corporate Debt Bailout." *The Wolf Street Report,* May 3, 2020. https://wolfstreet.com/2020/05/03/the-wolf-street-report-nothings-fixed-whats-behind-the-corporate-debt-bailout/

327 Andrew A D Burgoyne, *Hijacked—How the Banking Industry, Finance, and Corporate Interests Have Hijacked our Economy and Corrupted Democracy.*

328 Chuck Collins, Omar Ocampo & Sophia Paslaski, "Billionaire's Bonanza: Wealth Windfalls, Tumbling Taxes and Pandemic Profiteers." *Institute for Policy Studies,* April 23, 2020.

329 Wolf Richter, "Fed Cuts QE Helicopter Money for Wall Street Further. Still Hasn't Bought Junk Bonds or ETFs. Was Just Jawboning." *Wolf Street,* May 8, 2020.

330 www.Wolf-pac.com : The Free and Fair Elections Resolution.

331 https://indivisible.org/ We're a grassroots movement of thousands of local Indivisible groups with a mission to elect progressive leaders, rebuild our democracy, and defeat the Trump agenda.

332 George Monbiot, *Out of the Wreckage—A New Politics for an Age of Crisis.* Verso, 2018.

Becky Bond and Zack Exley, *Rules for Revolutionaries: How Big Organizing Can Change Everything*, Chelsea Green, 2106.